C000133966

"*Group Filial Therapy* is truly a masterpiece! Guerney and R of sage and practical information guaranteed to heighten p working with children and their families. Comprehensiv empirically supported, *Group Filial Therapy* is a compelling a must-read for any clinician, at any experience level, work groups of families. It features Filial Therapy as originally conceived and refined during the past 50 years by its founders, Bernard and Louise Guerney. This much-anticipated work will be a classic in the fields of Filial Therapy, play therapy, child psychotherapy, and family therapy. It is a fabulous gift from the authors, and it deserves to be read cover-to-cover."

—*Risë VanFleet, Ph.D., RPT-S, CDBC, President, Family Enhancement & Play Therapy Center and author of* Filial Therapy: Strengthening Parent-Child-Relationships Through Play, *Pennsylvania, USA*

Filial Therapy, co-developed by Louise Guerney, is the most significant happening in the field of mental health in the past 50 years because this innovative approach has the potential to improve a society. *Group Filial Therapy* is a long-awaited and much-needed book that provides insight into the dynamics of Filial Therapy and a practical how-to approach for implementing the intricacies of the process. Mental health professionals will want to return to this book again and again for helpful instruction."

—*Dr. Garry L. Landreth, Regents Professor, Counseling and Higher Education Department, University of North Texas*

"I am delighted that a very practical, step-by-step manual for conducting the Guerney model of Group Filial Therapy is now available! Kudos to Drs Louise Guerney and Virginia Ryan for preparing this comprehensive, clearly-written handbook which will serve to both improve the practice and strengthen the research base of Filial Therapy."

—*Charles E. Schaefer, Ph.D., RPT-S, Professor Emeritus of Psychology, Fairleigh Dickinson University, Teaneck, New Jersey and Co-founder of the Association for Play Therapy, Fresno, California*

"This book is a must-have for all clinicians who work with families. What a gift as a therapist to be able to assist and empower a parent to help and support their child as well as enhance their parent/child relationship via play. This book breaks down why Group Filial Therapy is advantageous for families, how to set up a parent group that is needs-balanced with the optimal number of children and parents, clinical goals, supervision issues to address, how to create play kits, etc. Essentially, the GFT clinician can use this resource from intake to group closure. Case illustrations connect theory with practice and the book ends with additional resources that the GFT clinician can seek out for further information. This will be the book that all clinicians want in their office for 2013."

—*Theresa Fraser, CYW, M.A., CPT-S, Trauma and Loss Clinical Specialist and President of the Canadian Association for Child and Play Therapy*

Group Filial Therapy

The Complete Guide to Teaching Parents to Play
Therapeutically with their Children

Louise Guerney and Virginia Ryan

Jessica Kingsley *Publishers*
London and Philadelphia

First published in 2013
by Jessica Kingsley Publishers
116 Pentonville Road
London N1 9JB, UK
and
400 Market Street, Suite 400
Philadelphia, PA 19106, USA

www.jkp.com

Library of Congress Cataloging in Publication Data
Guerney, Louise F. (Louise Fisher), 1928-
Group filial therapy : the complete guide to teaching parents to play therapeutically with their children /
Louise F. Guerney and Virginia M. Ryan.
pages cm
Includes bibliographical references and index.
ISBN 978-1-84310-911-2 (alk. paper)
1. Group play therapy. 2. Group psychotherapy for children. 3. Parent-child interaction therapy. I. Ryan,
Virginia. II. Title. III. Title: Complete guide to teaching parents to play therapeutically with their children.
RJ505.P6G84 20120
618.92'891653--dc23
2012041104

British Library Cataloguing in Publication Data
A CIP catalogue record for this book is available from the British Library

ISBN 978 1 84310 911 2
eISBN 978 0 85700 516 8

Printed and bound in Great Britain

From Louise:
To my co-author Virginia, for her dedication in shepherding us through the writing of this book, and with love to my husband, Bernard, and to my wonderful children and grandchildren.

From Virginia:
To Louise, who has made writing this book a privilege for me; to my husband, Michael, with all my love and thanks; and to our children and their families, for showing me the happiness families can bring.

We both wish to thank Bernard Guerney, Jr. who had the insight, vision and courage to create and advance the development of Filial Therapy, thus benefiting many families over the years.

We also wish to extend our gratitude to all of the families who have participated in Filial Therapy, and to our encouraging colleagues and friends, all of whom have enabled us to write this book.

Contents

Introduction

Filial Therapy (FT) is a very significant advance in the treatment of childhood problems. It is a highly positive and enabling approach for families, which has been practiced and researched for nearly 50 years at the time this book is published. An essential feature of this therapy method is that parents are regarded from the outset as partners in the treatment of their own children. Instead of considering parents as contributors to their children's problems, the task is seen as empowering parents to be more effective in carrying out their parenting role. It was a need to address this deficiency in understanding and managing children that led Dr Bernard Guerney to create FT. He thought that viewing parents' relationship and child management problems as products of pathology was not as productive as reframing the task as educating parents (Guerney B., 1964).

FT uses a psycho-educational framework to help parents learn to first play with their children in a therapeutic way under direct supervision from filial therapists, and then to apply therapeutic play skills and other parenting skills to their lives at home more generally. FT's strengths are that it delivers both therapy to children and parenting skills to parents, using an evidence-based method.

FT is designed to guide parents and give them practical skills, while simultaneously working directly on promoting and deepening parent-child attachment relationships within the entire family. While it can be used to prevent more serious problems arising within families, in this book we concentrate on Group Filial Therapy (GFT) for problems between parents and children that already have reached clinical levels and are more persistent. FT, because it is much more than a parenting program, offers help for a range of clinical difficulties, including children traumatized by life events, foster and adoptive families composed of children with more serious emotional difficulties, and families where continuing conduct problems are evident. All of these areas of clinical practice are of great concern to professionals and FT provides them with an effective way of working with families on these difficult problems.

FT by now is a well-established approach to children's and families' emotional problems in North America, and it is becoming better known worldwide. There is a solid body of both theoretical and research evidence to support FT's claim for effectiveness as an approach (e.g. Bratton *et al.*, 2005; VanFleet, Ryan and Smith, 2005). Dissemination of FT is gaining momentum because it fits well with the current mental health emphasis on empowering families to solve their own problems with their children, rather than relying primarily on professional help. It also is making advances because its research base demonstrates its power in increasing family cohesiveness and attachment relationships, and decreasing childhood problems.

This book draws on Dr Louise Guerney's extensive experience conducting GFT programs with children and their families. Louise Guerney, the co-creator of FT, has written this book along with Dr Virginia Ryan, after a long career training mental health professionals in FT. She and Virginia have written widely on non-directive, child-centered play therapy (CCPT), and Louise has written often on FT. However, she has not yet written down her approach to GFT step by step and in detail. This book is intended to fill this gap. It distils and formalizes her method for professionals who have not been able to access her training directly. It provides enriched guidance on many different levels on how to lead FT groups, and how to improve practice when using the Guerney 20-week model. The following chapters also give insights more generally into group processes, working with individual families, and FT and play therapy practice and theory.

The book begins with background on the FT method, and moves on to setting up GFT programs, including general considerations about the composition of the group, the length of the program, intake interviews and assessment, and the basic skills needed to be an effective FT group leader. Another chapter gives the reasons behind the CCPT skills taught to parents in the program, then the chapters follow the process of the 20 weekly meetings in the program for readers. Extensive examples from practice on issues arising in each group meeting illustrate vividly each phase in a 20-week GFT program. The last chapter gives examples from clinical practice of adaptations of this 20-week model, in order to help readers think about what their particular groups and circumstances may require. The appendices to the book have a practical aim. They give leaders forms to download for their use, including the Parents' Training Manual developed by Louise, and other practical advice for GFT program organizers and developers.

CHAPTER 1

An Overview
of FT and GFT

This book is devoted to GFT; many aspects of it are also highly relevant to FT with individual families and with one-to-one parent-child dyads. In this chapter, GFT is set within the context of FT more generally. The chapter first provides a brief overview of FT, including its history, theoretical and research bases, goals, aims and rationale. We then turn to GFT, highlighting FT's strengths as a group intervention and introducing the structure of a 20-week GFT program. General issues that arise for leaders when starting programs, including the two-leader model advocated here, the skills and professional needs of leaders, and general considerations for setting up groups, are then discussed.

Our definition of FT is the following:

FT is a well-established method of providing therapy to children with their parents or other significant adults serving as primary change agents.[1] Typically children range from 2.5–12 years of age, with adjustments in play session format at the higher and lower ends of the age range. The adults are trained and supervised in (CCPT)[2] by trained professionals. In addition, the adults learn relationship development principles derived from the play sessions they deliver for use in daily life. FT combines affective, behavioral and cognitive methods of therapy into a cohesive approach. Because this method involves the active participation of family or family surrogate members, including younger and older siblings, FT can also be considered a form of family therapy. FT can be delivered in a group format, individual family format, and individual parent-child format, and may be used for both therapeutic and preventive purposes.

---

1   The term "parent" is used generically in this book to refer to the main caregiver in the family, regardless of biological status.

2   The term "Child-Centered Play Therapy (CCPT)" is used instead of the more generic term "Non-Directive Play Therapy (NDPT)" in this book.

The history of FT

FT's development as a well-recognized method of therapy for children and families gathered momentum into the twenty-first century. Its beginnings are described first.

The original idea

When Bernard Guerney originated FT in the early 1960s in the USA, he saw it as addressing a number of ineffective practices of US mental health providers working with children and their families that were prevalent at the time. These practices arose from both theoretical and practice positions that were long-standing. Behavioral and emotional problems in children were often viewed as reflections of, or reactions to, similar, existing, overt or unresolved and unconscious behavioral and emotional problems of their parents. Their therapists' task was to work with the parents' intra-psychic issues underlying the maladaptive ways they interacted with their children. It was assumed that the children would benefit in turn. Some general parenting advice might also be offered to parents by therapists (e.g. "Be more consistent with your children.").

Guerney had a different explanation for the etiology of problem interactions between parents and children. He assumed that in the majority of cases, rather than parental pathology causing children's problems, parental lack of knowledge and skills of how to interact with their children were the bases of parent-child interaction difficulties. Parents needed to be taught how to motivate their children to make them feel loved and respected. In turn, children would benefit because they try to please parent figures, which is the basis for their appropriate socialization. Children's misbehaviors and emotional maladjustments, except of course when there was some organic or neurological complication, seemed to result from this lack of synchrony between parents and children. Thus, Guerney wanted to find a way to help parents, particularly mothers originally, to learn to interact with their children in positive, supportive ways that would still maintain the necessary control that children need.

Because Guerney was a practicing child-centered play therapist, he turned to play sessions for direction. Wasn't the CCPT session a kind of idealized parenting situation? (E.g. "idealized" because the demands of real-life parenting, which would require parents to leave the role of play therapist, do not exist in CCPT play sessions.) Perhaps if parents could be taught to conduct play sessions with their children, they could learn to relate to them in more positive ways? There had been isolated reports of parents holding "play sessions" in the literature by two therapists, Baruch (1949) and Moustakas (1951), with both reported as beneficial. However, those parents had been trained to do play sessions only with children no longer troubled with problems. Other early work with a parent was briefly reported by Rogers' daughter, who played with her own daughter under the direction of her father (Fuchs, 1957). And much earlier Freud had directed a father to carry out a form of playful therapy with his son, but not play therapy *per se* (Guerney B., 1964). However, these isolated cases of parents working therapeutically with their children had not become common practice before FT emerged.

FT was therefore one of the first models to make systematic use of family members as primary change agents. The essence of FT, and its most unique feature, is that parents serve as the change agents for their children. Guerney (1964) provided the rationale for this then radical approach. He reasoned that therapeutic change would be more likely and lasting in children if their own parents served as therapists. By taking on the play therapist role, parents would not only be given positive skills, but this role also would create a new perception of their parents on the part of their children. These behavioral and attitudinal changes required of parents in order to conduct play sessions then would be generalized to parent-child relationships in daily life. Simultaneously, the children would experience the positive benefits that accrue from CCPT sessions, as they would from any valid therapy. Guerney stated: "Every bit of success the parent achieves in successfully filling the prescribed role should have an effect many times more powerful than that of a therapist doing the same thing" (Guerney B., 1964, p.307).

Working with family members together

In addition to the idea that parents could serve in a therapeutic capacity with their own children, Bernard Guerney was also addressing another accepted practice of the day. This was the tradition of seeing individual family members, even when it was believed that more than one family member needed treatment, or at least inclusion. Seeing family members together was just beginning to be introduced by family therapy pioneers (e.g. Ackerman, 1966). However the idea of seeing family members together generally did not extend to younger children; usually it was confined to parents, other relatives in the home, and adolescents.

Guerney's idea of having family members deliver therapy to other family members was an extension of this new thinking. He saw family members as resources who could both assist in mental health service delivery, discussed next, and at the same time gain greater adjustment for themselves and their families. Guerney had believed for some time, and before conceptualizing the teaching of parents to play therapeutically with their children, that parents deserved greater recognition and respect in their children's treatment. Bypassing them as possible therapeutic resources seemed inappropriate to him. Mothers were typically the parent involved in their children's clinic attendance in the 1960s; therefore Guerney originally concentrated on them. But as FT developed, he felt it was appropriate to include fathers, and even other relatives living in the home, to participate in bringing about change in their children and the family as a whole.

Changes in service delivery

The practice of an individual therapist seeing an individual client was also being challenged at the broader level by US leaders in the mental health profession. For example, Nicholas Hobbs believed that a mental health system "…that is built on a 50-minute hour…is living on borrowed time" (1963, p.3). These leaders recommended that psychology should not be reserved for the most highly trained professionals, but shared via educational programs and prevention activities that would allow members of the public to utilize psychological knowledge for their self-growth. Also advocated was the use of paraprofessionals and other non-professionals to carry out psychological tasks via peer support groups and other forums (Hobbs, 1962). Guerney's thinking fitted in well with calls at the time for these proposed changes in service models. It was self-evident that professionals alone could not begin to match demand for a range of services in the community and institutions. Training and supervising parents and others to conduct play therapy with their children had the potential to significantly increase the leverage of highly trained mental health personnel, thus making it possible to reduce waiting lists and over-burdensome caseloads (Guerney B., 1964).

The term "Filial" Therapy

It should be mentioned that along the way FT has been referred to by more than one label. "Filial Therapy" was the second title, after the original title was claimed by someone else for a very different kind of therapy, and it is now the term commonly used. "Filial" is a word that conveys succinctly that this therapy refers to parent-child relationships. However, it is not a commonly used word and may make FT a little less easy to relate to initially. As a consequence, Bernard Guerney did try to change the name to Child Parent Relationship Enhancement Family Therapy (e.g. Guerney L. and Guerney B., 1989, 1994). The term "Filial Family Therapy" is also still used at times because ideally both parents, as well as multiple children, participate in FT at one time.

The educational model

Bernard Guerney, as mentioned earlier, conceived of the task as educating parents in better understanding of their children and better management of everyday parenting issues. In order to do this, he advocated teaching the skills of the play therapist as the way to involve parents meaningfully and directly in the therapy of their children. Guerney thus introduced another element into the FT method, that of skills training. FT was the first program representing this educational model.

More broadly, FT and other later educational models take the position that the task of mental health professionals is to educate clients in skills that would further their knowledge of good personal mental health principles, and the specific behaviors to express them. In this model, mental health professionals become primarily educators for clients who want or need to learn positive life skills that will enhance their functioning in specific skill areas. Using the best teaching and training methods currently available, mental health educators design programs that can be replicated by other educators who have the same clientele. Anger management, self-esteem building, and assertiveness training, represent the kinds of products possible using the principles of the educational model.

FT put into practice

Guerney found the opportunity to put FT concepts into pragmatic form at the Psychological Clinic at Rutgers University where he was the director. He assembled a team to work on methodology, including Jay Fiddler, community psychiatrist, Michael Andronico, Lillian Stover, and Louise Guerney—wife of Bernard Guerney and this book's first author—all clinical psychologists. Because FT fit into the goals of the new Mental Health Movement, the US National Institute of Mental Health (NIMH) took interest in it and funded research in FT for a number of years. This enabled the team to carry out extensive research on the process and outcomes of this new therapy.

The acceptance of FT was slow in the mental health community, although selected professionals, mostly psychologists, did studies and conducted groups in other settings, such as schools (Guerney B. & Flumen, 1970; Kraft, 1973; Levine, 1977; Stollack, 1968). It has been only since the 1980s in the USA, when play therapy was resuscitated, that FT began to be seriously pursued by the larger family service community. Prior to that time, various factors appeared to work against its growth, such as the low interest in play therapy *per se*, and questions about the ethics of parents serving as primary change agents for their children, even though they were trained and supervised throughout the therapy by knowledgeable professionals, usually psychologists.

Growing acceptance of FT

It was crucial for FT's acceptance that Louise Guerney, who is recognized as the co-creator of FT for her work, worked steadily on refinement of its methodology, such as "optimal parent groupings," a shortened version of FT, instructional methodology, training techniques for parents and professionals, and research on process outcomes. These efforts led to an increased number of graduate students across psychology programs at Pennsylvania State University, and much wider dissemination to agencies and private practice.

FT began to become more familiar and more accepted in the mental health community over time. The revival of interest in play therapy in the USA was accompanied by a parallel interest in family therapy, the development of skills training in several areas, including assertiveness training and parent effectiveness training (PET) (Gordon, 1970), and the use of paraprofessionals (Carkhuff, 1969). Each of these changes seemed to contribute to the acceptance and desire to practice FT. Psychologists trained under the Guerneys (e.g. Nordling, VanFleet) have since extended supervision and training in FT to structured programs for professionals. In addition, more empirical support for its efficacy using a 10-session model of GFT, outlined in the last chapter of this book, was generated most notably by Landreth and his former student and colleague Bratton (e.g. Bratton *et al.*, 2006; Landreth and Bratton, 2006), and their doctoral students.

While the original articles published on FT described a group format, single families whose needs did not synchronize with their group were from the outset taken aside for individual FT work as required. Practical considerations then led to further development of the use of FT with single families and single parents (e.g. VanFleet, 2013). Therefore, the effectiveness of FT with these other family constellations was always practiced from the start; however, the group format was the most researched. While this book focuses on GFT, other formats of FT are accepted and empirically shown to be successful as well. Thus, at the current time, GFT and FT are widely practiced in the USA with families from diverse ethnic backgrounds in a variety of settings, including hospitals, schools, and family centers. They are also becoming established in the UK and better known in scattered places throughout the world, including Ireland, Denmark, Australia, Hong Kong, Taiwan, and South Korea (Guerney, L., 2000; Ryan, personal communication).

The theoretical underpinnings of FT

FT: a cohesive theoretical approach

FT is unique in crossing theoretical lines to combine affective, behavioral, and cognitive theoretically based methods into a cohesive approach. The FT method is also supported by psychological perspectives on parenting, child development, and play in particular, as well as being a form of family therapy. It appears to derive much of its robustness and effectiveness from its incorporation of several different methods of therapeutic change, taken from several theoretical bases, within one intervention.

The affective component

Emotional changes in children as individuals, and in parents' and children's relationships with one another, are addressed in FT. The principles of Rogerian person-centered therapy were recognized from the start of the development of FT. Over time, the importance of FT in supporting changes in parent-child attachment relationships was more fully appreciated.

PERSON-CENTERED THERAPY

An important theoretical model incorporated into FT is person-centered therapy, on which CCPT is based. This method of therapy was originally practiced with adult clients (Rogers, 1951), then adapted to children (e.g. Axline, 1947; Dorfman, 1976), and now has a long history of application both to play therapy and to FT.

Person-centered practice is based on the self-actualizing principle that each person strives to live fully and well within their own abilities and circumstances. Another principle is that people are unique and valuable in themselves, and have their own developmental and life trajectories. Both assumptions are essential to FT, alongside the principle that, when life circumstances or intrapersonal issues interfere with functioning, facilitation by professionals may be required to restore individuals to positive functioning and to further growth. These person-centered principles resonate with the current approach to children's and adolescents' emotional difficulties of developmental psychopathology, which views emotional problems as part of children's more general, yet unique, developmental trajectories (Wenar & Kerig, 2006; Wilson & Ryan, 2005). These theoretical underpinnings enable both clinicians and researchers to look more closely at, and value, individual variations in development.

In order to bring about self-chosen, positive changes in clients, it is assumed that professionals must set up well-established and well-researched conditions for bringing about psychological change. These core conditions are acceptance, unconditional positive regard, and genuineness. Acceptance is expressed primarily through empathic responding. If these conditions were to be rated in order of necessity to bring about client change, acceptance (empathy) seems to be the most critical of the three. Empathy, along with the other core Rogerian conditions, is referred to often in this book, both as an attitude for leaders to show towards and model for parents, and as a skill that is actively taught by leaders to parents with their children in play sessions, and then extended to daily life.

An important feature of FT is teaching parents CCPT skills. One essential skill is that parents enable children to play with them in a non-directive way. This feature, in and of itself, aims to have a facilitative effect for children and their parents, promoting children's cooperative behavior with parents, and decreasing their negative behavior (see, for example, Parpal & Maccoby, 1985).

ATTACHMENT THEORY

Well-conducted play sessions by parents with their children seem to be the main source of powerful changes in relationships within families when using FT. As attachment theory and research have increasingly been applied to parent-child relationship patterns and therapy over the last 40 years, FT also has recognized that alteration of attachment patterns has always been at the heart of the FT method of therapy. Currently in the UK, FT is gaining acceptance as an effective attachment therapy for children and parents, especially for those in foster, adoptive, and reconstituted families (Ryan, 2007a, 2007b).

Attachment theory and research have demonstrated that when highly insecure children and/or their parents have entrenched and very insecure attachment strategies, more intensive therapeutic help may be required in order to change these strategies into more age-appropriate and adaptive styles of interaction (Ryan & Wilson, 2000; Wilson & Ryan, 2005). Filial therapists can be viewed as parents' "secure base" in this process of change. FT, in a very direct and professionally supervised way, helps parents become more highly attuned to their children's emotional expressions and accepting of their underlying emotional issues, with filial therapists' guidance. FT also increases parents' ability to effectively use their parental authority and parental experiences to support the development of their children's more secure attachment strategies (Ryan & Bratton, 2008). Children themselves, in feeling valued and contained, are enabled to grow more secure in their attachments to their parents, and in turn become less divisive in interactions with their siblings and peers.

The cognitive component

Cognitive therapy principles (Beck & Emery, 1985) are also prominent in the FT method. Learning and applying play therapy skills and then generalizing skills to daily life involve parents' active cognitive engagement, as we examine throughout this book. FT, similar to cognitive therapy, stresses that parents—as well as their children—are active collaborators in therapeutic change. As parents become more independent, they deliver play sessions at home (FT's unique approach to "homework"), and learn increasingly to self-monitor, once they have achieved a basic level of competence.

The educational model inherent in cognitive therapy is also prominent in other ways throughout the program. The program itself is a structured one, moving from one planned stage to the next as parents increase their skills. The explanations of and rationales for the principles of child-centered play sessions, and therapeutic change agents' attitudes and actions, are presented in both written and oral forms to participants. Reasons for avoiding negative communications are taught, along with an emphasis on parents' learning adaptive responses, and effective ways to problem solve at home. Children's ability to problem solve in age-appropriate ways for themselves, both in play sessions and in daily life, also is stressed in FT. Throughout the teaching of the principles of CCPT to parents, there is a continued emphasis on the expected positive outcomes of parents keeping these principles in mind when relating to their children. In addition, FT uses shared, direct experiences in play sessions, and then examples from daily life, as the basis for increasing participants' cognitive capacities as parents.

The behavioral component

Another key influence is behavioral theory and practice (Lazarus, 1971; Wolpe, 1969). FT assumes that, by concentrating initially on the positive aspects of parent-child relationships, and enhancing these relationships by means of play, the negative features of relationships between children and their parents recede and become less overwhelming. Skills training is the primary method of teaching; it utilizes reinforcement, modeling, and behavioral rehearsal to teach parents how to actually conduct the affectively oriented play sessions. There is also an emphasis on observational learning throughout the FT program, with parents observing and learning from one another's play sessions. In addition, the FT method relies on principles of shaping and rewarding approximations to desired behaviors, both when parents are learning CCPT and parenting skills, and behaviors to adopt at home in their interactions with their children.

Family therapy

Family therapy and its principles are significant aspects of FT. As stated earlier, FT embraces the systemic principles of family therapy, including the principle that altering one part of the system sets off changes in the system as a whole. FT ideally focuses on all the parent-child dyads in the family, with each parent offering play or special activity times to each of their children weekly. Filial therapists also aim to form strong therapeutic alliances with the significant parental figures in the family, helping them to work together harmoniously and competently in their parental roles with their children, and offering them therapeutic support with their own emotional needs in relation to parenting issues.

Family therapy and FT also aim to help families grow towards more effective communication with one another of their emotion-laden messages, both verbally and non-verbally. Children become more aware and more articulate of their internal responses, and parents learn to accept and reflect their children's needs, wishes, and feelings empathically, first during their play sessions and then in daily life. FT therefore is a comprehensive and integrated approach to child therapy in a family therapy context because it provides the structure and methods that allow both children and their parents full access to therapeutic resources. Ideally all family members participate in FT. Nonetheless, even when only one child and one parent participate, FT is a family intervention because as the single parent and child relationship changes, effects are felt through the whole family (Guerney L. & Guerney B. 1987).

Theoretical assumptions about play and other child development principles

In addition to attachment theory, other child development principles also have a prominent place in FT practice. We refer to them frequently throughout this book, particularly in chapters discussing the rationales offered to parents for the skills they are learning (Chapter 4), and when discussing how to help parents generalize their skills to daily life (Chapter 14). Because the assumed functions of play are essential to CCPT, and therefore to FT, the main principles about play are outlined here.

FT assumes that play helps families relax, laugh and enjoy being together, thus deepening their relationships with one another. In addition, children's play during special play sessions based on CCPT skills also is assumed to have therapeutic power. With parents providing a therapeutic environment in which their children use spontaneous play to address and resolve emotional issues, play can be restorative and life enhancing, enabling children to try out new ways of making choices and mastering their inner and outer experiences (Ryan, 2009; Wilson & Ryan, 2005).

Research on children who experience emotional regulation and attachment problems argues for therapy that is both play based and relationship enhancing (O'Sullivan & Ryan, 2009; Ryan, 2004). And neurological findings with traumatized children and adults show the need for therapy that works not just on a cognitive level, but on an experiential level (Gil, 1991). CCPT fits these criteria, since it encompasses children's bodily, perceptual, and emotional levels of expression. In CCPT, for example, children are helped with traumatic memories they have incompletely processed (see Ryan & Needham, 2001; Wilson & Ryan, 2005).

After this brief review of FT's theoretical foundations, the next section examines its research base.

Research in FT

Early research

From its inceptions in the early 60s, the originators of FT, Drs B. and L. Guerney, have always had a strong commitment to research on the method in order to demonstrate to professionals and clients that this (then) unorthodox approach was on a solid footing. As stated earlier, a psycho-educational approach was little known, if not unknown, in the early 1960s. Furthermore, a psycho-educational approach that utilized parents playing therapeutically with their own children was not immediately apparent to either the professional or the lay communities as a viable method.

In order to support the potential value of the filial approach, it was necessary to first develop instruments for measuring whether parents were able to conduct successful play sessions (Guerney B., Stover, and DeMeritt, 1968). Proof that parents (mothers only in this study) could be trained to conduct CCPT to a standard of effectiveness was gathered by assigning mothers to training or no training conditions (Stover & Guerney B., 1967). This study's measurements discriminated among parents' behaviors in actual play sessions on empathy, attentiveness, and permissiveness.

The study was able to demonstrate that trained mothers employed CCPT skills significantly more often than untrained mothers in the actual play sessions (Stover & Guerney B., 1967). The untrained mothers responded to their children in their customary ways. In addition, the children of the trained mothers displayed more positive behavior in the play sessions than the children of the untrained mothers. This demonstrated that the training was effective, and that using parents in a therapeutic role could be productive. Moreover, the comparison between the untrained mothers and trained mothers revealed that children and mothers merely sharing time together was not sufficient to bring about desired change—training was needed. Once it was determined that parents could learn play therapy skills, it was possible to train parents to actually apply FT with their children, and to teach this method to other professionals.

Refinements of this study's measure were made (Stover, Guerney B., and O'Connell, 1971) and used for succeeding studies of GFT that were conducted over a period of five years sponsored by the USA's National Institute of Mental Health (NIMH). Mothers and children in these studies were representative of typical outpatient clinic populations. Complete data about the children, parents, and filial application measures and outcomes appear in the final report to NIMH, Report 1826401 (Guerney B. & Stover, 1971). In one NIMH sponsored study of GFT, 51 mothers and 51 children were observed through one-way mirrors during mother-conducted CCPT sessions. Ratings of both the parents' and children's behavior were made every 15 seconds (Guerney B. & Stover, 1971). Weekly sessions ranged in number from 9–51. Post-treatment ratings were made on average 38 weeks after the pre-treatment ratings.

The ratings indicated that positive changes in both parent and child behavior took place over the treatment period. Mothers rated their children on three different types of child behavioral checklists (uncorrelated), including the Filial Problem List (FPL), revised from Leventhal and Stollack (1965). These ratings showed significant pre to post differences on all of these measures. All children in the study showed a marked reduction in problems as rated by parents. Parents experienced a reduction in their own parent-child difficulties. The method used for the study also permitted the researchers to chart the process of treatment, to be discussed in a later section.

Oxman (1971) conducted a quasi-control study approximately one year later, comparing the 51 GFT children with 77 non-clinical children with carefully matched demographics. The 77 children had never evidenced any behavioral or emotional problems. Oxman was able to demonstrate that GFT children made significant positive changes, while the non-clinical children did not show significant changes from the beginning to the end of the year. Thus it can be inferred that GFT, as the only significant factor that distinguished the groups, was responsible for the change in the clinical children. These results suggested that time alone did not account for the changes that occurred in GFT children, and indicated that placebo and "thank you" effects were not responsible for the changes.

A follow-up study of the same 51 children 3–5 years after the conclusion of therapy was conducted by L. Guerney (1975). This revealed that only one child required further professional psychological help. No other children were dysfunctional, and, according to their mothers, they had maintained most of their gains from the GFT program. Encouragingly, not only were the children functional, but some had exceeded expectations.

Extending research on GFT[3]

A number of academics began to study the effects of GFT on populations in other parts of the USA. Chief among them is Garry Landreth, who, with a core of his graduate students at the University of North Texas, was particularly active in research on his 10-session adaptation of GFT (see Chapter 16), offering it to a wide range of families. Landreth and his students focused on trying to determine how broadly FT could be used effectively. They targeted a wide array of parents, including single parents (Bratton & Landreth, 1995), incarcerated mothers (Harris & Landreth, 1997), incarcerated fathers (Landreth & Lobaugh, 1998), divorced parents (Bratton, 1998), custodial grandparents (Bratton, Ray, and Motif, 1998), and non-offending parents of sexually abused children (Costas & Landreth 1999). Additional research on GFT was conducted by others, including Ginsberg with foster parents (1989), Celaya with teen mothers in foster care (2002), and Walker on parents court-referred for child maltreatment (Walker, 2008).

FT, involving both parents and children, showed therapeutic effects for both. Regardless of the primary target, both children and parents in GFT research studies showed meaningful, positive changes on most variables. In many instances researchers chose to target the parents. Cultural barriers, such as immigration from a foreign country, discussed later, put some groups of parents at a disadvantage. Thus, focusing on parent-child relationships and parenting seemed particularly pertinent. At other times, children themselves were the primary target because of special issues in their lives. Some such studies targeted children with chronic illnesses (Glazer-Waldman *et al.*, 1992; Tew *et al.* 2002; VanFleet, 1992;), children with learning difficulties (Kale & Landreth, 1999), and children with clinically significant emotional problems (Sensue, 1981; Sywulak, 1979).

Research on representative cultural groups

Research has been conducted on families who have immigrated to the USA and Canada from other countries to test the effectiveness of GFT with parents from different cultural backgrounds, including Hispanic/Latino parents (Ceballos, 2008), Chinese parents (Chau & Landreth, 1997; Johnson, 2006[4]), immigrant Chinese families in Canada (Yuen, Landreth, and Baggerly, 2002), African-American parents (Sheely-Moore and Bratton, 2010), and Native American parents living on an isolated reservation (Glover and Landreth, 2000). Positive changes were found in all of these groups.

Research on teachers as therapeutic change agents for their students

GFT has been extended to educational settings, since teachers are significant adults in the lives of the children they teach. There is encouraging research on GFT in schools, beginning with Guerney B. & Flumen's (1970) study with elementary school teachers conducting

---

3   The following sections are intended to give readers the flavor of further GFT research over many years. Due to space limitations, this discussion does not include qualitative studies or case studies that occasionally appear in the literature. Only a selection of quantitative studies is included.

4   Chinese families in New York's Chinatown were trained in GFT over a four-year period, with positive feedback from agencies and parents. Empirical analyses are not yet complete.

play sessions with withdrawn students. More recently, Morrison Bennett & Bratton (2011) conducted a pilot study with preschool, disadvantaged children with clinically significant behavior problems. Teachers using Landreth and Bratton's 10-session Filial Therapy model for teachers, Child Teacher Relationship Therapy (CTRT), were compared with a matched, active control group of teachers using the method of "conscious discipline." The CTRT group showed significant, positive results. Landreth and Bratton's (2006) article discusses their own study, and refers to several other GFT studies in educational settings, for interested readers.

Research conducted outside the USA

Studies began to be conducted outside of the USA, for example in Korea (Jang, 2000) Germany (Grskovic & Goetze, 2008), and Israel (Kidron & Landreth, 2010). In a study that had experimental and control groups, Korean parents were trained at Namseoul University in Korea. 32 parents and 33 children comprised the four groups, two training and two controls. The Porter Parental Acceptance Scale (Porter, 1954), Parenting Stress Index (Abidin, 1997), the FPL (Horner, 1974) and the behavioral measure of parents playing, Measurement of Empathy in Child-Adult Interactions (MEACI) (Stover et al., 1971) were used. The program was shortened to eight weeks from Landreth's 10-week FT program (child-parent relationship therapy [CPRT]) (Landreth & Bratton, 2006; Landreth, 2012). Results indicated that for the treatment groups parent-child relationships were strengthened. Changes in parental acceptance and allowing children self-direction were significant on play session behavioral measures (MEACI). Also the non-behavioral measures showed positive changes for the experimental group, such as the FPL where significant fewer child behavior problems where evidenced in the experimental group at post-test. The conclusion was that this program of filial concepts and procedures transferred well to a population of parents living in Korea. Cultural differences did not seem to present problems in reaching the goal of improving parent-child relationships among these Korean parents.

Grskovic and Goetze's German study included 33 mothers attending a two-week health retreat, divided into two groups. The control group received the standard mother counseling program offered during the retreat. The second group was offered an 18-hour FT program conducted within the same two-week period, which included at least five play sessions per child, feedback sessions, and group discussions. Results indicated that German mothers using the filial model, in spite of its brevity, showed significant positive gains in parenting behavior, and the children similarly gained as a result of their FT. These changes were most significant and most observable in the play sessions themselves. The positive results of this study indicate that the program again seemed to transfer well to another country, and can yield positive changes in a shortened format.

Kidron conducted an Israeli study with a treatment group of 14 parents and a control group of 13 parents. The treatment group received two sessions per week for five weeks of CPRT (Bratton et al., 2006; Landreth & Bratton 2006). Non-behavioral measures were administered to the treatment and control groups pre and post, and the MEACI behavioral measure was administered to the treatment group pre and post. At the end of the treatment, trained parents showed improvement on the MEACI and on the non-behavioral parent measures. The control group showed no significant change pre to post. A year later the members of the treatment group reported that they continued to conduct special play sessions with their children, and that the most helpful skill in daily life was limit setting. (Parents from all cultures seem to truly appreciate the limit-setting skill.) Again the shortened time span for the program, the use of a control group and a population trained in their native country are all notable. Therefore, these studies from other countries suggest, once again, that GFT has a robustness that allows modifications, and still yields positive changes in trained parents and their children.

Outcome studies with controls

The use of control groups showing significant differences from treatment groups suggests that it is the FT training that is responsible for measured changes, as opposed to the passing of time alone, or time spent with the parent. The results of these control group studies have added strength to the evidence base for FT. A very significant meta-analysis was conducted by Bratton et al. (2006). It was based on the analysis of 93 control/treatment play therapy and FT studies that had to meet several research criteria for inclusion. Their results indicated that play therapy in general was an extremely effective approach (effect size = .80) for dealing with child emotional and behavior problems. And when parents conducted play sessions, the effect size was an even more impressive 1.15. VanFleet et al. (2005) also evaluated research studies of FT in their critical review, again finding positive results.

Deserving special mention out of the many outcome studies in FT reported over the years are several that used active control/comparison groups matched to treatment groups, in addition to pre- and post-FT outcome measures, since this is one of the most important ways to demonstrate treatment effectiveness. The first of these was Wall (1979), who compared three interventions: the first was CCPT conducted by mothers (FT, labeled "Guided Play Therapy" by Wall), the second was CCPT conducted by graduate students, and the third was a free play condition conducted by untrained mothers. Significant positive changes were found only in the FT group, both in the children and in their mothers, when compared with the other two groups.

Another study using both an active control group and a no-treatment group was conducted by Clark (1996). Clark used three groups, one with mothers who simply played in their own way, one with mothers trained in FT, and a no-treatment control group. Children in the FT group showed significant reductions in "conduct behavior problems" on the Eyburg Child Behavior Inventory (ECBI; Eyburg & Pincus, 1999). No similar reductions in problem behavior were found in the children of the other groups. Two months after treatment, Clark found that only the FT children showed further significant gains.

Two other small studies with active controls are Morrison Bennett & Bratton's (2011) comparison of Landreth and Bratton's 10-session GFT model for teachers (CPRT) with a matched, active control group of teachers using the method of conscious discipline and Smith's study (2000) with families residing in a shelter for domestic violence. Smith used results of previous CPRT studies to provide data for comparison with her five-week intensive CPRT program. She found significant pre- and post-FT changes on both the behavioral measure (MEACI) and other parenting and child measures (CBCL) in her shelter group. Smith then compared her results with those obtained by two previous researchers who provided other intensive treatments with populations who had also experienced domestic violence (Kot, 1995; Tyndall-Lind, 1999). The first study (Kot, 1995) compared intensive FT with intensive individual play therapy. No significant differences were found between the two groups. The second study (Tyndall-Lind, 1999) compared intensive individual play therapy with sibling group therapy. Tyndall-Lind also found no significant differences between the two groups. When Smith compared the results of these two studies with those of her shelter group, she found her shelter group had results that were significantly better on the Joseph Preschool and Primary Self-concept Screening Test (Joseph, 1979) than those obtained by the researchers using the other treatments. No differences were found on the other measures.

Process studies on FT

In the study and development of therapy approaches, including FT, process studies are not nearly as common as outcome studies. Outcome studies generally are done first, and in greater numbers, in the development and validation of a therapy. Yet process studies are very important in understanding the contributions of the respective components of a therapy method. However, they are done less frequently for two rather obvious reasons. First, until a treatment can be demonstrated as effective, there is not much gain to be had by understanding its processes. Second, process studies usually take more time and resources than outcome studies, which can frequently be adequately investigated via only pre- and post-FT and hopefully follow-ups.

Nonetheless, there are several process studies that have been conducted in FT that are useful to summarize here. These studies have been selected because they are both outcome and process studies, making them particularly valuable. The very first was a study by Guerney B. & Stover (1971), mentioned earlier, which investigated not only the effectiveness of FT, but also many of the processes that brought about the positive results demonstrated. Play session behavior of the 51 mothers included in the study were observed on a regular basis, and tracked throughout the course of GFT. Thus, the researchers were able to show that mothers improved in the use of their play therapy skills. Using 49,000 data points during 600 play sessions, it was revealed that mothers showed significant gains in their ability to employ acceptance, empathy, and allowing self-direction to their children in the play sessions.

These observations also revealed changes in children's behavior from early to later play sessions. There were significant statistical changes in the children over the weeks of therapy in ratings of affection, aggression, dependence, leadership, contact with their mothers, and role-playing. Leadership and contact with the mothers increased, while aggression and dependence decreased. Demonstrations of physical affection declined as more social egalitarian interactions with the mothers increased. Children's use of role-playing decreased in later sessions, and reality play increased. When reality play increased, the children seemed to have fewer conflicts to express through role-play, as their adjustment seemed to increase. This finding was reinforced by gains measured in mothers' attitudes and their ratings of their children's behaviors in daily life. These results helped clarify the ways in which the process of change occurred for children and parents in reaching the end result of successful FT.

Another investigation of the FT process, along with outcomes, was conducted by Sywulak (1979). Sywulak used a waiting list control design and administered tests to potential participants on perceptions of their children's problems, including FPL, and measures of their own attitudes. Half of the 32 parents (19 children) were assigned to the waiting list, and the other half to treatment groups. (Waiting list families were then offered GFT.) Comparing the results of parent measures for treatment and control groups, Sywulak showed that changes in GFT parents were evident at two months, and these changes reached the level of significance at four months. No such changes occurred in the waiting list control group. Changes in the children participating in FT also were evident by four months. The study concluded that the process of change on parent variables begins earlier than was known prior to this study, and that parent changes precede significant changes in children's behavior.

Sensue (1981) studied families that had participated in Sywulak's study 3–5 years after they had finished GFT. Sensue found that on the Des Moines Child Adjustment Scale (Moore, 1964), normed for age, many parents reported that their children had better adjustment than they had at the end of treatment. (Maturation alone, therefore, would not account for their noted improvement in reported behavior.) Sensue also found that more than half the parents continued to have some kind of "special time" with their children, primarily at the insistence of the children. Sensue created a quasi-control group of children, matched to the post-treatment sample on age, socio-economic level, and gender, who had never been identified with any problems. She compared this match sample with the post-treatment GFT children. Sensue showed that the post-treatment children did not differ from this comparison sample of non-clinical children, suggesting strongly that GFT had helped achieve appropriate age-level behaviors.

Eardley (1978) completed a unique process study. In addition to examining the parent-child change process, he focused on GFT leader behavior. Using a waiting list control group (which later became a treatment group) and two treatment groups, Eardley was able to present FT to one treatment group of parents using only the didactic piece of FT. (The didactics Eardley used were systematic and accurate.) The other treatment group received GFT. Every effort was made to avoid discussions involving empathy and parent-child family dynamics in the didactic group. Positive changes in parent and child participants were not supported in the didactic treatment group, but they were in the standard GFT treatment group, Eardley (1978) concluded that without the empathic, dynamic portion of GFT which the leaders contribute to the training and group process, the gains typical of GFT were unable to be attained.

Conclusion

The extent of research conducted on group and individual FT over 40 years by many researchers in numerous settings shows that this method is a valuable tool for bringing about desired changes in parents and children. It appears valid, reliable, and most outstandingly robust. The plethora of populations who have participated in the research using a range of program lengths, from very intensive compressed time frames, through the traditional five-month length, should assure clinicians and providers that the use of FT is productive, and may be more effective than other possible treatments, particularly those without solid research bases.

A special note on the consistency of the research measures employed

One unusual and outstanding feature of research conducted on GFT is the quite consistent use of measures that were employed in the original GFT studies (Guerney B. & Stover, 1971) and the studies conducted by Landreth *et al.* through the University of North Texas (see www.cpt.unt.edu/research). The replication of results is much more meaningful when the same measures are used for various studies. This makes it possible to compare the results across experimental groups. Unfortunately, this sophisticated measurement touch is not seen much in social science research, including clinical research. Many researchers prefer to modify measurement scales for their own purposes, making cross comparisons of treatment and other study results hard to generalize meaningfully from study to study. The GFT studies have added strength because of the general consistency of results that have been replicated by measuring the same variables in the same way.

An overview of the rationale, goals, and aims of FT

FT is a well-structured method of therapy, with its own rationale, goals, and aims, as set out here.

The main rationale for FT

The main basis for FT is that parents are the most important people to their own children, and are nearly always present in their children's lives on a daily basis throughout childhood. Many professionals, by contrast, relate to children for a limited time and generally for a limited purpose (Guerney B., 1964). The depth and continuity of the relationship between parents and children, and its critical significance to children's psychological and emotional development, means that therapy offered by parents is most likely to have greater impact than therapy delivered by professionals. FT seems to be a more direct and faster way of addressing family problems. Because parents are frequently involved in managing and understanding troublesome issues for their children in FT, the presence of their parents when children are working through emotional issues tends to speed up the process. Children do not have to take the additional steps of generalizing from their therapists to their parents.

Three goals of FT

As we mentioned earlier, the parents' role as primary change agents in FT is the key to therapeutic change in families: for the children, for each parent-child relationship, and for the family as a whole. Therefore, the first goal of FT is to teach parents to be competent at playing with their children using CCPT methods under direct supervision by filial therapists. The second goal is to teach parents how to conduct play sessions at home under indirect supervision. The third goal is to help parents generalize their play session skills to daily living, and integrate these skills with other effective parenting strategies.

The main aims of FT

FT aims to do the following:

- Guide parents to work directly on promoting and deepening parent-child attachment relationships.

- Change children's emotional responses to their parents to enable their parents to become sources of emotional security for their children.

- Change children's perceptions of their parents on a cognitive level. With parents in the role of therapists, and with the helpful, positive elements inherent in that role, FT aims to enable children to perceive their parents more positively and modify their misperceptions of their parents (Guerney B., 1964).

- Enable parents to model the role of the "good parent" with their children. Such parents are identified in research as warm and nurturant, but at the same time exerting needed controls (i.e. the "authoritative parent" [Baumrind, 1971; Baumrind & Black, 1967]; the "effective parent" [Coopersmith, 1967]; the "securely attached parent," [O'Sullivan & Ryan, 2009; Ryan and Wilson, 1995; Wilson and Ryan, 2005]). Parents first model this role when using CCPT skills in play sessions, and then generalize skills to daily life, modified as necessary.

Group Filial Therapy

FT in any form has significant advantages in its own right, but we have chosen to write about Group Filial Therapy (GFT) in this book for two main reasons. First, it was the original form in which FT was first delivered, and it has been researched more than any other forms. Second, FT co-creator Louise Guerney's expertise in delivering GFT has not been fully specified until now, despite her numerous publications on FT over many years.

The GFT format, then, is generally composed of multiple families, and aims to include all the members of each family, with each parent learning and delivering individual child-centered play sessions under supervision to each child in their family. The length of intervention we describe here is approximately 20 weeks, depending upon the number of children involved, and the degree of difficulties the families are experiencing. GFT also can be conducted within shorter time frames, while still adhering to its basic features, as illustrated in the final chapter of this book.

GFT is much more than a parenting program. Instead of having a primarily educative function, as parenting programs do, it is a therapeutic program delivered within a psycho-educational framework. It is particularly useful for families troubled by more persistent, clinical levels of distress that affect their daily lives. In addition to its therapeutic purpose, GFT can also be used to prevent more serious problems arising, especially in families who are more vulnerable and at risk. A few of the adaptations to the GFT model presented in the last chapter reflect this approach.

The model of GFT developed by B. and L. Guerney is a well-structured approach, as this book demonstrates. Its psycho-educational framework is skills oriented. It therefore does not aim to be a form of group therapy for parents, but nonetheless provides strong emotional support for parents, as discussed often in this book. GFT may be seen as less emotionally threatening by parents than some other group programs, particularly by parents who may feel criticized in some group programs that do not empower parents with close supervision as they develop their skills.

Advantages of FT in a group setting

The group format for FT has several distinct advantages. The positive aims and goals listed earlier are most readily attainable in groups. In a group format, families can help one another to achieve common aims and goals. Groups can offer the following:

- *A supportive atmosphere:* Parents in groups can convey understanding and acceptance of one another's joys and difficulties embedded in family life. The advantages and the value of supportive group experiences are well established (e.g. Solomon, Pistrang, and Barker, 2001). We adopt the position, and hope to convince this book's readers to do the same, that groups are the most satisfying form of FT, because they more easily offer peer support and insight into others' problems that cannot be fully provided by professionals offering individual families an FT program.

- *Common therapeutic and educational goals:* Parents learning with others in a group about children and about how to learn a new, therapeutic role with them have the benefit over individual FT of mutual acquisition of new information and skills by parents together. However, it is important not to see GFT as primarily an *instructional* group. Indeed, as illustrated frequently throughout this book, if leaders are too intent on *instructional* goals, they can lose sight of the program's therapeutic goals.

- *Pragmatic reasons:* Because GFT has an important therapeutic aim, as well as parenting and relationship enhancement aims, it can be used as a means to deliver a much-needed mental health service to more people than individual family work can achieve. These egalitarian and inclusive aims are important to keep in mind for both practitioners and funders because of the obvious efficiency and cost-saving benefits of the group format.

- *More research support:* All the theoretical underpinnings of FT, especially the psycho-educational approach, are enhanced when a group format is used to conduct FT. While there is much supportive evidence for the effectiveness of FT with single parents and couples, the group format has been investigated more frequently and found highly effective.

The overall structure of a GFT program

We turn now to the GFT program itself. It is designed with the goal of enabling parents to conduct play sessions at home and generalize the parenting and therapeutic skills they have learned in these play sessions to daily life. Therefore, the first part of the program has a training structure that enables parents to learn to conduct child-centered play sessions effectively. Parents first observe group leaders demonstrate these play skills with each of the children in the program in turn, and listen to leaders explain the principles and skills they used in these play demos to the group.[5] Cognitive understanding on the part of parents is the primary goal at this stage. Leaders empathically respond to initial parental concerns, such as questions about the validity of these CCPT skills for helping children improve behaviors, and parents' initial worries about their ability to employ these skills. As CCPT skills are taught to parents, affective and behavioral components follow on from these introductory cognitive principles.

During training, parents are asked to simulate adult-child play interactions and appropriate child-centered responses in role-plays with fellow group members and in mock sessions, all under the guidance of group leaders. The parents then are asked to conduct shorter play sessions themselves with their children, which are directly supervised by the leaders and observed by the other group members. Once these skills are mastered at a basic level, the next step is moving play sessions into the family home. At subsequent weekly meetings, supervision of play sessions continues, either live or via videotaped home sessions (or a combination of both), along with more general discussion of home sessions. Last, there is input and discussions on generalizing these skills to daily life, before the program comes to an end. Optional support meetings may be added to the program after its formal conclusion.

Table 1.1 (see p.34) gives general time lines for conducting a 20-week GFT program. This 20-week model can easily be varied, depending upon the number of participants and the needs of families. Ways to cover all phases in the GFT program in relation to different numbers of participants, without loss of quality, is addressed in several places in this book.

The time lines shown for demos by leaders, practice play sessions by parents during group meetings, and in-depth supervision of home sessions during meetings will be largely a function of the number of children participating in the program, and, to a lesser extent, the number of parents. Two-parent families with one child require the minimum number of practice play sessions, whereas groups containing single parents with multiple children participating could take slightly longer. However, it is largely the number of children in the group that determine the number of meetings needed for demos, practice, and supervision of home sessions. For example, half the number of demos are needed for a group of five children, as opposed to a group with ten fully participating children. (Parents are encouraged to include very young children and older teens in their home play sessions, but they usually do not participate in practice sessions during group meetings. How to arrange demos with different sized families is spelled out later in this book.) Nearly always, adjustments can be made in the number of demos to meet the needs of both children and their parents, without undue extension of the length of the group.

---

5   The term "demo" is used by leaders when addressing parents during GFT, instead of the full term "demonstration." This usage is followed in this book.

Table 1.1 Typical distribution of sessions in a 20-week GFT program with 8–10 fully participating children and a maximum of 10 parents

MEETING 1 Introductions to the program and one another. Summary of GFT's aims and objectives. Brief demo (live or video) of CCPT with a non-participating child. Overview of basic child-centered play skills.
MEETINGS 2–5 Demo of a play session with each participating child by leaders. Discussion of the skills used and feedback from parents. Skills training with parents. "Mock session" training.
MEETINGS 6–10 Directly supervised practice play sessions by parents. Feedback by group leaders and discussion. Additional skills training.
MEETINGS 11–12 Planning for home play sessions. Processing of each parent's first home session.
MEETINGS 13–15 Continued practice play sessions during meetings by parents (optional). In-depth supervision of selected families' home play sessions. Group reports of home play sessions. Discussion of play themes.
MEETINGS 16–19 Continued practice play sessions during meetings by parents (optional). In-depth supervision of selected families' home play sessions, including themes. Group reports of home play sessions. Generalization of skills to daily life.
MEETING 20 Ending and evaluation of the program by participants.
OPTIONAL FOLLOW-UP MEETING(S) Discussion of issues for parents who continue home play sessions/special times.

Note: CCPT, child-centered play therapy.

Clinical issues when starting a GFT program: leaders

Leaders' roles in delivering the content, form and process of a 20-week GFT program is set out in detail in subsequent chapters, including how leaders use an "empathic responding," "unconditional acceptance," and "learning new skills" approach with parents. First we consider the attributes, roles, and needs of leaders who deliver GFT programs.

The two-leader model

This book is based on a two-leader group model; this is the most preferred leadership model for the GFT program and very commonly used. Benefits of two leaders are: first, they can serve a greater number of parents and children; and second, they can enhance each other's contributions. Before embarking on the GFT program, two leaders need to have developed a strong, professional partnership and to have already resolved issues of compatibility, therapy styles, and methods of interacting with clients. Resolving any conflicts in personal style that may impede the close coordination leaders require in delivering a therapeutic program to participating parents is essential.

For inexperienced leaders, co-leading is essential. While FT in a group format is a superior experience in our opinion to individual FT, it is a more complex intervention. GFT therefore makes multiple demands on leaders' skills and energy. Leaders need to simultaneously observe and process multiple parents' practice play sessions, instruct parents in developing therapeutic skills, and remain responsive to multiple parents' emotional needs during feedback and discussion times. For example, balancing the two basic leadership tasks of empathic support and instruction, and their subcomponents, can be more easily done by two leaders, so that neither component is relatively neglected.

The division of labor and mutual support of a second leader is very important and enhances the GFT experience for everyone involved, even for experienced leaders. Setting up a group and having it function effectively can be demanding tasks, particularly for newly practicing GFT leaders. Leaders themselves need to support one another with a variety of logistic issues, which we discuss in detail later, as well as with issues related to group dynamics. These issues are in addition to the main psycho-educational tasks of the group. However, once new leaders have run one group successfully, they typically find themselves buoyed up by the changes that families have achieved with their help, and often quickly begin to plan when their next group will take place, and how their next one can be further improved.

When only one leader is available

Two leaders are always preferable, as stated earlier. However, when only one experienced leader is available, it still is possible to conduct a full-length GFT program. With careful planning and allocation of time, a single leader can cover all phases of the full 20-week program adequately. The authors recommend strongly that, if a single leader is planning to conduct a group, the group comprises only four to six parents and no more than six children in total, with two auxiliary children for home session inclusion. Timing must be especially well planned out, so that all parents and children receive enough input and practice prior to home sessions. For smaller one-leader groups, the length of the program can be shortened accordingly.

Leaders' needs and attributes

As we emphasize throughout this book, GFT leaders are delivering a structured and complex therapeutic program for families. The group format is more demanding than delivery of services to individual families. Therefore, leaders need to think carefully about their own professional needs when conducting GFT. Recommendations on leaders' personal qualities, professional experience, and supervision needs are discussed next.

PERSONAL QUALITIES NEEDED IN GFT LEADERS

All clinicians working with troubled children and their families need to have an ability to show easily to parents that they are sincere, convinced of the effectiveness of the approach they are advocating, and have generally good judgment. Because GFT is a relatively unfamiliar approach to child and family therapy outside of North America, and because managing group participants' experiences positively and productively can be more challenging than working with individual families, GFT leaders must establish themselves as credible practitioners quickly. Similar to other therapeutic work, GFT leaders often have the least trouble establishing their credentials when they have "face validity" for the group they are working with—that is, when group leaders are older and experienced professionals, and of similar background and ethnicity to group members, their credibility may be easier to establish.

Clinicians who appear less familiar with participants' daily lives may have to work harder at establishing their places as leaders of the group. But afterwards it may be these leaders who must prove themselves to groups more fully, who also may feel an increased sense of accomplishment when they have successfully "earned" their credibility. In the first author's experience, such leaders are helped in earning their credibility when they realize that their use of genuine, accurate empathy for group members can very effectively fill the reality gap between clients' life plights and leaders' own experience. This is similar to the way grief counselors may use empathy to join grieving clients, by drawing on more general feelings of loss, but without having necessarily experienced the same kinds of losses themselves. Empathy facilitates powerful joining of any two people in therapeutic encounters, and in groups it facilitates this joining between leaders and parents, and of parents with one another.

PROFESSIONAL EXPERIENCE NEEDED BY GFT LEADERS

Due to the nature of GFT programs, training and experience in certain therapeutic skills by leaders are needed.

First, advanced training, experience and expertise in CCPT are essential for leaders. Leaders need to competently give a live demonstration to group members on how to conduct play sessions with each of their children. In addition, parents are non-professional therapists with their own children in FT and need support and specific help from leaders to address common (and sometimes uncommon) issues that arise in CCPT, and in child therapy practice more generally.

Second, sufficient clinical experience in working with families on underlying emotional issues, and an awareness of family dynamics is essential. This is because one of the goals of GFT is to alter family dynamics and help parents and children create more adaptable patterns of interaction with one another.

And third, because GFT is a structured and complex intervention, direct training in FT that is intensive and participation based is required in order to practice and learn this approach beforehand. (See Appendix 1 on suggested training opportunities and certification programs in FT for trained professionals.) We suggest that, after this specialist training, professionals gain experience in FT with individual families, including two-parent families, before undertaking to deliver a GFT program. This is because groups of families are often more challenging; delivering FT first to single families can ease the process of learning GFT for leaders.

Teaching experience with adult learners, who often have higher levels of performance anxiety than younger people, also can prove helpful for GFT leaders, as can experience in delivering psycho-educational group programs such as parenting and anger management programs. With two-leader groups, leaders' training and experience may supplement and complement one another. When one leader is highly experienced in all the components needed for leadership, that leader can train a second less experienced leader in an apprentice-like capacity. However, this arrangement is able to work very well for training GFT leaders only where both leaders are well trained in CCPT and have already had direct, participatory training in FT.

SUPERVISION AND SELF-CARE FOR GFT LEADERS

Clinical supervision requirements for therapists vary from country to country, and from one professional group to another. Good practice in GFT has similar supervision needs to supervision requirements for general child therapy practice, with leaders having access to qualified supervisors whose work and judgment they respect and value (see Drewes & Mullen, 2008; Wilson & Ryan, 2005). Because GFT is a complex intervention, specialist supervision from more experienced GFT leaders is vital for leaders to access. This is because leaders need help managing more challenging group and play session issues effectively. For sole leaders and co-leaders with less experience in training adults and group processes, these leaders need more intensive, specialist, clinical supervision from experienced GFT supervisors.

Experienced GFT co-leaders do not usually need such a high level of specialist supervision, unless a group presents new or unexpected challenges for them. They are more able to provide co-supervision to one another on a planned basis, in addition to their regular supervision by an experienced GFT supervisor. We highly recommend that experienced (and, of course, inexperienced co-leaders, even more so) build in co-supervision time after each GFT meeting. Co-leaders need to go over their videos of each meeting together and give feedback to one another on how they responded, in addition to planning the next meeting and how they will divide the work next time. Solo leaders are more dependent upon self-supervision, which should include videoing each meeting, viewing the video, evaluating their effectiveness as a leader afterwards, and then adapting their delivery to group needs for their next meeting.

For every leader we recommend that their experienced GFT supervisors have opportunities to view and discuss videos of selected parents' play sessions and videos of the group process with their GFT supervisees. For professionals who are newly practicing GFT, we suggest having regular, scheduled times with their experienced GFT supervisor at least once every three sessions, with the additional proviso that more supervision is available when needed. Until GFT practitioners have had enough experience to identify and bring issues to supervision on an "as needed" basis, and are experienced enough to begin the solo delivery of GFT with small groups, this level of supervision is highly needed. Webcam and other internet facilities for transmitting video materials currently make live supervision viable over great distances. These options ensure that specialist GFT supervision is accessible for leaders even in circumstances where face-to-face supervision may be impossible (e.g. in countries starting to offer GFT, and for professionals who do not have the time or funding to travel).

In addition to specialist supervision, other forms of supervision—for example, group peer supervision—may play a useful role for GFT leaders. However, it is important that the peer group itself has sufficient experience of GFT or FT to provide a knowledgeable sounding board for GFT leaders. Finally, occasionally while delivering GFT, similar to other forms of child therapy practice, leaders may find that more intensive personal reactions and experiences are activated that interfere with their clinical work. Leaders may decide to undertake personal therapy under these circumstances, sometimes deciding on this course of action themselves, or after discussion with their supervisor, co-leader or supervision peer group.

Clinical issues when starting a GFT program: families

It is well recognized in current clinical practice that children and their families are part of a closely knit system and children's emotional problems and treatment options are highly dependent upon their parents' views and motivation. As mentioned earlier, FT is an ideal way to strengthen family relationships and has been researched and practiced for a wide variety of children's problems.

Common referral problems

There are three common reasons why parents are motivated to attend GFT programs.

First, clinical populations of children already experiencing more serious mental health problems, such as high anxiety, more serious attachment, conduct and/or attentional problems, and other mental health difficulties that adversely affect school and family life, motivate parents to seek help and are suitable for referral for GFT. It is this population of children and their families who commonly have funding priority because of their overt levels of distress. The GFT program is suitable for this population because it offers child therapy, along with parenting and relationship-building skills. Earlier research was done on this population, from which empirical evidence was generated supporting the GFT approach.

Secondary prevention also can be a motivation for participants and referrers to access GFT. Families at risk of more serious emotional problems—such as those who have a mentally, cognitively or physically disabled family member (child or parent), those who have had separations or been reconstituted, and those who have undergone difficult life events (for example, fostering, adoption, living in a war zone, immigration, or imprisonment)— have all been participants in successful GFT programs. The final chapter of this book on adaptations of the 20-week GFT program gives a few examples of programs tailored to the needs of particular groups.

Third, primary prevention may be a goal. Some parents want to increase their parenting capacities, and attend Filial Therapy to enhance their children's emotional development, and to prevent problems arising in their current and future lives together. However, given funding constraints in most countries, primary and secondary prevention goals often are not adequately funded because clinical populations are prioritized over prevention.

Organizing the GFT program and recruitment of families

FT has been shown to be successful in helping parents and children positively change their emotional lives. But parents who do not attend the program cannot change. Therefore, the first task for leaders is organizing the GFT program and recruiting families to attend. Appendix 4 provides leaders with a prototype for designing their own general information leaflet for families. Appendix 2 gives detailed steps for starting up GFT programs, especially those offered within organizations. This appendix may be of particular relevance to leaders where GFT is not a familiar method of therapy within their organizations. If a GFT program is a new undertaking, leaders need to allow additional preparation time and sharing of information with parents, professionals, and managers, in order to ensure sufficient uptake of places in their group programs, over and above the usual time frame for recruiting new participants for the next GFT program on an ongoing basis.

It is important to begin a group with a larger number of parents than leaders intend to see through the program. This is because some families who agree to participate may be unable or unmotivated to attend. These families usually identify themselves at the early stages in the program in our experience, and waiting list families may be slotted in fairly easily. However, sometimes the number of clients is not sufficient for a waiting list, or the program is being newly offered. In these instances, leaders may decide to fill the group to capacity, assuming there will be one or two non-attenders. This strategy is an effective one, but the risk, of course, is that the group will be at very full capacity, if everyone does decide to attend. Leaders then need to be experienced and adept at slotting in all aspects of the program, in order to deliver it without a loss of quality. Some of the adaptations of GFT suggested in the final chapter may also be worth considering under these circumstances.

Planning issues arising in GFT programs

Leaders need to start making practical plans for running the program before intake meetings for GFT with individual families. These intake meetings and the general characteristics of parents and children suitable for GFT are discussed in the next chapter. In this section, we explore more general planning issues for leaders and their agencies when setting up GFT programs.

GROUP COMPOSITION

It is important for leaders to select families that complement one another in the group itself. Parents from different socio-economic and family backgrounds, educational levels, and ethnic groups are suitable for inclusion within one group in our experience. Indeed, an egalitarian emphasis is essential for group leaders to foster in participants, regardless of the composition of the group. This attitude, in fact, is made easier in GFT because all participants are initially equal in their need to learn how to conduct child-centered play sessions with their children.

Another criterion when leaders consider their group membership is that participants are able to take part in a group without undue stress for other members. Similar to any group with a supportive aim, leaders should ensure that they do not include parents with extreme views that are highly threatening to other group members (e.g. extreme xenophobia). The supportive aim of the group can be easily thwarted by one very extreme member. Members' defensive responses can be raised if they are subject to verbal attacks, and other members' caretaking responses towards a threatened group member can also be easily activated.

Other features of group membership also need to be taken into account by leaders. Parents with ongoing, more serious emotional, attentional and/or addiction problems, even though meeting the criterion of being able to focus for limited time spans on their children, may not be best served in a group setting. And parents whose mental capacities are significantly below average may not be best served in a group setting because of the longer than average time they usually need to learn play skills. Parents who cannot focus sufficiently on their children's emotional responses in play sessions, or ones who feel that they continually have to fight for status on all fronts, are likely to be unable to keep up with the group program because participants are required to learn child-centered play skills at a relatively equal rate. However, families unsuitable for GFT are frequently suitable for individual Filial Therapy, where group learning is not a feature of the intervention.

ADVANTAGES TO DIVERSITY OF CHILD AGES AND PROBLEMS IN GFT GROUPS

In our experience, groups seem to work well with families that have varied reasons for referral, and children who have a variety of emotional issues. A range of problems and ages is helpful in a group in order to increase the diversity of issues addressed within group meetings, and in order to prevent group members over-identifying their own problems with other group members. For example, groups may have adoptive families, and families whose children have high anxiety levels, along with families whose children have disabilities, and families where conduct problems have arisen.

Groups also can be successfully run where children come from the same referral source. For example, charitable agencies and schools often have specialized referrals that are suitable for GFT programs. Groups can be formed with parents who share one characteristic, such as having fostered children, adoptive children, bereaved children, and children with chronic illnesses, to name a few. These kinds of referrals are feasible because the children referred from one source, say a bereavement service, do not present exactly the same problem behaviors. Therefore, the parents are not dealing with the same kinds of parenting issues related to those behaviors. Yet, these families do come with a common history that allows them to join together quickly and easily, and to advance into working with the children's individual differences, as well as the commonalities shared by their respective children.

Therefore, we recommend, where possible and particularly for inexperienced leaders, that several families with serious conduct problems not be placed together in one group, but be dispersed among parents with children showing varied problems. We suggest that often families with children who display serious conduct problems seem particularly suited to being placed with families whose children are withdrawn and have somatic difficulties.

Groups composed of families with children of the same age (e.g. same grade level in a primary school) also can be successful. Other groups may be formed on the basis of common ethnicity, or on the basis of shared adversity (e.g. GFT following a natural disaster). What allows these groups to work better in our experience than groups where the children share a common, more serious, pathology, is that the common experience is essentially external to the family (e.g. a disaster, ethnicity, or bringing a foster child into the family). It is when conduct disordered, highly depressed or extremely withdrawn children share common behavioral issues that, at least theoretically, their presentations could be heavily associated with difficult family relationship patterns. In a group, the process of identification and reinforcement of these patterns by parents tends to get in the way of reasonable progress, and the groups become significantly more challenging for leaders to manage. In addition, with such commonalities, little in the way of other perspectives or alternative behaviors may be offered by group members.

Finally, because GFT is a family intervention, leaders should aim to include both parents in two-parent families in their groups wherever possible, and as many children as possible in the family, from toddlers to teens. But we have tried in this book to recognize the reality for leaders of engaging only one adult in the family, despite their best efforts, and only some of the children. We offer suggestions and caveats for these circumstances elsewhere in the book.

NUMBER OF PARTICIPANTS TO SELECT

As stated earlier, the number of families selected for a group is highly influenced by the number of children in each family, and by the length of the program, which is discussed further later. The program presented here is a 20-week one, but it can easily be adapted to a somewhat shorter or longer time frame, as we discuss later. However, there always will be program constraints on the amount of time group leaders can take to conduct demonstrations with each child, and the time each parent has to do practice play sessions with each of their children during group meetings.

OPTIMAL NUMBER OF CHILDREN

Experienced leaders in a 20-week program with two leaders, with meetings lasting two hours each, plus a half-hour break, are able to comfortably schedule a maximum of ten children for demos and practice play sessions during the initial training phase of GFT, before home sessions begin. While the program is typically for children aged 2.5–11 years, 12–13-year-olds also may be appropriate to include, given suitable adjustments in the materials used for sessions (see Ryan & Wilson, 2005). With ten fully participating children, for example, leaders would be required to have turnaround times of 15–20 minutes per child for demos during Meetings 2–5, in order to accommodate ten children. Sufficient time for discussion of demos and skills learning also needs to take place during each of these meetings. For meetings with demos, then those with practice sessions, and in-depth supervision of home sessions, ten children is the most comfortable maximum for leaders to accommodate, with approximately three additional, "auxiliary" children. Auxiliary children include toddlers and teens in participating families who receive shorter play sessions or special times at home, and siblings without identified emotional problems who are offered play sessions at home, both groups of whom do not need as many demos, practice sessions, or supervision of home sessions by leaders during meetings.

Large families referred for GFT remain highly suitable, but leaders and parents may need to agree that only some of the children are prioritized during the first stages of the program, before the transition to home sessions when more children can be included. Alternatively, if several children in the family need immediate intervention, or if siblings have intense and enmeshed relationships with one another that would preclude this staged approach, individual FT may be more suitable than a group program.

OPTIMAL NUMBER OF PARENTS IN TWO-LEADER GROUPS

We recommend ten parents as a maximum for two leaders. These parents should ideally be a mixture of single-parent families with one child, along with other family combinations, when the maximum of ten parents attend. Leaders need to remember that two-parent families with more than one child, and single parents with several children, necessarily take more group time than a one-parent family with one child. Numbers of parents are determined by the requirement that each parent have two directly supervised play sessions during Meetings 6–10, before home sessions start. A likely group formation would be two couples and three singletons attached to ten children, with three auxiliary children who participate in the program primarily via home sessions.

When leaders find that the proposed numbers of parents or children get higher than suggested here for a group they are considering assembling, they may need to make adjustments in the composition of the group. If at intake, leaders have an unmanageable number of couples for a group, say five couples some with more than two children each, rather than trying to stretch GFT resources to cover this number, we strongly recommend that a few of these couples are assigned to a second group composed of both couples and singletons, and that a couple of singletons are added to the first group, in order to ensure that the numbers come out right.

MINIMUM NUMBERS FOR GFT GROUPS

At the lower end, a group of, say, three parents, one of which is a couple, is possible, but it may end up with only one family attending the entire program, rather than two families. Frequently, if one parent in a family does not attend (e.g. due to the weather, a conflicting appointment), the other parent also is less likely to attend. Of course, the one remaining person who attends ends up feeling very special, but does not benefit from the dynamics of the group. Should the non-attendance of this couple continue, and the single parent is alone at meetings frequently, the single parent might stop feeling special and begin to feel abandoned. Therefore, individual FT from the outset may be a more useful intervention with very small numbers.

Because of the kinds of attendance problems mentioned here, in actual practice it is unwise for GFT leaders to try to conduct a group of fewer than six parents (but see Chapter 16 for an exception to this rule with foster parents). Starting with six parents who are suitable for GFT permits one or two parents to drop out or miss meetings, and still maintain a functioning group with all the attributes necessary to further parent development. The option of having individual FT can always be extended to a family when numbers do not reach this minimum. It is also possible for parents whose problems are not urgent to wait until a large enough group can be assembled. However, the latter is the least desirable method of management in our opinion.

LENGTH OF THE GFT PROGRAM

The anticipated length of the program should be decided at the outset, before families are recruited. Leaders need to reserve space and resources for the group, and inform parents at intake, so that everybody can plan on, and commit themselves to, the length of the program. As already mentioned, this book presents a 20-week GFT program. While shorter GFT programs exist, as the final chapter attests, and the 20-week program detailed here can be adapted to a shorter 10-session one in certain circumstances, for many populations and purposes, adhering to the 20-week program we present is the best option. We have found that 20 weeks provides the optimal time to cover all elements of the program, without undue time pressure, for an average size group.

However, there is some flexibility in the number of meetings planned. The program, as presented here, may run from 15–24 weeks, with 20 weeks as the most frequent number. Leaders can adjust the number of meetings offered, either expanding or contracting them. The number of weeks depends on how many demos, practice play sessions, and processing of home sessions are needed, which varies with the actual number of parents and children participating in the program, and the number of optional follow-up meetings (usually 1–4 meetings).

The length of the program also can be altered based on the seriousness of families' problems, discussed next.

LENGTH OF PROGRAM IN RELATION TO SERIOUSNESS OF PRESENTING PROBLEMS

Another factor that affects the length of the program is the characteristics of the children and families who are recruited. The standard 20-week program presented here for a group of average size is the appropriate program to address common clinical issues in sufficient depth. We also recommend the 20-week length of program when families reach the secondary prevention level, if practicable. Short group programs, and programs that only offer indirect supervision on one parent-child dyad in the family, may be less likely to address entrenched emotional problems, or to develop new relationship patterns for the entire family group with clinically significant problems.

For primary prevention, and for secondary prevention when necessary, leaders may want to consider other, shorter GFT models instead, some of which are presented in the final chapter. However, leaders forming 20-week groups with families who have entrenched problems at a clinical level also should consider including families in 20-week groups whose issues place them only at high risk for future problems, particularly when leaders do not have sufficient numbers of clinical cases to run a full 20-week group program. These less troubled families often have a high level of motivation and less distress, both of which have a favorable impact on other group members with more serious clinical issues to address. For example, newly adopting families may be highly suitable for inclusion, even though the adoptive child is not presenting with serious emotional/behavioral problems. GFT usually resonates with new adoptive parents' need to be highly involved in their children's emotional care; it develops their parenting skills, and enhances their newly forming attachments (Ryan, 2007b; Ryan & Bratton, 2008; VanFleet, 2013). While these adoptive families would generally be expected to contribute more positive elements to the group's exchanges, leaders also must be cautious that the benefits to the adoptive families are not overwhelmed by the greater problems of the clinical families.

PARENTAL MOTIVATION AND LENGTH OF PROGRAM

Finally, and crucially, in determining the length of their programs, leaders have to judge the level of motivation of families to be selected for their groups. In our experience, there is a tendency for parents who are not committed to resolving underlying problems to feel finished when superficial problems have been solved, and not go on to deal with more deep-rooted problems that require attention. 20-week groups, rather than shorter group formats, may give these parents the structure to make more enduring changes in their relationships. However, leaders also need to select participants who are sufficiently able to be self-motivated to attend GFT meetings and carry out home sessions. Sometimes in our experience, individual FT may be more suitable for less motivated parents. Or, it may be more appropriate to start with play therapy as the first intervention, followed by a shorter GFT program. Parents may become highly motivated to learn FT once they have seen the positive results of the children's play therapy first. Overall, when motivation or predictable ability to carry through with the 20-week program appears to be minimal, a shorter program with more limited therapeutic aims may be most realistic.

POPULATIONS BEST SUITED FOR THE 20-WEEK PROGRAM

The next chapter gives more details on the types of families and children suitable to participate in 20-week GFT programs. Several examples are given here of types of families and children who can benefit from a 20-week GFT program:

- Families presenting with more serious, entrenched family and child problems.

- Children with early onset conduct problems.

- Parents and children with moderate relationship difficulties.

- Children with more serious anxiety problems.

- Children on the autistic spectrum.

- Children with cognitive deficits who are exhibiting moderate emotional problems.

- Families whose issues place them at high risk for future problems (e.g. inter-racial adoptions).

- Children who are fostered.

- Children who are late adopted.

- Children who have been maltreated, and are not currently at risk.

For these families, the parents' ability, both emotionally and cognitively, to learn new skills, change their emotional attitudes during play sessions, then generalize these to their home life, may require more time than would be available in a shorter program, and/or their children may need more time to make therapeutic gains.

Shorter versions of GFT, presented in the final chapter, may be more suitable for other families, including those with the following attributes:

- Families with primary prevention goals (e.g. families with early adopted children).

- Reconstituted families.

- Families with children having chronic and/or terminal illnesses (e.g. juvenile diabetes).

- Families with parents who want to optimize their parenting abilities and skills.

- Families with limited socio-economic resources and/or schedules that make attending longer programs problematic.

- Families with lower motivation.

Scheduling weekly meetings

This section explores some general considerations for leaders in setting up GFT schedules and making provisions for running the program.

Administrative support

It is highly advantageous for leaders to have good administrative support for practical help with logistics (e.g. babysitters, reminders to parents, answering general queries). The administrator's positive and encouraging manner during contacts with participants also is essential. It is very important for leaders to have briefed the administrator on the types of questions and comments from parents that may need clinical input, and which need to be referred on to leaders to address. These clinical issues can include parents expressing doubts about the program, giving reasons for absences, sharing family difficulties, or discussing the contents of home play sessions. If it is necessary for professionals to conduct GFT as single leaders, as well as adhering to the smaller group format recommended earlier, skilled administrative support becomes even more vital.

Holiday and school vacation breaks

We advise that no group meetings are held during major holidays, since this is family time for both participants and leaders. For lesser holidays, and when leaders are available and have the flexibility, the group should be given the option to decide whether to hold a meeting. As with any therapeutic program, it is most useful if holiday and vacation breaks coincide with natural breaks in the program. In deciding on what holiday breaks are required, leaders need to work these out during their planning. Leaders need to consider how disruptive to learning, detrimental to continued motivation for attending the group, and how anxiety provoking having a break will be for participants.

For GFT, a natural break of a week occurs when home sessions have become established, and before generalization gets under way formally. It is also possible to have a week's break during the training period, or once practice play sessions during meetings have been under way for a while, if a break is essential. We do not recommend ever having a week's break immediately prior to participants' first practice play sessions, or prior to and after the first home sessions.

Childcare provision

Providing good childcare during GFT meetings is necessary. Each child's direct involvement in meetings takes up only part of any meeting times, and childcare is needed for the remaining time. Good childcare also is important in order to ensure that parents are certain that their children are well cared for while they attend meetings. Parents find it much easier to concentrate on their own learning while in the group, if caregiving has been competently managed elsewhere. These principles of caregiving and learning are captured well by attachment principles showing how activation of parents' caregiving system (e.g. such as hearing their child cry) blocks the activation of their exploratory/interest sharing system, the latter of which is necessary for their learning (Heard & Lake, 1997).

It is equally important that children view their childcare arrangements as enjoyable. Childcare that is something for children to look forward to, and easy to return to once they have had their turn with their parents during meetings, is essential to the success of GFT. Again, attachment theory and research show that separations and reunions, such as those that are built into the GFT program, can activate children's care seeking and defensive systems. Therefore it is important for leaders to ensure that childcare arrangements are both pleasurable and relaxing for children. One adaptation of the 20-week model discussed in the final chapter, Chillery and Ryan's model, shows how combining GFT with a parallel, weekly, informal children's group can provide opportunities for children to increase their prosocial skills, as well as provide childcare. Children can help their parents to be motivated to attend weekly meetings when they look forward to their own children's group.

Premises

The "ideal" premises consist of a kitchen area for breaks, a room for childcare, a meeting room for leaders and parents for training and discussions together, and a separate room for holding demos and practice play sessions with parents and their children. This separate room ideally is linked by either a one-way mirror to an observation room in which all parents can fit, or by a video link to the group meeting room. Current multiplication of wireless technologies has made it more possible for leaders to create an affordable observation scheme that can accommodate a full group of parents.

Yet it is worth keeping in mind that experienced leaders have managed to run successful groups under far from ideal conditions, and have used ingenuity and resourcefulness in adapting to what they have available. As a last resort, when space and/or funding are very restricted, leaders may consider holding demos and practice play sessions with parents observing in the room, if the number of parents is small enough. However there are obvious drawbacks to this arrangement. First, it can be overly inhibiting for parents and children, particularly older children, to have an audience in the room. Second, it can be difficult for observing parents to remain completely silent during the play session.

For these "same room" observations by parents, when they are necessary, we offer the following guidelines:

- The room should be big enough to separate parents from the play space by at least ten feet.

- Temporary barriers (e.g. a bookcase, chairs) should be made between the observing parents and the play section of the room, to create an artificial division in the room itself.

- Lights in the parents' part of the room should be turned off. The part of the room with the child and leader/parent should be the only part of the room that is lit.

Even with these temporary aids, leaders still have the additional task of ensuring that parents are particularly quiet, and do not distract the children during their play by any comments or larger movements.

Meeting times and meeting breaks

The decision on the time of day for the group is based on multiple considerations. Among them are when the participants are most readily available (e.g. working parents often cannot attend during the daytime), when the children are amenable and not too tired to participate in play sessions, when the leaders are available, when the facilities can be used, etc. It is important to remember that, if an evening slot is decided on, both children and parents are more tired and therefore usually less able to adjust themselves to new situations rapidly. Therefore, a scheduled break during the meeting is essential. However, an advantage is that often both parents in two-parent families are able to attend meetings, when they are held in the evening.

For all the meetings, regardless of time of day, we advise leaders to schedule meetings for 2.5 hours on the same day each week, with approximately half an hour at midway point allocated for a break with a snack and drink. These breaks are important for several reasons. Breaks encourage participants to chat informally, thus promoting both group cohesion and the building of individual supportive relationships among group members. Breaks also are times for participants to relax and not be expected to take in new information and learn new skills. This change in tempo is especially important when parents are learning to do play sessions and having their first practice play sessions. And finally, breaks enable leaders to model for parents that structuring and attuning to people's needs is an important part of the attentive caregiving they are trying to facilitate in parents with their own children, both in play sessions and later in their daily living.

The next chapter addresses the intake process and selection of participants in more detail, including further discussion of whether individual FT, GFT or another intervention is the preferred option for a family.

CHAPTER 2

The Selection of Suitable Participants and the Intake Process for GFT[1]

The selection process in GFT

Selection of suitable participants and the intake process is an important task for leaders when setting up GFT programs. This chapter begins by discussing in general terms the types of families and problems that are suitable for GFT. It then explores the kinds of intake information to collect that are specific to FT, and the importance of preliminary discussions with families on their possible participation in GFT.

General selection issues
General characteristics of children suitable for GFT

Almost all children are highly motivated to participate in play sessions with their parents. (See Table 2.1 for a summary of general characteristics of children to consider when deciding on GFT.) Families rarely need to be excluded from GFT due to their children's lack of motivation to participate. Children ranging in age from 2.5–12 years are suitable, with some adjustments at the higher and lower ends of the age range in the play session format. For example, with older children, materials for sessions may include a couple of structured games and more complex activities. And for very young children, the length of the usual half-hour play session may be decreased, in addition to modifying the toy selection. Adaptations also can be made in play sessions, once parents have established play sessions in their own homes with selected children, in order to fully include younger

---

1   The American term "intake" has been chosen here, rather than the British term "assessment," which has a narrower meaning in the USA.

and older siblings who are at the edges of the 2.5–12 age range. Parents can be helped to respond to their babies' and toddlers' more rudimentary play interactions in briefer play sessions, and to their teenagers' more advanced requirements in special times together. These variations are discussed in more detail later in this book.

Table 2.1 General characteristics of children to consider in decisions on GFT

1. Motivational factors: Are the children able to play? (Most commonly, children 2.5–12 years are eager to participate in play sessions, with some adjustments at the higher and lower ages—e.g. materials, length of sessions, "special times.")
2. Practical factors: Do children have a very high level of other commitments professionally (e.g. health or mental health interventions) and/or personally (e.g. shared care) that do not allow time for regular play sessions?
3. Attachment styles: Are the children sufficiently non-defensive to play with their parents? Do children have a very high level of aggression towards their parents? Do children have very serious attachment disorders?
4. Inherent characteristics: Do children have difficulties that may reduce their participation in special play sessions (e.g. severe learning difficulties, psychoses, profound autism)?
Other questions to consider: When siblings choose not to participate in FT, and they have significant emotional distress, are such families suitable for GFT? Can the decision on the suitability of this family for GFT be reserved until after the family play observation?

FT has been found to be effective for children with more serious mental health and relationship difficulties. As described in Chapter 1, delivering therapy for children with a wide range of problems through mainly playful, rather than verbal, means has a long history. Play sessions are especially suitable for children who are unable to express themselves adequately through verbal means (e.g. children who have multiple emotional issues). Children with hearing, cognitive, language, and other disabilities, including those on the autistic spectrum, also can benefit. Group leaders have some experience and skills needed to work with these special populations.

Parents of children with special needs already have developed means to communicate with their children and know intimately how to interpret their non-verbal responses. These features of their relationship make these parents the natural choice for therapeutic interventions with their children. However, in some cases, children with more serious impairments may not be able to play with their parents, even on a rudimentary level, which may preclude their participation in the play sessions inherent in GFT. A "learn to play" program, such as Stagnitti (1998), prior to FT, for children who have rudimentary ability to respond playfully, may be helpful. In a few other cases, children may have highly complex emotional needs, or respond with severe aggression towards their parents in a playroom situation. Again this limits the ability of their parents to conduct play sessions with their children initially, as discussed further next.

General characteristics of parents suitable for GFT

As mentioned already, motivational factors are important to consider in selecting parents for GFT (see Table 2.2). Parents need to agree to attend and participate in a group program, sharing the strengths and difficulties of their parenting with other parents. Therefore, parents who for practical reasons (e.g. shift work) are unable to attend group meetings on a regular basis, or those who are extremely reluctant to share their thoughts with others, or those who exhibit more extreme, unsociable behaviors may not be suitable for GFT. However, they all may be candidates for individual FT.

Table 2.2 General characteristics of parents to consider in decisions on GFT

1. Motivational factors: Are the parents committed to actively helping their children? Do they have a general desire to relate more effectively with their children? Does one of the parents in a two-parent family strongly object to the purpose or delivery of FT? Are other professionals delivering therapeutic or parenting programs that may actively interfere cognitively or emotionally with participation in GFT for the parents?
2. Practical factors: Can the parents participate in the intervention or will other commitments (e.g. shift work) interfere?
3. Attachment styles: Are the parents sufficiently non-defensive to share their thoughts and feelings regarding their children with leaders and with other parents? Do the parents have a highly antagonistic attitude towards one another?
4. Inherent characteristics: Do parents have mental health, addiction, and/or learning difficulties, at a sufficient level to preclude their ability to learn FT skills and remain child focused during special playtimes?
5. Child protection issues: Are these issues ongoing and serious?
Other questions to consider: • Do extended family members need to be included in the intervention? At the first intake meeting? For the next two assessment phases? (Note that families' ethnicity and family dynamics may influence these decisions.) • Where parents do not want other siblings to participate (especially older and younger siblings), is this in keeping with the filial therapist's clinical judgment? Can judgment be reserved until after family play observation (FPO)? If one parent in a two-parent family does not want to participate in FT, can judgment on the suitability of this family for GFT be reserved until after the FPO?

In general, parents need to have an overall desire to relate more effectively with their children. Very infrequently, parents and children whose levels of anger and resentment towards one another are extreme may not be able to participate initially in play sessions together. Parents may be unable to maintain positive attention on their children, even for shorter periods of time, and their children's spontaneous, angry responses may be too difficult for their parents to manage. In these more extreme cases, a program such as the College Park program, presented in the final chapter on adaptations of GFT, may be more suitable. In this program, a play therapist offers play therapy initially alongside more intensive parent consultations. GFT is offered to suitable families as the second step of the intervention.

A few referred families may already be receiving ongoing mental health input or attending parenting programs, some of which may be incompatible with FT principles. In such cases, therapists have to decide whether these families are able to commit themselves to GFT practically, emotionally and cognitively. Parents who have mental health difficulties or cognitive difficulties that still allow them to attend to and respond to their children during play sessions, and to participate in group discussions *are* suitable for GFT, as are parents with histories of addictions/alcoholism that are now managed and do not currently preclude their ability to parent. However, parents who currently have moderate to severe, untreated mental health difficulties and/or current and significant drug or alcohol dependency that would prevent them from being able to focus and learn from the program are not suitable candidates for FT, nor are families where there are significant and/or ongoing, more serious child protection concerns. Very occasionally, parents in two-parent families who have highly antagonistic relationships with each other also may be unsuitable for GFT, as well as families in which one of the parents is committed to FT while the other parent is strongly opposed. All of these areas are important to screen for by agencies and therapists during their initial intake step, which is discussed in the next section of this chapter.

Aiming for an inclusive therapy

Ideally, GFT includes the entire family, with parents and all children in the family participating. There are several reasons for including all the siblings, as well as the referred child or children, in play sessions. The inclusion of siblings is intended to enhance the family's individual parent-child relationships and prevent additional sibling rivalries developing, which can occur when one child is singled out for attention. Another reason for inclusion of siblings is to ensure against pathological responses emerging in the other children, once the referred child's presenting symptoms reduce. A further rationale is that parents often find it easier to practice new play session skills with the less distressed children in their families, with whom they often think that they have better relationships. Finally, parents commonly realize at intake that their time and energy have been disproportionately given to the referred child, to the detriment of their other children. These parents often welcome an opportunity to redress this imbalance.

When all family members do not plan to participate

NON-PARTICIPATING PARENTS

In some two-parent families, parents may decide that work, personal or family commitments preclude one of them from participating fully in GFT. In our experience, it is well worth leaders exploring creative solutions to these dilemmas with parents at intake. Sometimes it is possible to alter these commitments by working on the issues together, rather than leaders accepting difficulties with attendance immediately. For example, we have found that some employers can be persuaded by a letter or email from the GFT leader to release their employees on the basis that the skills they learn as parents in GFT have positive applications to their jobs. The second author has persuaded employers that the skills of empathy, structuring, and limit setting benefit employers by enhancing their employees' management skills and cooperative working relationships with other employees.

If some commitment, rather than full participation, is viable, we suggest leaders encourage the overloaded parent to attend as many of the meetings as possible with their partner. This parent may be able to have sufficient attendance to conduct play sessions with their children under direct supervision during group meetings, and still find some opportunities for home sessions, albeit less frequently than their fully participating partner. Another option that has been used is assigning each parent to separate groups that meet at different times. This variation permits parents to provide childcare for their non-participating children.

However, sometimes it is not possible for one of the parents to participate in GFT, even on a more limited basis. In these cases, it is very important that the non-participating parents understand the aims of GFT and are supportive of the participating parents, their children's participation, and the program's values. In our experience, when one parent attempts to participate in GFT with active opposition from other powerful family figures, increased family tensions, failure to engage fully in the group process, and dropping out of GFT are more likely. Therefore, we suggest in these circumstances that another intervention other than FT is considered.

The participating parent, in addition to carrying out the program, has the very important role of conveying information about it to their non-participating partner on a personal level, including their own and their children's responses to the program. Leaders need to be attentive to the influence of non-participating parents on the participants and their children, and try to deal with them effectively. Leaders should play a proactive role, arranging to have telephone or email contact with non-participating parents if at all possible, and supplying written information on the program for these parents. This close attention to non-participating parents by leaders is crucial because, in order for GFT to be effective as a family intervention, parents attending the program need a supportive home atmosphere. This support should be both practical and emotional, in order to enable parents to attend meetings, learn skills, conduct home play sessions, and change their relationships with their children during the program.

Additional physical support may need to fall to non-participating parents, such as practical help in childminding during the other parent's group attendance, and keeping the other children occupied during the other parent's home play sessions with each child.

Where a partner is not available for active support, leaders should consider other adults who may provide an invaluable supportive role for participating parents from the family's wider support networks. Again, these support figures need to be able to provide both practical and emotional support, while they themselves do not participate in the program actively.

During FT, similar to child therapy generally, children need supportive and emotionally available parents, including any non-participating parents, in order to effect changes in their family relationships and daily lives. When there are doubts about the ability of couples to successfully support one another, or about single parents' ability to accept support, an objective measure, such as the Attachment Style Interview (Bifulco, 2003), which assesses adults' current emotional supports and attachment styles, may be useful to administer during the intake phase by professionals trained in its use.

NON-PARTICIPATING SIBLINGS

In other families, it is sometimes siblings, particularly older siblings, who choose not to participate in the program. Other times parents, despite leaders' presentation to them of the value of all family members' participation, decide that one or more of their children are not in need of play sessions. In these cases, we suggest that leaders follow the parents' lead, where such decisions do not seriously compromise their clinical judgment, and either omit these children, or decrease the amount of time devoted to practice sessions for these children during group meetings. A timely suggestion by leaders that parents may want to reconsider and begin play sessions or special activity times with non-participating siblings later in the program seems more effective in our experience than insisting on participation at the outset.

However, leaders do need to carefully monitor these non-participating siblings during the program. Sometimes parents' and siblings' initial reluctance disappears once play sessions have been established (e.g. during meetings after practice sessions begin, or when home sessions begin), and once parents have more confidence in the value of play sessions overall. In other cases, parents begin to report deterioration in their non-participating children's behavior, once their referred child's behavior and emotional reactions become less distressing for the family. In both sets of circumstances, leaders are then in a stronger position to encourage full participation.

Leaders also need to be open to the possibility that the family's initial decision that certain family members will not benefit from the intervention can be a valid one for some families. In some instances in our experience, non-participating siblings do remain able to maintain close attachment relationships with their parents and participating siblings, while also maintaining their own emotional well-being.

The roles of extended family members and close friends

Because GFT is intended as a family intervention, we caution leaders to limit direct participation in the program to family members, rather than, for example, to extended family members or friends of the family. However, it is important for leaders, depending on family dynamics or families' ethnic values, to consider including extended family members in the GFT program in certain circumstances. These issues should be explored at intake. For example, either before or during the intake process, it might become apparent to leaders that an extended family member (e.g. grandmother, head of extended family household) is the key to making the decision on whether nuclear family members participate in the program. It is then important for leaders to either meet with or provide these family members with sufficient information about the program for consent to be given.

In other families, adults other than parents (e.g. grandmother, grandfather, aunt) have primary attachment relationships with referred children and their siblings. In these cases, leaders may decide to include these significant adults in the intake and give consideration to whether to include them as participants in GFT. For example, for Chinese American families (Johnson, 2006), grandmothers who played a significant caregiving role with their grandchildren fully participated in GFT programs offered to these families. Adult siblings who take on major parental responsibilities for their younger siblings during childhood also may be suitable for inclusion, given that sufficient family support is available to the entire family.

For reconstituted families or separated/divorced families where more than two parents are significant to the children, it is possible to consider that all significant parental figures fully participate in GFT. In these cases, leaders need to discuss this option with all parties, and use their clinical judgment on whether the estranged parents/step-parents have a relationship that could accommodate to a group setting. Otherwise individual FT, with separate training and supervision of each parent would be more suitable. Another option chosen by the first author, which has been successful, is placing estranged parents in separate, concurrent groups.

The intake process for GFT

The three steps in the GFT intake process are the initial intake meeting, the family play observation (FPO) and the final intake meeting.

Steps in conducting the intake process

This section summarizes the three steps in the intake process, before more detailed discussion of each step.

STEP 1

The first step in the intake process described here is written from the viewpoint of agencies where GFT leaders are not part of the initial intake team. This stance is taken in order to demonstrate that the initial intake process by non-filial therapists is a very important preliminary that should not be overlooked by leaders in recruiting and selecting families for inclusion in GFT.

Agencies often have multi-professional intake/assessment teams and usually have their own intake protocols and interview formats at the first step in making a clinical decision on whether GFT is suitable for a referred family. Therefore, as discussed in Appendix 2 on introducing GFT to organizations, it is vital that GFT leaders have already provided the agency, and particularly the initial intake staff, with sufficient information on GFT for agency staff to be confident about conveying this information to families. A suggested handout for agency professionals, which can be adapted by readers to meet their own requirements, is included in Appendix 3. This appendix gives suggested information for staff including, briefly, FT's history, research base, the goals and types of problems addressed by GFT, general inclusion criteria for participation in the group, and practical details about delivery of the program, its structure and contents.

STEP 2

When initial intakes result in recommendations for child and/or family-based interventions, the second step of the intake process with an experienced GFT leader begins. At this step, a leader observes a family play session and meets with parents afterwards to discuss the observation.

STEP 3

At the third step, a leader meets with parents to recommend GFT and helps parents understand and commit themselves to the GFT program.

   The second and third steps of the intake process are described more fully in the next section of this chapter. When GFT leaders are the professionals involved throughout all three steps in the intake process, leaders usually provide more information about GFT at the initial meeting than this section indicates.

   We strongly recommend that each of the steps outlined here for the intake be a separate meeting. Each step has unique demands and works best if those can be satisfied. If time constraints require that any two steps be covered in one meeting, extra time should be allowed to complete the double agenda. This doubling of agendas is not optimal for families to process and share information fully, and can result in the families for whom doubling was done having less grasp of their own roles and that of the leaders. This may make the tasks of the family and GFT leaders more difficult during early group meetings. All three steps are summarized in Table 2.3 below.

Table 2.3 GFT intake steps

Step 1: Interview and GFT pre-measures.
a. Initial interviews to take the family's and referred child's histories, their descriptions of their difficulties, results of any psychometric tests that were administered earlier, administering any GFT pre-measures needed for evaluation purposes, including those relevant to GFT (e.g. PSI, PPAS, FPL), and initial recommendations for the family. (Preparatory information on GFT for intake professionals is required beforehand, if they are not GFT leaders.)
b. When GFT is being considered for families, interviewers provide preparation for the family play observation (FPO) to be conducted by the GFT leaders. If Step 1 has not been conducted by a GFT leader, a phone call to parents from a leader is highly recommended before Step 2.
Step 2: FPO. Where initial intake information indicates a possible GFT recommendation, the next step is observation of a family play session by a GFT leader, and a meeting with parents immediately afterwards to discuss the observation and relate the contents to GFT.

Step 3: Meeting with parents by a leader to recommend GFT and to emphasize that the features of GFT typically lead to positive behavioral/emotional changes in the child and in family relationships. Leaders also emphasize that participating in a group enhances the experience for parents.

Note: FPL [Filial Problem List]; PPAS, Porter Parental Acceptance Scale; PSI, Parental Stress Index.

Step 1: the initial meeting, Meeting 1

The initial step of the intake process is an important one in the GFT program. It serves several purposes. One of its main purposes is for agencies to collect information on referred families and to offer services tailored to each family's requirements. Another purpose is for families to receive information on what is available and how suitable these services are for them. A third important function is to provide families with a means of expressing their emotional needs to skilled and supportive professionals, and for professionals in turn to understand and helpfully respond to families' emotional distress. This emotional component of the intake process should be emphasized when leaders prepare other professionals to conduct initial intake interviews. It is equally important for leaders to keep in mind throughout the entire intake process. Sensitivity to family emotions has implications for developing group cohesion and skills learning during the first part of the GFT program, as discussed in the next chapters of this book.

In the first step of the intake process with referred families, we assume here that agencies and organizations follow their own intake procedures. This initial meeting usually includes taking the family's and referred child's histories and their descriptions and understanding of their difficulties, administering any psychometric tests needed, and giving initial recommendations for the family. Agency information and procedures for families, including permission forms for data collection, confidentiality, data storage, and mandated reporting requirements are also commonly addressed here. This section therefore concentrates on the types of evaluation measures specific to GFT, and the ways in which GFT can be introduced to families by agency professionals.

INITIATING PROGRAM EVALUATION

GFT pre-measures, also used for evaluation purposes after the intervention, begin during this initial intake step. Questionnaires and checklists for the parents to complete prior to their first face-to-face meeting, or alternatively during this meeting, are common practice. Collecting standardized information on families permits pre and post comparisons for evaluation purposes.

A useful measure, particularly for research purposes, originally developed at Rutgers University for GFT (Guerney B. & Stover, 1971), is the Measurement of Empathy in Adult Child Interactions (MEACI), which requires specialized training for its use. The data from the MEACI is based on actual observations of parental behavior as they interact with their children in play sessions. There need to be at least two observers of these interactions whose ratings are in sufficient agreement to obtain the necessary inter-rater reliability for the results to be considered reliable. This measure has been modified at the University of

North Texas (see Bratton *et al.*, 2006, for their revised protocol). In general, behavioral measures such as the MEACI are superior to self-report measures. However, in agency settings, training behavioral raters and using the behavioral scales can be time consuming, especially if the behavioral ratings are to be used pre and post intervention. Therefore, in agencies, except when research is being conducted, we suggest leaders opt for the self-report measures described next.

The Parental Stress Index (PSI) (Abidin, 1997) and the Porter Parental Acceptance Scale (PPAS) (Porter, 1954) have established reliability and validity and, short of actual behavioral measures like the MEACI, are well worth using for pre and post intervention. The PSI provides parents with many sources of personal stresses related to the family, asking them to rate themselves on each stressor. This measure has empirical support for distinguishing parental stress in pre and post treatment situations. The PPAS provides parent-child situations that parents are asked to respond to. Responses have been found to discriminate among varying degrees of parental empathy, an important skill developed in GFT.

For GFT, as well as the usual assessment tools, or instead of one of the commonly used child behavior checklists, it is highly useful for parents to complete the more specialized FPL (Filial Problem List) (Horner, 1974). The FPL does not provide norms for child ages and other qualities; however, this checklist has the advantage of being filled out quite easily by parents in a relatively short time, and has gradations of a problem. It allows parents to differentiate between minor problems and problems that are very difficult for them, of both internalizing and externalizing types. One of the advantages of using the FPL is that it is easily scored by clinicians without outside help, and thus is convenient and cost effective. Statistical studies of the FPL (Horner, 1974) indicate that it differentiates between families with more serious problems and those with minor ones. It also can discriminate between pre and post administrations, indicating what changes have taken place through the GFT intervention. Assessors need to make plans, and mention to parents at intake, that they intend to collect post-intervention results on this measure, as well as on the other measures used by their agencies; this is discussed further in Chapter 15, devoted to ending the program.

PREPARING FAMILIES FOR THE FAMILY PLAY OBSERVATION

At the end of the initial intake meeting, professionals may indicate to families that GFT is being considered as an intervention to offer them, and that the next step in the intake process is a family play observation (FPO) conducted by a GFT leader. (Occasionally another agency professional may observe an FPO, with the family's and GFT leaders' agreement, but would not conduct the FPO.) Therefore, agency professionals conducting initial intake meetings need to have been briefed on the purpose and structure of both the FPO and the follow-up discussion after the observation, in order to explain these to parents before ending their first meeting. Intake professionals also need to be briefed and explain to families that there will be contact from a GFT leader before the next part of the intake process. Appendix 5 gives a sample letter to parents from leaders. We also highly recommend an introductory telephone call from one of the leaders prior to the FPO, in order to answer any further questions parents have before they attend. (For GFT leaders who conduct their own initial assessments, this will already have been covered at the initial meeting.)

For this telephone call and the next two meetings, we recommend that one leader, rather than two leaders, even in two-leader groups, takes responsibility for a family. In addition to being an effective use of staff resources, meeting only one professional helps families manage their anxiety more easily in an unfamiliar situation. It is helpful for two-leader groups to have each of the two leaders conduct these intakes with half of the families, where possible, in order to familiarize families who form the group with both leaders from the outset.

THE PRE-FPO CONVERSATION WITH PARENTS

In their initial meeting, intake professionals provide preliminary information to families about the observation and its purpose. Leaders of the GFT group are informed by intake professionals about families who are candidates for GFT. Leaders then contact these families to set up the FPO. In their telephone conversation before families' FPOs, GFT leaders should check that families have had all of the information discussed next, and show empathy towards any concerns they may have.

The purpose of the FPO is to try to see how children interact with each other and their parents when not engaged in a structured activity like taking a test, or following instructions from a therapist. Professionals should tell families that the whole family participates in an FPO, that it lasts about half an hour, and that it is an open, free-flowing time of play and interaction. The parents should be told that, if their children refuse to stay for the entire half hour, they should not force them to remain. However, a few requests on the parents' part to try to persuade their children to stay in the room should first be made.

After the FPO, therapists discuss the family play with the adults who participated for about half an hour, while their children are looked after nearby. The purpose of the discussion is to talk together about the playtime and see how it is the same and different from regular family life and the referral problems of concern to the parents. Leaders stress that all immediate family members should be prepared to come, including grandparents or other relatives who live in the home and take responsibility for child rearing. If not all of the family members can or will attend, the observation can still be conducted, with the therapist discussing with the adults who are present what they think the missing family members would have done, had they seen the kind of play and interactions that took place.

The family is told that in the FPO they can do just about anything they want—together, in pairs, or separately. They are not expected to demonstrate their talents and skills, such as writing well or singing a song. The observers would like to see how everybody interacts, or does not interact, with each other. It is important that all family members know they are being observed and by whom—*needed permissions should have been obtained during the initial intake meeting*—and that a video is being made (if that is the case). Should there be any hesitation on the part of the family as to why everybody should attend, and why they should be videotaped, they should be told that seeing the family interacting in a relatively "natural" way provides very useful information to confirm the suitability of GFT. It also is useful for leaders during the therapeutic process.

Sometimes parents say in response, *"We're never together"* or *"We never play together"* and therefore argue that the situation would not be natural. Therapists can say, *"That's OK. We'll all find out how it would be, if you had an opportunity to play together."* Leaders can emphasize with parents who are reluctant, that it would be very interesting for them to see how the children interact, and may mention that children tend to forget very quickly that they are being observed, and reveal a lot about how they deal with interpersonal situations.

Parents also should be made aware of any rules that must be followed during the FPO, such as not throwing things at the observation window, not leaving the room to go elsewhere in the building, and not playing with cameras or telephones. Awareness of these limits helps the parents know what to tell their children about what they can do and cannot do, as the need arises while they play. We also recommend repeating the reassurance that all information about the families from FPOs remains confidential to the agency, except under the circumstances referred to in agency guidelines.

Professionals need to help parents with a simple way to explain the FPO to their children. Children will want to know what is going to happen at the FPO. Parents should explain to them that the whole family will be together and have a free playtime together. Children will be able to play with all the toys in the room and do pretty much what they would like—with each other, or alone—whatever they would like, and there will only be a few rules. They do not need to perform in any way. Parents should add:

> Nobody else will be with us, but they will be able to see what we do through the observation window [if available], or on a video tape. They would like to see how we do things as a family. Whatever we do will be fine with them. They will not be giving out any grades or thinking that certain things are better than others. They hope we enjoy playing with their toys.

Step 2: the FPO, Meeting 2

As well as providing leaders with direct information about family relationships and individual dynamics in order to decide whether GFT is suitable, FPOs also help leaders develop understanding and rapport with parents who go on to participate in the GFT program. Many times children reveal in the FPO the behaviors that parents have reported as problems for them at home (e.g. a child who refuses to respond to parents' repeated requests). Parents feel validated when leaders have witnessed this behavior. But even when children do not replicate the behaviors that are reported to happen at home, productive discussions occur as leaders and parents try to figure out why the children's behaviors were different in this instance. The extended example at the end of this section illustrates a FPO and the following discussion more fully.

On a practical level, leaders need to ensure that the play space they have available accommodates families, including younger and older children, along with adults. Ideally the room would be fitted with a one-way screen and video facilities. Video is very useful to use both during the follow-up discussion afterwards with parents and, later, for the leaders' own review. One-way screen or mirror facilities ensure that leaders are not drawn into participating in the FPO. Where these facilities are not available, leaders can section off one end of the room and remain separate from the family, while taking written notes. If leaders use their own play therapy rooms for FPOs, they need to ensure that toys and activities are manageable for families to play with together, rather than presenting parents with too many situations that challenge their limit-setting skills (e.g. computers, test materials).

WHEN THE FAMILY ENTERS THE FPO ROOM

When leaders introduce families to the room for the observation, a short explanation should be given (e.g. *"I am looking forward to seeing how your family plays together."*) and leaders may wish to mention one or two minor rules (e.g. *"Mind the mirror."*). They also should remind families of the leader's role in observing them (e.g. *"I'll watch you from here."*).

THE LEADER'S ROLE IN THE FPO

The leader's main focus during the observation is forming working hypotheses about family dynamics and each family member's individual dynamics. These hypotheses should be tentative and open to revision. The ideas developed during FPOs, where relevant and clinically appropriate, are shared by leaders with parents during the discussion following the observation.

From a family therapy perspective, leaders may wish to form hypotheses about parenting styles, the parenting alliance, family structure, unresolved family dynamics issues, and the attachment styles in evidence among family members (Stollack, Barley, & Kalogiros, 2000). From a child therapy perspective, general areas to consider may include each child's attachment style, emotional/social, physical, cognitive, and language development, play development, and any evidence of neurological or unusual signs (Rye & Jaeger, 2007). More specific ideas about the dynamics that underlie a family's play behaviors also are useful to consider (Harvey, 2000).

Some leaders may wish to organize their observations by developing their own checklist, and we offer some general categories given by the authors just mentioned for clinicians to use to evaluate parent-child interactions during FPOs in Appendix 6. Checklists may be useful to leaders as a reminder to note behaviors of interest and behaviors specific to given children (e.g. tics, mannerisms). However, checklists are not appropriate for direct use by leaders during the discussion of FPOs with parents. The formal, limited form of a checklist may interfere with natural responses from parents, inhibiting the collaborative discussion process.

LEADERS' FEEDBACK WITH PARENTS AFTER THE FPO

Parents return with leaders to discuss the FPO while their children are cared for nearby. Leaders should aim for approximately a half-hour discussion. This discussion is intended to be a rich source of information and rapport building for both parents and leaders (see Rye & Jaeger, 2007, for an extended example). The leaders set the tone for the future by embodying the principles of the GFT program in their feedback.

The focus at the outset of the discussion is on what everyone observed during the play activity and what similarities and differences there were from regular family life and the children's referral behaviors (e.g. children behaving aggressively in the FPO and not at home, or vice versa). Often it is important leaders acknowledge that the FPO is artificial, but that there are always interesting things to discuss all the same. The leader then tries to elicit parents' reactions with open-ended questions such as: *"How did that feel for you?"* and *"What did you think your child/children made of it?"* Throughout this half-hour discussion, it is important that leaders empathize with parents' verbalized and non-verbalized feelings, as well as responding to the factual contents of the discussion readily. Video recordings made during the FPO can be used effectively to illustrate interactions and points discussed. We suggest that video contents, in the spirit of GFT, be used in a positive way to show attuned interactions between children and parents primarily. One or two instances of more difficult interactions can be used as well, but we strongly urge that leaders always keep the balance on the positive with parents and end with a positive example.

Leaders also try to help parents to relate their children's behavior during the FPO to the aims and goals of the GFT program. If a filial therapist happens to spot a parent behavior that is compatible with FT principles, this could be mentioned to the parent (e.g. following their child's lead in play, reflecting a feeling). Parents are often impressed that this behavior was regarded as positive, and tend to retain it, facilitating their learning of FT skills. It can also spark meaningful dialogue, even for parents who are highly reticent.

Leaders should take every opportunity to relate child behaviors seen in the FPO to the gains that can ensue from participating in the GFT program. For example, if in the FPO a child is afraid to leave the parent's side, the leader could explain to the parent how filial play sessions could enable the child to be less fearful in the future. Bringing forth such examples can motivate parents to wish to participate in the GFT program. This method of leaders helping parents to access and create more meaning in their children's behavior immediately after they have had play interactions is a key feature of GFT. This type of parent-leader interaction begins in the discussion after FPOs, and continues throughout the program, as later chapters attest. Leaders relate what they observed in the FPO to what can be gained or learned by parents in the GFT program, in order to motivate parents to want to participate in the program, as discussed next.

RELATING FAMILY CONCERNS TO THE BENEFITS OF GFT

One of the primary tasks of leaders in discussions after FPOs is to encourage families to attend a GFT program, when such a program seems suitable. Leaders can stress, for example, that one benefit of participating is that through GFT their child will be likely to become more confident. Leaders should take note that all potential benefits of the program they give to parents should always be expressed in terms of *likelihoods,* rather than certainties, since outcomes in interventions cannot be guaranteed. However in our experience, when parents see in a very concrete way the relationship between observed child behaviors in the FPO, and link them with what they will learn in GFT, they are more likely to see its benefits. We have found that the percentage of parents who reject the GFT program is very small when this approach is taken. Another example of linking behavior observed in the FPO to the advantages of GFT is a leader saying to parents:

> *We all saw together that Jay became rather aggressive when you had to tell him to stop throwing the toys at the one-way mirror. It seems as though it's very hard for him to deal with frustration without going on the attack. We have found that giving*

children an opportunity to play out their angry feelings in the special controlled environment of a play session helps children reduce this unacceptable response. If you participate in the GFT program, you will learn with other parents how to conduct these special play sessions with Jay. We expect that if things go as they usually would, that in time, this behavior of Jay's would be reduced to the point of it no longer being a problem.

For another child, the leader may say:

We all saw together in your family's play that Emily was really at a total loss to know what to do without you directing her. She virtually begged you to tell her what to do, even though you tried to sit back and let her go her own way. You have reported that in other parts of her life, she is also extremely dependent on you and seems fearful about initiating things on her own. The kind of play session that we will teach you to have with Emily has a long history of helping children learn to get in touch with their own feelings. They become more able to decide what they would like to do, and take leadership where it's appropriate. This seems a probable result for Emily too.

Two tasks for leaders before ending the meeting are, first, to inform parents that they will now look at all the intake information, collect other information where needed (e.g. school and medical input), and decide on a recommendation. Leaders should add that there will be a third meeting at which a final recommendation for GFT or, rarely, an alternative that would seem more appropriate to the particular family's needs, is discussed. In the final meeting, leaders explain more about the GFT program, and have parents talk more if they wish about their family life.

The final task before ending the discussion is for leaders to ensure that parents are able to process the FPO with their children afterwards in a positive manner. Leaders should take time to help parents prepare simple, positive statements about the FPO before rejoining their children. For example, Jonny, aged 10 years, asked his mother what she thought about their family playing together, and what she and his father talked about with the filial therapist afterwards. His mother replied: *"I enjoyed watching what everybody was doing, and thought that you had a lot of fun shooting the darts, and June (therapist) thought so, too."* As this example demonstrates, leaders should help parents only refer to what their children were doing, and not be evaluative in their comments.

Case illustration of an FPO and follow-up discussion

FAMILY MEMBERS
Mother, Amy, father, John, 10-year-old son Harry, and 4-year-old daughter, Susan.

BACKGROUND TO REFERRAL
This is the second marriage for the father, John; Harry is his only child with his first wife. After his first wife left when Harry was 3 years old, John had sole custody of Harry and

was a single father for one year, until meeting his second partner, Amy. Susan was born after they had been together for two years.

PRESENTING PROBLEMS

Both parents state that in the early days Harry was a "model" boy, outgoing and affectionate with both of them. During the last year he has become moody and irritable, is increasingly aggressive towards his sister Susan and will not cooperate with what his parents ask him to do. Harry's academic performance is suffering too, but he will not talk to them about what is wrong. He stays in his room and plays on computer games most nights after school, and there are escalating struggles with him to do his homework, eat his meals with the family, and go to bed at night. Susan, on the other hand, is very easy to care for and affectionate with them, just like Harry used to be at her age.

FAMILY PLAY OBSERVATION

Leader (showing facilities to the family): *Your parents have already told you that they want your family to get along better together, and they've come here to learn some ways that they can do that.*

I'll watch behind that mirror and video it, while your family does some playing together for about a half hour. Your parents and I will watch some of the video together afterwards and talk about it, while you are with X. (Leader shows the family the observation booth and camera, then the room.)

You can do most things in here and choose what to do. There are a few small rules in this room, like not throwing anything at the mirror, but you can do most other things. I'll knock on the door when the time is up. (Leader withdraws to the observation booth.)

The mother, Amy and father, John seemed excited with this opportunity to play with their children as they enter the room. Susan immediately goes over to the table and starts drawing; her mother follows her.

Mom: That's a great start, Susan. (Mother takes up felt tip pen and looks at Susan's paper.) *What shall I draw? Should I add some seagulls here?* (Susan and mother sit at the table and draw a seaside picture together.)

Harry looks around the room and then moves around from one thing to the next, looking but not touching or playing with anything. His father stands near the door, then moves over to Harry and says that they could play a game together.

Harry: Naw, that's boring. I don't like any of this kid stuff. (He continues to wander from object to object.)

Dad: I know, let's use those cars and build a ramp so we can race them afterwards.

Harry: You do it, I don't want to.

Mom: Harry, your dad just wants to play with you. Look, Susan has found something to do right away with me.

His father then starts building the ramp, talking to Harry as he does so about what he is doing. Harry sits down on a beanbag nearby and fiddles with a length of rope he picks up off the floor.

Dad: The ramp's finished, Harry. Choose your car.

Harry (in an irritable voice): *I said I didn't want to.*

His father takes two cars and races them by himself a few times, glancing at Harry, then quietly abandons his cars, and joins Susan and her mother at the table.

Dad: How about coming over here, Harry?

Harry moves near the table, walking around behind everyone's chairs, and starts looking at the drawings that were done by Susan and her mother.

Harry: What's that?

Susan: It's a dog on the beach with a stick.

Harry: That's a stupid drawing. It looks more like a cow than a dog!

Mom: Harry, she's only four. You do one, if you think you can do better.

Harry: I will, then. (He takes up a pen and starts drawing on his own paper.)

Susan drops her pen under the table and goes to look for it. She then says she can't find it and their father looks under the table.

Dad: Harry, the pen is under your foot. You were hiding that from Susan. Give it here.

Harry: I wasn't. I always get the blame.

Mom: You do tease Susan a lot, Harry.

The family continues their drawing together for a time, with Susan asking her mother for reassurance that her drawing is looking like a dog this time.

Mom: You're doing a great job Susan. You can't expect to draw as well as bigger people.

Harry: Mine's much better!

Susan reaches across to his paper and scribbles on Harry's paper.

Harry: Hey, cut that out! (Susan smiles to herself.)

Mom: Well, you were teasing her, Harry.

Dad: You know she's only little, Harry. Just be grown-up about what she's done.

Harry continues to draw with a sullen expression on his face.

Dad: Look at this cartoon I've done! Did you ever see anyone with that bulgy a nose?! I'm going to give him stick-out ears too! What do you want to add, Susan?

Harry: That's just stupid.

The family continues to draw until the end of the FPO.

(The leader was forming tentative working hypotheses about family dynamics and each family member's individual dynamics during the observation, some of which will be shared with parents during the discussion illustrated below.)

Discussion with parents

Leader: We'll talk together about the playtime now, and see how it is the same and different from your daily life. How did that go for you?

Dad: Well, it certainly was different from ordinary life! We all did something together, for a start!

Leader: That felt really good to you, to be able to do something with everyone.

Mom: Yes, but I've been thinking—how is it going to help to have separate play sessions with Harry, when most of his problem is not wanting to be with us?

Leader: You're feeling doubts about whether this is the right approach for your family.

Dad: Yes, we're trying to get Harry to do things with all of us.

Leader: So it seems pointless to have him get one-to-one attention from each of you.

Dad: You could see that he didn't want to play with me by himself at the start. He only started to get involved when we were all together.

Leader: You made a lot of effort to play with him at the beginning, and he rejected your efforts.

Dad: Yeah, it happens time after time.

Leader: This makes you feel bad, from what you've said. But in the Powerful Play Program [local name for GFT], it's not ordinary play. It's play based on therapy that has been shown to work. That's what you'll be learning. And from what I could see today, you both put a lot of effort into trying to help your children. In this program you have special one-to-one time with each of your children. I wondered if it usually works out in your family that Amy, you spend a lot of time with Susan, and John, you try to do things with Harry more.

Mom: Well that's natural, because Harry doesn't want to do the things that interest Susan and me.

Leader: You feel that Harry isn't interested in you and Susan so much. Let's just take a look at the video here for a minute. I thought it was very interesting to see how Harry behaved when you weren't looking at him, and he went behind your chairs. See what you think he was interested in. (Video excerpt of Harry looking intently at Susan's and Amy's drawings is shown.)

Mom: He spent a long time looking at Susan's drawings, didn't he?

Dad: Yes, and yours too.

Mom: But he was then just nasty about Susan's.

Leader: So you're seeing that he's interested, but then gets very critical of Susan.

Dad: They fight all the time. Then Harry goes to his room and stays there, when we tell him to stop it.

Leader: You've tried to set some rules for Harry on what he can and can't do, but they seem to be making him very unhappy. In this program, parents learn to set rules in ways that help children to respect their parents' authority over them, without having it undermine their relationship with their parents. I think that would be very helpful to you.

Mom: We have tried every way we can think of to get it right for Harry.

Leader: You both really care about Harry, and want to be good parents to him. This program has helped many parents and children to feel closer to one another. In the program, children can choose what to play with, and how to work on their own issues, with parents trying to understand what they feel. This helps children to trust their parents more and value their time with them.

Dad: I sure hope it works. Harry is really good at all kinds of things. You could see how good he is at drawing just now.

Leader: You're proud of him. You were very interested in what he was drawing. And so were you, Amy. Let's look at that part of the video together. This is what we'll be training parents to do more of during the program. You already have a start on this skill. (Parents and leader discuss the contents of the video clip.)

Leader: We haven't talked about Susan yet.

Mom: I think it would work for us and Harry, but I don't think Susan needs anything.

Leader: You think the program would be useful for Harry and both of you, but not Susan. We'll ask John his opinion in a minute, but first let's talk about why the program is designed for all the children in the family, not just the child parents are having problems with. In many families, it is hard for brothers and sisters to get along well together if they think that one child is receiving too much attention. In this program, parents' attention is fairly spread out among all their children wherever possible, so that each child gets special, regular playtimes with each of their parents.

Dad: Amy, that might work for you and Harry, and I wouldn't mind spending a bit more time with Susan. I don't seem to get a look in when you're around.

Leader: John, you can think of the positives of including Susan then. You sound like you're looking forward to being part of the program.

Dad: Yeah, I really like to play with my kids. I miss doing that with Harry, and would like to do more of it with Susan.

Leader: That's a very positive attitude.

Mom: I'll think about it more, John.

Leader: You're willing to think about it more, Amy. Before we end, I want to say that the program looks like a very good fit for your family from the family play observation you did today, but we'll need to look at all the information we have and contact Harry's school before all of us make a final decision. That won't take long to do, and we will schedule another meeting with both of you next week, so that we can all make a final decision on how to go forward. We can also talk about any more questions or worries about the program you might have then. Let's think about what you might say if Harry asks about your reactions to the observation. Can you think of anything he did that you might want to react positively to? And what about Susan?

Mom: Well Harry did do a good drawing. We could talk about that, and about Susan liking to draw too.

Dad: We could also say that we enjoyed playing all together as a family.

Leader: Those are both useful suggestions. Let's rejoin them now.

Comments on this case illustration

This example shows the way a leader introduced the FPO and her own role, as well as illustrating the way the she followed the parents' lead and feelings during the discussion, while weaving into the discussion ways in which GFT may help the family. A rich variety of information on the individual family members and their interactions with one another was obtained in the FPO, which was reinforced by the leader using selected video examples in an illustrative and positive manner. (See Chapter 10 for a further example of work with this family.)

Step 3: the final intake meeting, Meeting 3

Another appointment with the same leader should be arranged, in order to meet with the parents on their own and discuss recommendations at greater length. For this meeting, if GFT is recommended, leaders help parents understand and commit themselves to the GFT program. In our experience, Steps 2 and 3 should be scheduled in two separate appointments, if feasible. When the second and third steps are combined into one meeting, often the amount of time needed by parents in discussion with leaders is lengthier than waiting children can manage. A longer meeting, therefore, can lead to increased stress for the children and parents, and is counter to GFT's goal of helping parents become more responsive to their children's emotional needs. Longer meetings also are not usually conducive to parents' being able to concentrate as well, due to their potential concerns about their waiting children.

During the final meeting, leaders make recommendations to parents, clearly stating their reasons for the recommendations based on what was seen in the FPO and the other intake and assessment information. These recommendations are most helpfully stated in terms of what both the children and their parents need, rather than emphasizing referral problems. Some thought needs to be given by leaders to the wording of these recommendations, in order to make recommendations hopeful and helpful to families. When recommending GFT, it is best to formulate these recommendations in terms of what the program can offer families. For example, with children who have school anxieties, leaders can point out that children may choose to play out school experiences during their play sessions and adapt to school better as a result. Leaders also need to be highly empathic to parents' doubts and anxieties over their own therapeutic role in GFT, and doubts about how GFT can help their family's difficulties. While factual information about GFT is important to convey, we remind leaders that it is most important that they help parents air and manage their emotional reactions to the recommendation of GFT with empathy and respect.

At this step, leaders should explain to parents that GFT is a psycho-educational intervention, which means that parents will be educated in new ways of interacting with and helping their children therapeutically, as well as receiving emotional support during the learning process. Parents all learn to share experiences with other group members and learn with them the principles of GFT. The program is designed for approximately five months, with the option of continuing beyond should group members wish to have a few follow-up meetings.[2] Leaders can add that many groups have found the GFT program so satisfying that they have wanted to continue working together beyond the 20-week program, or in other ways outside of the group.

An illustrative example of a Step 3 meeting in which a leader explains GFT to parents is given next.

ILLUSTRATIVE EXAMPLE: EXPLAINING GFT TO PARENTS[3]

At their third intake meeting, the parents of a 10-year-old boy, Jay, described their worry and frustration that he would not obey them or listen to them. Jay was very defiant, aggressive with them and other children, and stole things.

> Leader: The kinds of problems you describe are ones that GFT helps with. Many children have such problems and they have been helped by our program. These children can be helped by having a special kind of play session. The play sessions give them opportunities to play out things that may be behind some of the behaviors you are describing. It's not just about telling children to stop hitting people, or stealing. In play sessions, you're getting down to the feelings children are experiencing that underlie the misbehaviors. Play sessions have been used for many years by professional therapists, and have served as a fine tool for children to acquire better behaviors.

---

2   Deciding on the length of the program is discussed in more detail in the next chapter.

3   This dialogue is adapted from Louise Guerney's commercial videotape on FT, with permission from the publishers.

Dad: We're interested in that, to have him change his behavior.

Leader: These play sessions have been used widely. In GFT the major difference is that, instead of a professional therapist, we train parents to conduct these special play sessions themselves. (Parents look surprised, skeptical and worried.)

Leader: You look really surprised by that.

Dad (skeptical tone): Our playing with Jay could solve his problems?

Mom: But we already play with Jay all the time.

Leader: It's hard to see how playing could help. You're already doing it and it doesn't seem to be helping.

Parents: Yeah.

Leader: Well ordinary playing may or may not have benefits, but special play is so different from ordinary life, and has a different effect. The sessions give children a lot more freedom to explore their feelings, and express themselves, but at the same time there are boundaries. They can express themselves in every way, but behaviors are limited and you are taught to set these limits and make certain they are effective. So that would help Jay with his control. The freedom he has to express and explore his feelings before he reaches those boundaries could be very helpful to him, getting at the kinds of behaviors that are difficult.

Parents give their children more freedom in play sessions; they don't have as many jobs as in real life. You aren't going to try to teach Jay any new behavior. You're going to be trying to give him time to express and explore his feelings in an atmosphere that is very accepting. (Parents continue to look skeptical.)

Leader: You're not sure. Maybe you have questions, or you want me to explain it more.

Parents: Yeah, please explain it more.

Leader: You don't judge Jay, or put him down, or say he shouldn't feel that way in play sessions. Children can play out the feelings that trouble them that are underneath the behaviors that you don't like. We teach you how to do this, and develop your skills so that you can conduct the play sessions the same way professional therapists do. All the group members will be playing with their own children, and you will learn together.

Mom: I don't think I'd like to do that in front of other parents I don't know.

Leader: That seems scary to you. (Mom nods.) We leaders build up support, and not criticism, among all the parents in the group. We find that, when parents are in a group, they seem to benefit from sharing experiences with each other, and that gives them a broader perspective on child behaviors. Observing each other playing with their respective children deepens parents' understanding of the principles and process that they are learning. Parents are being educated in new ways to relate to their children, which has therapeutic effects.

Studies have shown that, when parents learn how to apply these new skills correctly, it brings about psychological change. And the results are often superior to professionals alone attempting to bring about changes. After you learn to do play sessions in the group, then you take them home and come back to the group to talk about them, and maybe do more in the group. Towards the end of the program, the group is helped to apply their play session skills and other skills to daily life. That way the program is an efficient way to bring about lasting positive effects for your family.

Dad: It's a big commitment, but we are at our wits' end.

Leader: You've tried everything you can think of, and you're both feeling desperate.

Mom: Well, if you're sure it can help Jay...

Leader: I can't guarantee it, but it certainly has worked for other families who have similar problems to your own family. I can tell how important Jay is to you; you want so much for him to get on the right track.

Dad: Yes, we do love him and want what's best for him, but it's very hard to like him. He was great when he was younger.

Leader: You're thinking of good times you've had with him in the past, and want it to be good again. That's one of the aims of our program, to help families have good times together.

Dad: We'll have to try it.

Mom: Yes, we've run out of ideas ourselves.

Comments on the case illustration

This example shows how the leader accepted and empathized with the main issues and anxieties raised by Jay's parents, as well as giving explanations of how GFT works to address these concerns. Leaders should remember not to overload parents with explanations about the program at this meeting. As stated already, it is most important that leaders hear and accept parents' doubts about themselves, their children and the program itself at this point. Acceptance of parents' thoughts and feelings enables them to make informed decisions on whether to attend. Empathizing with parents' feelings on an individual basis also has positive effects on parents who then go on to attend group meetings, as discussed later. As demonstrated in the case example, it is important for leaders to get a firm commitment from parents to participate in GFT, and also to try to end the last intake meeting on a positive note, thereby giving added encouragement to parents to join the group. Once parents appreciate the value to be found in GFT, they should be asked to make a commitment to regular meeting attendance for 20 weeks, and to playing with their children as prescribed by the program. A brief summary of FT may also be useful as a handout for parents to take away at the end of this meeting (see Appendix 11 for a suggested handout.)

GFT consents for videoing group meetings, demos and play sessions

When leaders intend to video record the group meetings for their own use during the GFT program and for supervision purposes, and perhaps for more general training purposes, written consent forms for families need to be signed by parents by the end of the final intake meeting. (See Appendix 9 for a prototype form.) Recording permission is commonly asked for the meetings themselves, leaders' demos with participating children, and practice play sessions during meetings of children with their parents. Leaders can explain the professional purposes and uses of these videos verbally to parents, if required, towards the end of the meeting. Any questions parents may have also can be answered (e.g. *Parent: "What if my child objects?" Leader: "Either your child, verbally or non-verbally, or you can indicate that it is better not to record a play session. We will always respect that."*)

Parents' explanations of GFT to their children

Leaders should mention to parents in their final intake meeting that it is important that they give a brief explanation of the purpose of GFT to their children after it is agreed that the family will participate in the program. Leaders can point out that usually it is sufficient to say to children that their parents are learning a special way to play with them that will help their family. Parents also need to be informed by leaders that more detailed preparation of their children for participating in GFT will be given at the first meeting. Parents should be reminded that they can say, if their children ask questions about the program now, that they will be able to answer these questions after the first meeting.

Formulating goals for families participating in GFT

After the intake meetings with each family are completed, leaders need to more fully formulate their professional goals for the family for their own use. These goals are based on collected intake information and leaders' understanding of clinical issues. We suggest that these professional goals be formulated in terms of family needs, in keeping with the ethos of the GFT approach. For example, a goal for one family may be that the mother will come to have an understanding of her child's need to resist her excessive controls, and that the mother be able to reduce these controls in a way observable to the leaders. Another professional goal might be increasing family communication, particularly the verbal communication between a father and his daughter on both positive and negative topics. Leaders find these formulations useful as reminders to themselves, or useful as beginnings that are refined later in the program. Formulating goals at the outset also helps leaders' thinking when they review progress families have made as the program comes to an end.

Informing participants

Once families have been selected for GFT based on both their own characteristics and group composition criteria, which were discussed in the previous chapter, leaders then confirm places with families and give them practical information on the group. This includes location, dates and times, contact details, and an agenda for the first meeting. A sample letter for parents to confirm their attendance is given in Appendix 7.

Leaders also need to prepare themselves for running the GFT program. The next chapter gives guidance for leaders on developing successful groups in GFT.

CHAPTER 3

Guidelines for Conducting Successful GFT Groups

This chapter addresses issues that arise in GFT for inexperienced leaders and reviews considerations for experienced GFT leaders in running the program successfully. The first part of the chapter examines general leadership skills and their applications to GFT; the second part focuses on two particular challenges presented to leaders during GFT programs. Practice examples and possible resolutions of challenging issues are provided throughout the chapter.

General leadership skills required for GFT[1]

Because the structure of any group contributes to its success, leaders need to plan ahead to avert or minimize difficulties. Chapter 1 addressed some practical issues for leaders, such as childcare and venue, when starting GFT programs. Here we turn to leaders' tasks within the meetings themselves.

Creating a proper climate for learning

Experienced GFT leaders recognize that parents acquiring GFT skills and incorporating them into their behavior depends greatly on the relationship and credibility leaders develop with them. For this reason, building and maintaining a comfortable group atmosphere that encourages learning is essential, as we explore in detail later. The overarching element in creating this positive learning climate is leaders' ability to be verbally accepting of parents' attitudes, behavior and feelings. Non-verbal behaviors—good eye contact, head nodding, and total body position—are also essential in communicating acceptance. By acknowledging difficulties parents may have, and employing empathic responses, leaders show parents they see the world through their eyes. For example, rather than berating

---

1   The following sections have been adapted for GFT programs from Guerney L. (2013) *Clinician's and group leader's manual for parenting: a skills training program*, with permission from the publisher.

parents who have not collected toys for their home play sessions at the appointed time, leaders are more effective if they first recognize the difficulties these parents have in performing this task, and then try to help them solve the problems themselves with realistic deadlines. Leaders' acceptance of parents' viewpoints and difficulties in turn encourages open-mindedness in parents towards what leaders have to offer. The communication of leaders' understanding of parents via empathic responding encourages parents to be willing to listen to leaders, and models the empathy and openness that leaders hope parents will establish with their children in play sessions.

This mode of acceptance must be established at the outset, and leaders should continue to maintain an atmosphere of open communication and rapport throughout the program while dealing with parents' questions and apprehensions about using their skills. It is particularly important for leaders to recognize parents' concerns—even after they have accepted the principles upon which the program is built—when they are beginning to attempt to use the skills with their children in play sessions. Leaders need to empathize with the awkwardness parents report when first implementing the skills, and encourage them to express their feelings about this, as appropriate.

Empathy and acceptance towards parents also can have positive effects on the parents' attitudes towards themselves, as well as on their children and on their learning motivation. Parents frequently report greater feelings of self-confidence and self-esteem after having had their feelings accepted by leaders and other group members. This is particularly true if the feelings are not ones to which they readily admit. Self-examination and self-exploration are always best fostered in a non-threatening atmosphere.

Practical leadership skills

This section outlines the main practical skills GFT leaders need in order to run successful GFT programs.

PLANNING AHEAD

It is important before going into a group meeting that leaders have an organized plan of action worked out, something similar to a teacher's lesson plan. General meeting plans or agendas for each week in the 20-week program presented in this book are provided for leaders in Appendix 13 (Meetings 1–20). When using these agendas, leaders themselves need to decide on the specific points each group needs to cover, which ones to stress, and how to do this most effectively. In addition, leaders need to prepare a number of their own examples for use in training role-plays and explaining GFT concepts, including generalizing later in the program. These examples are used in exercises with parents or in illustrating answers to questions parents ask. We suggest examples in places throughout this book that may be useful for leaders to adapt to their own circumstances.

PACING

Pacing is the means by which leaders keep action moving quickly enough to maintain interest, yet not so quickly as to confuse participants and hinder the achievement of program goals. Leaders should ensure that there is sufficient variety in their examples, their use of two leaders, and their use of different training methods, yet simultaneously ensuring that parents' learning is at a speed that suits each group. Our agenda for each GFT meeting in Appendix 13 is given with pacing needs in mind. For example, we suggest that when parents begin learning play session skills, that they are asked to role play parent and child roles for only a short time, in order to accommodate to learning this technique for the first time.

ORGANIZATION OF TEACHING MATERIAL

As a general guide, we suggest that examples of each new concept are provided immediately following the presentation of the concept by leaders. In fact, in our experience any input to parents is most effective if it has short examples laced throughout it. Rather than postponing examples until covering all of the ideas, it is much more attention inducing and user friendly when examples are an integral part of teaching. Furthermore, points should be added one at a time, rather than several at once. Leaders should in addition summarize or "underline" important notions frequently. Finally, important points need to be returned to by leaders at different places in the program, as the context changes.

USING SUPPLEMENTARY MATERIALS

We remind leaders that, when they use supplementary materials like video, they should ensure that all of the necessary equipment is available and that they know how to operate it efficiently. This is in order to prevent lapses of attention by parents while leaders struggle with technical equipment. It facilitates the process if leaders set up the equipment beforehand, to be switched on immediately after introducing materials. If mechanical problems do arise, it is best to try to handle them in a casual, humorous manner, in order to avoid making the parents feel uncomfortable, and then to move the meeting forward.

BEING RESPONSIVE BUT FOCUSED

After deciding on the contents of meetings and how leaders will work with one another, it is important to keep to the agreed plan. However, leaders also need to keep in mind that they must be flexible and able to make use of opportunities as they present themselves, illustrating points and making good use of examples from information spontaneously presented by the group. At the same time, leaders must continually guard against long digressions into free discussion, or exchanges of childrearing notions, or problems among participants that may arise in the early stages of the GFT program. Discussions need to be directly related to the task at hand. Leaders can tactfully remind parents that the break is a very good time to talk about unrelated issues.

The early meetings are not problem-solving meetings *per se*, but have the aims of skills training, practice, and discussion. Leaders need to continually refocus on the task at hand, after they have provided a minimal level of satisfaction for any parent bringing up unrelated problems. Parents (and leaders too sometimes) may need to be reminded that parents will be ready later in the program to generalize their skills to daily life.

CREATING INTEREST IN FUTURE MEETINGS

During each meeting leaders usually have many opportunities to structure for future lessons by dropping hints about skills and issues to come later, while also stressing the importance of the task at hand when parents digress, saying something like, *"In a future meeting, we will talk about how you can best express yourself to your child. For now, let's stick to children's feelings."*

Leaders can also introduce basic points of future lessons. For example, during a meeting later in the program, when leaders began to introduce the application of play session skills to daily life, starting with empathic responding, a parent, Janet says:

> Janet: I tried structuring by having a time for Susie to talk to me about her homework right after dinner, instead of running out to me every two minutes while I am trying to prepare the meal. It has worked beautifully in gaining cooperative behavior from her.

> Leader: That's great to hear. Structuring worked so well for you, and we'll be getting to that very soon, right after we look at showing understanding of your children's feelings first. Let's see how that might work with Susie...

Here the leader is acknowledging that Janet was generalizing the skill of structuring into daily life, something that the group will learn soon. It also is often useful to tell parents that their successful, but premature, examples will be used when the topic is covered later. Of course, leaders will then need to remember to build these examples into the relevant meeting.

DEALING WITH DIVERGENT QUESTIONS AND TOPICS

Sometimes when performance anxiety is high for parents, they may raise problems or questions when, or right before, they are being asked to practice. We suggest in these cases that leaders either put these questions on hold until after the practice section of the meeting, or briefly answer one or two of the queries that are directly relevant to this practice. A brief answer about the rationale for the skill to be practiced can be sufficient; however, often leaders' empathy for parents' emotional messages can be more furthering than rational explanations.

For example, a leader was introducing the skill of showing understanding of children's feelings during an early meeting in the program, and asked parents to begin practicing this skill in a role-play with one another.

> Gemma: I'm not sure how it would work for me and my daughter, Helen. She keeps complaining about her teachers, one night it's one teacher and the next night it's another one. I feel like I should be doing more about it.

> Leader: You feel a bit overwhelmed by her feelings, and worry that she sounds unhappy. I will write this down on my list of examples for discussion when we reach that point in the program.

Comments such as Gemma's are important to acknowledge by leaders because they help motivate parents for the transfer and generalization stages to come. Overall leaders should exercise good judgment about what furthers current group goals and future interest in the program versus diversions and/or topics that are better postponed until later.

MAXIMIZING SUCCESS IN SKILLS TRAINING PRACTICE

In order to optimize parents' chances for success in learning and applying skills to their play sessions, leaders first "sell" them on the usefulness and importance of play sessions. This is done by presenting a clear rationale and then giving examples, ideally from what has already been a shared experience in the group (e.g. examples from the demos by leaders). Leaders also can build in opportunities for parents to be successful by structuring questions and exercises so that parents are more likely to answer them correctly and effectively.

Leaders need to give parents "multiple choices" frequently, because these responses concretize and illustrate skills, thus making it easier for parents to make more correct choices than they would with open-ended questions. If parents do not provide the correct answer very quickly, leaders should do so. It retards learning and is awkward for the group when they have to struggle to respond correctly.

For example, leaders may give the following types of choices when teaching parents to conduct play sessions:

1. *What would you say if your child asked you why they cannot run out of the playroom to check on their sister?*

    a. *Why do you think you should check on Beck?*

    b. *I told you before that you don't go running out when you feel like it.*

    c. *The rule is that you stay in the playroom.*

2. *What response would you give if your child said, "I don't like these toys"?*

    a. *That's what comes in the special play kit.*

    b. *What would you want?*

    c. *You wish you had some different toys.*

If there are several distinct steps involved in learning a skill, we suggest introducing each step one at a time. Leaders should begin this step-by-step practice by asking questions in order of difficulty. For example, when teaching the skill of "showing understanding," leaders can proceed from:

Step 1: "What is this child feeling?" and, if necessary, to:

Step 2: "Which is the better response: a) 'You're sad' or b) 'You're angry?'" (leaders always provide the choices) and then to:

Step 3: Eliciting parents' own statements in response to situations. (e.g. *"You're sad because you cannot go to the picnic."*). This step is more difficult and should be done only after a lot of practice by parents in identifying feelings and discriminating between more and less desirable responses.

USEFULNESS OF SUMMARIZING

Leaders should make clear, concise, positive summary statements during teaching that include a restatement of the rationale, but *without introducing* new examples or material. Summary statements should be repeated when necessary, because the summary helps to integrate learned skills for future use. It also reinforces the understanding of why the skill is useful and important, as the following example illustrates.

> *Leader: The opening statement to your children when bringing them into a play session appears very simple, and it is really, but it contains one particular word that is critical in setting children's expectations of what their play session will be. The statement is: "This is your special playtime, [name of child]. You can do ALMOST anything here. I'll let you know, if there is anything you cannot do." (This statement may include the optional statement: "You may say anything you like.")*
>
> *The word "ALMOST" lets the children know that they are very free, but not completely free, to do as they wish. The word allows you, the parent, to set necessary limits. Telling children you will tell them when a limit is reached lets children know they don't need to try to figure out what is "too much." It avoids what we used to encounter as play therapists years ago, when anxious or limit-testing children would ask continuously, "Is this OK?" This essential one word provides a clearer structure that tells children that you will keep them adequately informed, and spares them trying to anticipate what might not be allowed.*
>
> *Let's all say together two times: "In here, you can do ALMOST anything you want." (Leader laughs.) I apologize that it seems like kindergarten class, but saying things out loud helps learning. The mistake that is most often made by people introducing play sessions is to forget to include the "ALMOST." If forgotten, some children will be very distressed if you set a limit, because you did not tell them that there might be a limit on what they do.*

USING HUMOR EFFECTIVELY

As this example illustrates, throughout group meetings, and especially during early skills training, it is important that leaders make their teaching light enough and manageable for parents. Of course, new leaders find it more difficult to relax, because of keeping their mind on their new GFT tasks. But with practice, leaders are able to find their own delivery style and individual uses of humor. In our experience, after leaders run groups a few times, they are better able to focus on and appreciate the group and the individuals within each group. As they feel more competent, leaders also are able to use humor more spontaneously and effectively.

Maximizing success in skills practice

In addition to presenting didactic material, group leaders also are helping parents practice the skills used in play sessions prior to their beginning to directly play with their children. The following are general points to consider for leaders during the initial stages of GFT, when skills practice is most intensive.

Skills training goals

Leaders' training goals initially are to:

- convince the parents of the usefulness of particular skills

- make sure that parents understand how to use the skill and practice it in the training, and later in the supervised practice components of the program

- ensure that parents have realistic expectations with regard to the skills.

Later in the program additional goals are making certain that parents apply the skills in their home play sessions and, finally, that they generalize these skills to their daily lives.

Focusing

"Focusing" in the GFT program means that leaders need to concentrate primarily on skills training at the initial stages of the program, as mentioned earlier. Leaders should give highest priority to helping parents learn skills and apply them to working therapeutically with their children. Mastery of these skills produces more changes in parents' behavior and in their children's behavior over a relatively brief period than any other methods used over this period. Mistakenly changing the focus of the group from skills training to other methods or concerns can lead parents to misunderstand the program's goals and make it difficult, if not impossible, for leaders to fulfill them. Leaders must, therefore, keep their skill training goals in mind and remind parents, when necessary, that program goals are in their best interest because mastery of the skills enables parents to fulfill their own desires for change.

"Selling" the skill

In order to convince parents of the usefulness of the skill being taught, leaders must present a solid rationale accompanied by examples that graphically illustrate its usefulness. Rationales for all of the GFT skills taught are presented in the next chapter, Chapter 4. After this, leaders should demonstrate how and when the skill is applied in play sessions, as the next chapters in the book discuss in detail. The talk and demonstration by leaders should be brief and concise, in order not to "lose" the parents. We suggest no more than 15 minutes per skill.

Structuring

After this introduction, parents should move into practicing the skill in whatever way seems appropriate. This includes role-playing and open-ended responses to sample situations, which are illustrated in the following chapters. Leaders should initially explain to their group that they will practice in different ways at different times, depending upon what seems most effective in learning to use the skills.

Reinforcing parents' skills learning

Learning theory has influenced FT in several ways, as we briefly discussed and illustrated in earlier chapters. One major way is in how parents are helped to learn the skills needed for conducting play sessions. Positive reinforcement, used genuinely and respectfully, is a key response for leaders to use in skills training. We now discuss each facet of this learning theory approach in turn. This discussion is very familiar to professionals already practicing behavioral/reinforcement types of therapy. However it may seem more alien to person-centered practitioners, and is therefore summarized here.

Shaping

"Shaping" involves leaders positively reinforcing parents, both verbally and non-verbally, by comments such as "good," "excellent," "terrific," for moving in a positive direction during learning, no matter how slight their efforts. Any interaction by parents that shows they actively understand and/or are attempting to put new knowledge into practice is noted positively. Reinforcement is used deliberately to promote the behaviors needed, and the chances of those behaviors recurring is greatest when leaders give positive recognition to what is done correctly, rather than correcting inappropriate responses.

It is often necessary for leaders at the outset of GFT to commend actions that fall far short of the desired end result, because the smallest step in the right direction contributes to the acquisition of the desired final behavior. Reinforcing each small step in skills learning is a means of "shaping" the behavior parents ultimately need for their play sessions. Parents seldom learn the skills all at once, and there is variation in what skills are easiest to learn for each parent, as we discuss in later chapters. Parents acquire skills step by step over time—until all the pieces are put together in a final synthesis.

An example of shaping

John did not venture to use feeling words in order to "show understanding" with his child Martin during his first play session for fear of feeling awkward. During his second practice play session, John tried expressing understanding of Martin's feelings about not being able to draw a racing car the way he wanted it, by saying that Martin "must feel disappointed." But Martin then replied, *"No I don't care. I'll draw a house."* John did not respond and did not reflect any more of Martin's feelings during the remainder of their play session.

Leaders supervising the play session realized that Martin seemed more indifferent about his failed drawing than disappointed. Afterwards, when the leader provided feedback and supervision to John on his practice session, which was observed by the group, John mentioned that he got Martin's feeling wrong. It was important for the leader first of all to empathize with John's feelings—that he tried something he found difficult, and he thought the response was a bit off track—and that he in turn must be disappointed. It also was vital for the leader to reinforce John's first attempt to reflect a feeling—that is, instead of correcting John, the leader acknowledged that, although John thought the way he showed understanding was inaccurate, it was a good attempt at figuring out what Martin was feeling. This is an example of good shaping by the leader, with John's step towards learning to recognize and empathize with Martin's feelings being acknowledged and reinforced. Further help in showing understanding accurately could follow later, if needed. But it is possible that, on reflection, John will begin to label feelings more accurately for himself. This is the essence of shaping—pinpointing the major step forward, reinforcing it, and ignoring the lesser elements of the response.

DIFFERENTIAL REINFORCEMENT

Leaders can also reinforce differentially. For example, during her first play session with her daughter Jane, Kathy set a limit appropriately when Jane tried to use the intercom in the playroom. But when Jane ignored this limit, Kathy did not follow through in giving a warning of possible consequences, an essential element in limit setting.

In this situation, leaders should selectively reinforce the parent's positive action immediately after the play session—that is, praise Kathy for stating the limit. Leaders should ignore her failure to follow through with restating the limit and warning of the consequences for the moment, thereby neither reinforcing nor encouraging it. It is important in such situations to focus on positive components in order to reinforce parents for what they are doing right, and more or less ignoring the undesired behavior. Focusing on the undesired behavior, even after recognizing positive actions, could tend to create resentment or reluctance to attempt the skill again.

However, after the feedback to Kathy, whether or not the issue of setting limits is raised by other parents in the group, it is important for leaders to address this issue of when to warn of possible consequences as a group learning experience. This strategy of helping the group learn takes the focus away from Kathy's error and provides what could well be a needed review for the whole group. Leaders can mention that limit setting is difficult to do for everyone, when there is so much to remember in play sessions, and then rehearse the group in limit setting briefly before the end of the meeting.

Using examples during skills training

As advocated earlier, examples are crucial aids in defining the particular skill being taught. It is important that leaders not only explain the rationale for a skill and when it is to be used, but also give a number of appropriate examples of skill use. Examples are most effective when they are relevant to the ongoing concerns of the group members in play sessions. When using examples, leaders should, where possible, give a hypothetical example of poor skill use and follow this with a hypothetical good example, since people often learn more quickly through contrasts, and also tend to remember the last thing. It is very important, however, that the poor example is one that leaders have made up themselves. Parents may be very inhibited or embarrassed if an example was taken from, say, one of their play sessions, or they thought the example was based on parents' practice from earlier GFT programs.

For instance, when teaching parents to follow their children's lead during play sessions, leaders need to explain what this skill consists of, and then give examples of less effective and more effective ways to follow children's leads. Leaders may give a hypothetical example of a parent reminding her child to put away the pens before moving to the doll's house during a play session, then give a positive example of a parent following her daughter to the doll's house, even though her daughter had been doing a drawing that the parent was hoping to see finished. Leaders can then follow these contrasting scenarios with an example offering multiple choice answers to the question of which parent followed the child's lead, placing the correct answer last.

As soon as a response is correct and complete, leaders are encouraged to move on to another parent and another example. When using practice examples, one fully correct response from the group per example is usually sufficient. If leaders feel that an even better response would be quickly given by another group member or two, they could continue up to three. A good rule of thumb is to stop after a maximum of three parents have dealt with an example, regardless of whether it has reached perfection. Before moving on to the next exercise, leaders could reshape parents' responses into the best form and provide the reasons for the reshaping. Finally, leaders need to present parents with a summary statement about the components of and uses for the skill at hand that is realistic and does not exaggerate what the use of the skill can accomplish.

Trying to squeeze out full participation for each example slows things down and creates boredom. The same or nearly the same responses are often repeated in those instances. In order to be sure that different members are involved for different exercises, and thus provide opportunities to everybody in the group, leaders should use strategies such as saying, *"Well, this time we'll start asking those of you in the middle of the semi-circle to respond,"* or *"Those at the other end will start now."* (There is a tendency for leaders to start at one end or the other of semi-circles, which sometimes means that parents sitting at the other end are never asked to respond.) While leaders do not want a few people to dominate and others to be left out, neither do they want to embarrass parents, waste time or divert the group's attention by urging unwilling members to respond.

Using role-play as a skills training device

Role-playing is defined here as a technique whereby people take the frame of reference of others and pretend to be in a certain situation. Using role-play as a training device has certain advantages over lectures or straight discussions because it provides a variation in teaching methods—and using a variety of methods helps to hold attention. Role-play also is close to real life, and therefore is processed both cognitively and experientially. For these reasons role-play is used frequently in GFT skills training.

It is an ideal way for parents to acquire and give meaning to the skills they are learning and seeing demonstrated by allowing them to practice under controlled conditions. We suggest that leaders engage in role-play themselves first, before asking parents to role-play. This modeling by leaders enables parents to observe a skill being properly used. Leaders also should be aware that when parents take on the role of the child in role-plays, it is much harder for them than taking their usual parental role. Therefore leaders need to help parents to adapt to this "child" role initially, and not expect them to engage in more sustained role-plays.

Leading discussions in GFT

Another important aspect of delivering a successful GFT program is helping parents learn through group discussions. Group discussion can be used to create an atmosphere in which parents feel free to discuss issues of general concern to themselves and the group, and their reactions to particular skills or concepts. It is common at the beginning of GFT that participants want to share their distress and negative feelings about their children, and the impact on their own lives. However, we have already mentioned that group meetings are not designed to include lengthy discussions of participants' current and past lives.

Instead they primarily are intended to address here-and-now emotional issues as they arise during training and supervision of play sessions.

Group discussion is helpful in developing rapport between the leaders and the group as a whole, and also develops rapport among group members. In spite of the primary task of GFT, that of mastering the skills for conducting play sessions, the program provides many opportunities for parent discussions. For example, in the first meeting of the program, there are no skills to learn. It is an information session focused on discussion of the program and group development. Emphasis on discussion in this first meeting is intended to serve an important function, helping to build a "sense of group." Discussions also are generally scheduled to follow the use of videos, demos, practice play sessions, or spontaneously when either leaders or parents raise the appropriate questions during meetings. Because some of the ideas and behaviors of GFT are alien, even perhaps antagonistic, to many parents' beliefs or practices, a great deal of processing must go on for them. Feeling responses and feedback about their thoughts need to be provided. In these discussions, group members in time become as active, or more active, than the leaders, once the group is well under way. However, leaders are the ones to take ultimate responsibility for the understanding and interpersonal comfort of parents.

How to facilitate discussion

GOALS FOR LEADERS

Leaders' goals in leading discussions are to:

- isolate the most important elements in the situation under discussion and to focus on them

- to encourage maximal group participation and input

- to identify any consensus that has been established by group members through discussion.

There are numerous ways of facilitating the achievement of these goals, and we examine these next.

ORGANIZING AND BUILDING

It is important that leaders keep up the pace of the group in order to foster anticipation and to cover issues thoroughly. At the same time, experiences and feelings during meetings from different group members also need to be responded to empathically. After showing empathy, leaders should summarize the views or feelings of those involved. Then leaders should move on to new and related areas, using the previously stated opinions as take-off points, until the leaders are able to lead the group to an acceptable consensus. The following example illustrates this skill in GFT.

ILLUSTRATIVE EXAMPLE

Observed by the other parents, Jim was receiving feedback from the leader after one of his practice play sessions during a meeting towards the end of the program, when skills were beginning to be generalized to daily life by parents. Group cohesion is evident in the comments that follow; the group has a well-established attitude of helpful comments, rather than criticism. The example shows how the leader giving the feedback first responded empathically to Jim's frustration, and then asked him what he wished he would have done. The leader then invited other parents to join in the discussion. (Jim is relating an unsuccessful interaction at home in daily life.)

Jim: It worked pretty well here in the play session when I responded to DJ's feelings, but boy, when I tried it at home the other day, it didn't work at all. She was complaining about not being able to get a new case for her cell phone and I said, "You just got one." And she said, "I know, but it doesn't fit right, so I need a new one." And I said, "I can't afford to buy new cases every week." Then DJ said, "It doesn't cost that much, and my friends have that kind." And I said (trying to show understanding of her feelings), "It's very frustrating to you when you can't have what you think is the right thing." And she said, "Duh." It just ended there, for the moment, but I knew it was not a success. I didn't know where to go from there.

Leader: You tried to show understanding, and instead you got a big put down.

Jim: Yes, I would have been tempted, if I had not been trying to show understanding, to give DJ a lecture on how it was wrong to have everything and spend money that we don't have on all these silly things.

Leader: You thought you were sparing her a kind of scolding, but it didn't seem to make her feel like you were doing her any favors.

Jim: No. Sometimes she'll react well to my showing understanding, say "Yeah," with real feeling. Other times, she says something fresh, or just looks at me funny.

Leader: It's hard when you're trying to do something better, and it doesn't work.

Mary [another parent]: Yes, our kids don't appreciate how hard it is to try to do things better for them.

Al [a third parent]: I'm wondering if you had said first how much she really wanted that and let her know that you could see that it was important to her—if you had, it may have been easier for her to appreciate where you were coming from?

Leader: Do you have any ideas, now that we are thinking about it, Jim, about what you might have done differently?

Jim: I guess Al's suggestion is a good one. I could have tried that, maybe.

Leader: Yes, it sometimes does help if you first acknowledge more of the child's position, so let's see how you might have done that. Do you want to have a try, Jim, to come up with some words to use?

Jim: I'm a bit stuck. Maybe someone else might help with this.

Leader: This can be difficult for most parents, Jim. Maybe other parents have some examples themselves and can mention them later. Before we hear about them, let's all try together as a group to construct some responses that would show DJ that we appreciate her feelings about this cell phone case. It requires empathy on our part, because probably none of us think that this is a really important thing ourselves. We have to put ourselves in her shoes.

(The group then provides a number of possibilities, which the leader reinforces when they are useful ones, always ensuring that Jim is fully involved and his opinion is highlighted.)

Comments on this example

This example illustrates how leaders aim to build on shared group experiences. Once a number of different experiences have been given by other parents in a discussion, leaders need to summarize them by isolating the elements that make for successful, rather than unsuccessful, experiences. Leaders also must be quick to inject stimulating and pertinent questions, if the discussion lags or veers off course, and present a wide variety of possibilities and examples, with sample responses where required for parents to elaborate on, if they themselves do not have any.

After isolating the most important elements in successful responses (e.g. the child's feelings, the parent's feelings, the context), the leader may then go back to Jim, asking if he has ideas about what made his particular experience unsuccessful in his own mind. Perhaps Jim says he should have put his values, ones he wants DJ to learn, to the side and instead reflected her feelings. If this is suggested by Jim, the leader can use this comment to point out that there will be more input soon on this issue, or use this comment, if time permits, to introduce an additional skill needed for generalization.

Leaders should also remember that it is important to help parents with positive comments after a parent volunteers a problematic example. In Jim's case, the leader will need to help him with positive feedback on his interactions from his play session with DJ during the meeting. Leaders also should follow this feedback by giving other group members opportunities to suggest what they think worked well for Jim during his play session. The leaders can then encourage Jim and others who have had unsuccessful experiences with showing understanding at home to try again during the next week, taking into account the additional ideas they now have.

Establishing a consensus

In general, leaders should try to build from one point to another in this way, by extracting points from the discussions and emphasizing and underlining the important ones. Then leaders need to summarize, so that parents have a general idea of the structure of the process, skill, or interaction involved. Leaders should note that a successful discussion does not always require that a complete consensus be reached. Sometimes a diversity of views is expressed and adhered to. However, when a broad consensus does develop, it is important to state what it is in clear terms with such leader statements as, *"So it seems that most of you agree (feel, believe, etc.) that..."* The leader can then move onto a new point, but not before testing the limits of that consensus by saying something like, *"It seems we all agree that showing understanding can best be used when..., etc."*

A premature consensus is usually met with resistance on the part of some of the participants. If everyone seems to agree, but leaders suspect that they are doing so with even slight reluctance, leaders may wish to present them with a new aspect or possibility. This will test the firmness of the consensus. For example, a leader might say, *"Mary's experience with showing understanding seems to indicate that it might work under different circumstances than those you've agreed upon."* If the group simply agrees with the leader's statement, the consensus is probably firm, but, if a new round of discussion follows, the consensus was not genuine.

The criteria for recognizing a truly acceptable consensus are as follows:

- Usually there is not a single, simple, specific explanation agreed upon.

- The consensus is tempered by one or more conditions.

- Most people have participated and/or expressed agreement.

- The consensus does not represent the views of a sub-group, like young versus old, or men versus women, but rather nearly all members agree.

The leaders are the ones responsible for challenging an unrealistic consensus. If, for example, after a discussion about whether it is safe to let children shoot a dart gun at their parents during practice play sessions, and the group concludes that it is safe to do so, the leader would introduce new information. For example, *"I have heard of both parents and children who were hurt when a dart was fired into their face, etc."* If the parents hold firm to their unrealistic notions, the leaders must then be prepared to deal with parents' feelings. Leaders should accept their feelings without endorsing them, even when they are not viable (e.g. parents feeling that their children *should* be able to manage firing a dart gun away from the face). Leaders should remember that acceptance of feelings is not equivalent to supporting the actions that might stem from those feelings. Rather, acceptance is a first step towards desirable self-change.

In any discussion, leaders should try to avoid relating their own personal experiences, except where it is necessary to get the group out of a bind. Leaders' best contribution is to facilitate the participation of group members and have them give their own examples. Furthermore, if leaders do give their own experiences, they tend to model and reinforce the behavior of any group members who wish to indulge in an exchange of anecdotes that do not serve to further the stated purpose of the group. *The fulfillment of the goals of the training program can be severely hampered by allowing meetings to degenerate into cozy chats.*

Overall, leaders should try to focus on positive aspects that have been discussed when summarizing and concluding the discussion. A focus on the positive reinforces what the group members should take away with them from the meeting. And it serves to focus attention on those things that best prepare parents for future meetings.

Drawing in reticent members

If some parents seem especially reluctant to talk, leaders can try to discover whether they really have nothing to say, or are afraid to participate for some other reason. Leaders can do so by questioning them directly, but should structure their question in such a way that it will be easy for them to answer. For example, a leader might say, *"Sam, I know that you have a child of about the same age as Jim's. Have you experienced..."* If Sam responds with only one or two words, the leader can assume that he really does not want to talk, or has nothing more to say.

Nevertheless, leaders should continue to try to involve reluctant group members through such structured questioning in the future, both to show them that leaders care about them and their ideas, and to continue to "test" their silence. But leaders also should remember that it is not necessary to push a non-participant into participation. A leader's goal is not to persuade every group member to achieve the same degree of expressed involvement, because some people are just not talkers, or they may have ideas and experiences to share only in relation to one or two topics of exceptional interest to them. Leaders need to remind themselves that they should not gauge the degree of verbal participation by individual group members on a meeting-by-meeting, or topic, basis. Instead, leaders should consider parents' participation over the entire program period and expect a large degree of variation from week to week, person to person, and topic to topic. It is important not to slow down the group by trying to involve everyone, once it is clear that one group member or another does not choose to contribute after a leader's discrete, structured attempts to involve them. These parents may learn best simply through passive absorption. Evaluations of parenting skills training groups over the years by the first author demonstrate that most relatively quiet members have as positive results as the more expressive group members.

Creating group openness

Discussion should be an open process that encourages challenging of program concepts and openness about parents' cherished practices. Regardless of how much these practices may not be compatible with program principles, parents should feel safe to share them in the group setting. Empathic responses from group leaders—and later by other parents—show acceptance of their comments. While some views are not condoned in GFT, it is important to accept expression of them in order to assist parents in evaluating their own attitudes and practices. For example, some parents report "quick and dirty" control techniques, which are questionable, based on their imperfect understanding of the application of limit setting in play sessions to other aspects of their lives. First of all, it is important that parents should never be made to feel blamed or stupid for sharing such examples. Leaders should help the self-disclosing parent feel acknowledged and accepted, even if not agreed with. The leader might comment: *"You want very much to be able to help your child accept the consequences of his behavior, so you decided to try out a punishment that you heard from a friend."* Overall, the leaders' goal is not to agree with parents' ideas that conflict with program principles, but to acknowledge their motives and feelings empathically.

Dealing positively with advocates of unacceptable parenting behaviors

In open discussions, a parent might reveal a parenting behavior in real life that is of such an undesirable nature that leaders do not want to let it go unchallenged. Leaders then need to suggest that another way of handling the situation would be preferable. It is important that it is the leaders, rather than other parents, who suggest a more acceptable action. This is done in order not to undermine the supportive relationships parents develop within their groups. After making a suggestion, leaders should point out the negative components of the parent's behavior in the least accusatory manner possible.

There are two main reactions that should be avoided by leaders to a parent's highly negative behavior with their child, because they may be detrimental to both the group and the parent involved. (This assumes of course that the behavior is not so extreme as to warrant reporting this behavior to child protection authorities.) First, leaders should avoid extreme emotional reactions, such as panicking, or becoming outraged and angry with a parent. Some parents who mention their disciplining strategy at home reveal such behavior in order to test leaders' reactions. If leaders react strongly, the "tester" may try to goad leaders further, and a full-scale power struggle can ensue. Second, leaders should always avoid engaging in power struggles with group members. Leaders need to find a comment that avoids a head-on clash. For example:

> Parent: At home I don't have time to deal with feelings with four children to take care of. I just react, and smack them, and that's that. They know not to go on, or they will get more.

> Leader: You have found that works for you. You are satisfied with it. Here we are trying to learn skills that involve certain principles. Let's see, as we move on to applications of skills at home, if we can come up with a way that will be more consistent with these principles.

In general, if leaders try to convince parents that they are wrong in a direct way, this approach usually results in failure, and can create an atmosphere in the group of power testing. Tactfully confining comments to the skills' learning during play sessions, particularly in early GFT meetings, enables leaders to avoid power struggles and reinforce the aims and methods of the program itself.

Dealing with argumentative parents

We urge leaders *never* to get involved in an argument with a group member. It is essential for leaders to remember it is not the task of the leader or the group to solve conflicts of opinion, but rather to help participants to master skills and accept different opinions. If a group member insists upon a point leaders cannot accept, they should say something like: *"Let's try to continue with the new methods we are learning. We are sure that you will see that they work for most of you..."* It also is important that leaders do not talk down to group members. Anything that creates tension, control issues, or resentment only hinders the achievement of leaders' goals. Power struggles and resentment are detrimental to learning, which is best promoted in an accepting atmosphere. Above all, leaders need to remember that *in FT parents are the paths to their children's healing.* Therefore, willing, contented and motivated parents are critical in order to further this therapeutic process.

Handling put downs between group members

If a group member puts down the offering of another member, be it a program-appropriate response or not, the leader should say, *"Marilyn doesn't agree with the suggestion made by Jane. How do you feel about that, Jane?"* The parent who was put down should be provided with a specific chance to be heard. Leaders never want self-disclosure or unique opinions to result in "punishment" for a parent. Leaders should always remember that contributions given to the group by a parent are part of a process that should be encouraged. They permit leaders to examine issues and specific behaviors in a way that promotes critical evaluation of parental approaches, and helps parents come to grips with their parenting values. To create a positive learning climate, critical comments need to be addressed immediately, but without leaders adopting a critical tone themselves.

Inclusiveness and group dynamics

Sometimes one parent wants to discuss their reaction to a teaching point or interaction in detail. Leaders should guard against the temptation to have a ten-minute mini-therapy, or learning, session directed at one parent only. Instead, leaders can say that they will go back and review this teaching point or difficulty again later. If it is clear to leaders that this parent has a personal reaction, rather than a learning need, and this response is one that requires more than a few minutes to address, one of the leaders may need to say that a time can be arranged at the midway break to talk later about that parent's personal issue. If the parent persists in trying to discuss their personal issues at length in a way that does not enable the group to move forward, the leader needs to be clear that *"you and I will have time to talk later."*

There are two additional important ways that leaders might respond when a parent requires more time for their individual issues. First, rather than singling out the individual in the group as having difficulties, leaders may direct their responses back to the learning needs of the whole group. For example, the leader may say: *"Let's review the opening statement for the children when starting a play session"* rather than, *"John, you need more help with your opening statement."* And second, leaders have to be effective in setting limits for individuals in the group, while at the same time avoiding comments that activate individual group members' defensive responses.

Leaders would not be effective in saying:

> Louis, we already covered that. I don't think we should be dealing with that now. We have other points we need to cover.

Instead, it would be tactful to say:

> We have so many things to cover in here, it would be best if we moved on now to our next points. If anybody wishes to have us discuss something, please talk to us at the break, or at the end of the meeting.

In our experience, this type of limit setting for an individual is important at the early stages of the group process. By later meetings, participants are aware of the kinds of responses that are helpful to them, as well as to the group.

In general, leaders should be constantly alert to where parents' needs really lie and where these needs are dealt with during meetings. Co-leaders need to be alert to each other's responses, in order to be sure that a leader's responses are not skewed towards any one individual, to the detriment of the group. On the other hand, leaders also should examine whether their responses are too focused on the whole group, and do not sufficiently address individual needs. Clinical supervision, as discussed in Chapter 1, can be very useful for leaders to guard against these types of imbalances.

Additional group inclusion issues for leaders

In our experience, the following issues that arise in a few groups are more difficult for leaders, particularly new leaders, to respond to effectively.

Expressions of strong discomfort with other group members

Very occasionally, the intake process does not reveal strong negative attitudes and prejudices in parents that would question their group membership. Very occasionally, a parent may reveal a strong antagonism towards another member of the group during an early meeting. Leaders should be equipped with a strategy for handling this. For example, if a parent confided in a group leader during the midway break that they "hated" some feature of another participant, thus displaying a strong prejudice, we suggest that the leader try to respond empathically, stating that this participant sees this as difficult to deal with. It would then be important for the leader to offer to spend one-to-one time outside the regular group meeting with this parent, in order to discuss ways to handle this parent's attitude, without causing offence to the named participant. This extra meeting would be especially important if this attitude had been detectable by other members of the group, since this parent's negative attitude could affect the comfort of the entire group.

Other issues may arise in groups in a covert, rather than in a direct way. These too need to be acknowledged by leaders in order not to disrupt the group process. For example, a mother in the group may not give a single father, the only male in the group, any credit for knowing how to deal with his daughter's day-to-day care. In such instances of covert discrimination, group leaders may decide that these issues do not need to be addressed directly; instead they can be productively ignored and the father given a higher level of positive attention when it is appropriate by the leader, in order to offset and compensate for this unspoken attitude. However, some situations cannot be managed with indirect tactics, and planned, individual input with the parent who is making covertly critical comments may be required.

Non-attendance

Non-attendance is dealt with in different ways, depending on the reasons for it, the point in the group at which it occurs, and the length of time it persists. As a general rule, it is difficult for parents to be active and integrated group members if they miss more than two meetings at the beginning of a group. If parents miss the first two meetings, it is essential for a leader to hold individual "catch-up" times in lieu, before these parents join the third meeting. Leaders first should contact them directly by telephone or email to explain the importance of their attendance and arrange for catch-up times (given that this is possible for the leaders and parents). If this catch-up time does not occur before the third meeting, we suggest that a letter is sent to the parents, giving the reasons for their not being able to join the existing group (e.g. other parents missing their input, inability of the leaders to catch parents up). Parents may be offered either an alternative date and contact information for joining another group, if other groups are planned, or another option. The options suggested will vary, depending on the referral issues and the involvement of other professionals with the family.

If parents unexpectedly miss meetings later in the group process, leaders have to make clinical judgments about whether these parents are able to catch up with the ongoing group process, and are able to take part in one-to-one work with a leader prior to rejoining the group. Leaders' judgments may be influenced by whether the parents have sufficient focus to concentrate on participating in the group again, particularly if a serious life event (e.g. a parent's mother having a stroke in a distant location, and now needing a high level of nursing care) has intruded on planned participation. If such an event is responsible for unplanned absences, the leader should discuss the consequences for further absences with these parents directly.

Supplemental skills development for an individual participant

Additional, one-to-one input can be offered by leaders as emotional and/or skills support, if this seems necessary in order to maintain the pace of the program for the majority of parents. The leaders' aim for the few parents needing this extra input is to help them relax, lessen their performance anxiety, and adopt an open learning attitude, where emotional support is required, or to attain an adequate competence level on a par with other group members, where skills support is required. These latter parents' practice play sessions with their children should be scheduled at the end of the training phase in GFT, before these parents' practice play sessions are scheduled, so that they can gain from observing the other parents, as we discuss further in a later chapter.

For example, Harvey was worried that his work had precluded him from attending two meetings that concentrated on learning the skill of limit setting, a skill he would certainly need when he had his play sessions with his unruly 7-year-old son. One of the leaders decided to give Harvey a half-hour of skills training on limit setting, including role-plays, prior to the meeting in which Harvey was to have his first practice play session observed by the other parents. This additional input had the dual purpose of enabling the group to move along together, and enabling Harvey to fully participate in the program.

Dealing with "slow to learn" parents

When parents are slow to grasp FT skills, leaders need to be prepared to structure skills learning more fully for them. This usually includes:

- presenting them with some alternative responses from which they choose the appropriate one

- additional role-playing and/or

- some other means of concretizing the skills for them (e.g. charts, supplementary videos, or diagrams).

As soon as leaders see that a parent is unable to respond without leaders' probing or prompting, leaders should provide the correct answer to these parents at once. It is very useful to then role-play the correct response, or use some other teaching method as described earlier to indicate the correct response. Hesitation and "wrong" responses should clearly tell leaders that parents need more input and shaping of responses. If leaders try to pull out correct responses by giving hints one after the other, but without offering additional structure, the learning process is usually slow, fragmented, and unrewarding for both parents and leaders. It does not yield results that endure in the minds of the parents.

Responding to emotionally burdened parents

Parents who have experienced more serious past maltreatment, and those with entrenched emotional blocks, are commonly identified during the intake process before the GFT program begins. Leaders may recommend an option other than GFT to these parents, or recommend that they receive psychotherapy themselves before individual FT or GFT commences. However, occasionally these parents' emotional distress is not prominent at intake; it is in actually practicing therapeutic skills during GFT that traumatic memories may be triggered for them that create serious blocks to learning to conduct play sessions. Leaders need to rely on their clinical judgment in cases where the burden feels too heavy on the group, and the particular emotional issue seems to be confined to one individual.

When leaders have indications that a parent is preoccupied or overwhelmed during a meeting, they need to arrange a time to talk further with this parent after the meeting. Leaders usually suggest that these parents may wish to observe, rather than participate actively for the remainder of the meeting, while leaders continue with the meeting's agenda for the rest of the group. (Very rarely, if a parent reacts strongly and is unable to continue during a meeting, one leader may need to leave with this parent immediately, while the second leader continues.) Leaders may say:

> It's pretty clear Barbara, that this is a very important issue for you. It is going to require some time to discuss it in full. I do not want to rush you. Therefore, I want to schedule another time to talk about it further, either after this session, before the next session, or at another time that will work for both of us.

During discussions with any emotionally distressed parents after a meeting, leaders use their clinical judgment about what these parents require. A key question is whether the parents need additional therapy over and above what GFT leaders can provide during meetings. If these parents' issues seem tractable over a short time frame, leaders may recommend that parents see another therapist for brief therapy, and maintain their attendance in the GFT program. If leaders are experienced in individual psychotherapy, able to manage professional boundaries well, and have a schedule that would permit it, in the authors' opinion there would be no role conflict in theory if they helped parents in individual psychotherapy for a few sessions, until they worked through a problem. However, most GFT leaders rarely have time to add individual psychotherapy for group members to their caseload. It is essential, therefore, that leaders have a constant alertness to where parents' emotional needs really lie, and where they need to be taken, including using outside referral sources. In most cases, motivated parents are able to work on their personal issues separately with a therapist, alongside maintaining their group attendance. In some circumstances, leaders need to supplement these parents' skills development with an individual catch-up time or two. However, leaders should consider in exceptional cases recommending that parents wait until a later date to attend GFT or FT.

Two particular challenges for GFT leaders

While the rewards for leaders are considerable, there are two important duties of leaders that are particularly challenging, to be discussed next. The cooperative interplay between two leaders can ease the pressure involved in continually remaining vigilant in meeting these responsibilities, and also be very beneficial for the group. The first task is the practical one of fitting everything into the time frame of the meetings. The second is remembering to make empathic responses first, before moving on to any other type of response, such as answering a question. Both of these responsibilities are critical to the management and quality of the GFT process. Continued empathic responding on the part of leaders distinguishes GFT from other group therapies and parenting programs. In our opinion, this is what makes GFT especially effective.

Apportioning time effectively

Time management begins for leaders before the group itself starts and continues to be a priority for leaders during all meetings. Time keeping by leaders is an important factor in setting the pace for the group, and including everyone in the introductions and discussions. This task needs to be done without rushing participants or making them feel unimportant or unheard. For example, usually some group members arrive earlier than others for meetings, resulting in those group members getting into informal conversation while waiting for others to arrive. It may be tempting for leaders to allow the (sometimes fascinating) discussions to continue after the agreed start to the meeting. Because they are very engaging, leaders sometimes find these conversations difficult to stop, resulting in time lost for other meeting components. This lost time is especially detrimental during meetings with scheduled demos and play sessions. Keeping play sessions as the top priority helps leaders in their efforts to keep the time distribution optimal for all the necessary components of GFT meetings. A tip that has worked for the authors is for group leaders to stay apart from waiting group members, busy themselves with preparations for the play sessions, and then signal the time to start.

Other places in meetings also are prone to overextending the time. For example, generally watching and discussing play sessions generates excitement in parents. This raises the energy level of group members, tending to make them more talkative. As shown throughout the book, group discussion is a necessary feature of GFT. However, the time for this valuable component needs to be limited, so that the group meeting time is distributed appropriately to cover play sessions and didactics, as well as time for group members to air their feelings and reactions, as examples in this book demonstrate.

Using empathy in GFT

As stated earlier, in order to help parents to be motivated to participate in the program and to help one another, it is essential that leaders demonstrate sincere empathy for each participant's feelings (Andronico et al., 1967; Eardley, 1978). Group leaders need to demonstrate and practice the skills that they want parents to use with their own children, and *empathy is the foremost skill to use*. In addition to knowing when to convey empathy to parents from intake onwards about their feelings regarding their children, leaders also need to demonstrate empathy for parents' feelings about the group process and the new skills they are acquiring.

MOVING FROM TEACHING TO FEELINGS

Knowing when the moment has arisen in a group for leaders to make a shift from didactic to empathic responses is crucial to achieving excellent results with parents. An example of a leader addressing an "empathic moment" during a group is as follows:

The leader is giving examples to parents during early skills training of how to follow their children's lead in play sessions and use tracking comments:

> *Parent: It's too hard. I can't do it. And my son won't stand for it either.*
>
> *Leader: You just don't see how you and your child will be able to learn to do this. (Not: "Let's go over these ideas again, and then you may see how it will work with your son.")*

In this example, the leader recognized that this was a moment of emotional resistance for a parent, and stopped the teaching for the moment. Flipping over to a dynamic/ feelings role was required here. This empathic comment by the leader helped this parent feel understood. In our opinion, which is supported by other clinicians, but not as yet by empirical evidence, if opportunities for making empathic responses at crucial times for parents are seized by GFT leaders, parents experience firsthand for themselves the power of empathy. It is likely that there will be this qualitative shift in their own parenting style later. They are likely to feel better about their own feelings and thoughts, and be more willing to substitute empathic understanding of others, as appropriate, instead of more typical responses such as asking questions, challenging, and making critical responses.

It can be difficult for leaders to remember not to plough on with teaching points when a parent's feelings are the main issue. Often when new leaders are presenting teaching material, they understandably have more anxiety than when they develop greater experience in GFT. New leaders may fear losing control over their teaching when a parent "interrupts," or else they can be overly preoccupied with teaching points. In both cases, new leaders may not be sensitized sufficiently to what is happening at a feelings level in group participants. Leaders may then perceive a comment as a challenge to a teaching point, and not as a feelings issue. However, not recognizing a parent's feelings and continuing to teach is counterproductive. Feelings will get in the way of learning. If not attended to at first, feelings will persist and continue to interfere with learning. A rule of thumb for leaders is that when parents do not learn, or they resist learning a new behavior, leaders should look for a feeling(s) that has not been fully aired. Once these negative feelings are recognized and explored empathically, these learning problems generally disappear.

Yet leaders should guard themselves from the expectation that, if they reflect parents' feelings accurately, then parents will immediately be able to use this comment to shift towards a more effective parenting style. It is important for leaders to guard against this unrealistic expectation. More realistically, leaders' comments may be needed at crucial, receptive learning points three or four times at least for parents to make this shift, rather than once or twice. Also, the role of other supportive group members in valuing the struggles of their peers, and their dedication to their children's well-being, should not be underestimated.

ILLUSTRATIVE EXAMPLE

Mary Jane did not set limits on her daughter Anna's aggressive behavior in her practice play session during a meeting, as she had been instructed to do on more than one occasion. Anna had hit her mother with bean bags twice, and her mother responded, *"You want me to have those."* When the leader provided feedback after the play session, Mary Jane's struggles over setting limits were acknowledged:

> Leader: We've gone over how to set limits in play sessions together a few times. But it seems like it was really hard for you to see where to do this, and to enforce limits on Anna's aggressive behavior in your play session.

> Mary Jane: Well, the bean bags didn't hurt me, and I do have trouble telling her to stop in the play sessions and at home. Anna takes any correction from me as an insult, and becomes very difficult. I really can't deal with that...it makes me feel so guilty.

> Leader: If Anna becomes negative to you in any way, you feel like a bad mother, that you have done something really bad.

> Mary Jane: Yes! I can't afford to have Anna feeling like I'm not a good mother. It's very important to me that she loves me and feels that I'm doing the right things by her.

> Leader: You wouldn't want to destroy that by scolding her.

> Mary Jane: Well, you know that she is adopted, and that we went to great lengths to get a girl, since we already had two boys. And I believe that if you adopt a child, it's necessary to be especially giving and accepting because you've volunteered to make a good life for this child. An adopted child doesn't just come along like some other babies, whether you're ready for them or not [in tears].

> Leader: When you go out of your way to get a child, you have a special obligation to be sure that this child's life is happy, with as few restrictions as possible.

> Mary Jane: That's right. I like to give Anna whatever she wants. Let her do whatever she wants, whenever she wants. Unfortunately, as you know, this hasn't really stopped Anna from having problems. So, I guess I really do need to think about trying to do things a little differently to help her.

> Leader: You've done every possible thing that you could do that you thought would make Anna happy, including sacrifices to her yourself. And, it really hasn't worked they way you'd hoped. Now you're feeling like perhaps doing some things differently might help her in the end.

> Mary Jane: Yes.

Leader: It would be hard for you to change all at once. One small thing you could do that might give Anna a better notion of the need to control her feelings would be to set limits in the playroom that she understands, that there are boundaries there that she needs to live within. So, let's go over the incidents of hitting you with the bean bags in tonight's play session, and rehearse a way for you to deal with that according to the playroom rules. We'll also talk about how you think you might feel when you enforce the rules. It's pretty clear that your feelings need to be addressed in order for you to place this restriction on Anna.

Mary Jane: Yes, I would feel pretty harsh and mean, but I can see that it might help Anna if she knew that she couldn't push me all the time as far as she feels like.

(Future play sessions became easier for Mary Jane because she had cleared away the feeling barrier that was stopping her from conducting play sessions according to the rules. In time, Anna began to demonstrate more respect for her mother in the playroom, and eventually at home.)

COMMENTS ON THIS EXAMPLE

This example shows that it is often both necessary and appropriate to empathize with parents' feelings when they show learning blocks. This mother was able to openly acknowledge her difficulties, and move towards learning how to set limits as required in play sessions. It also seemed essential that the leader concentrated afterwards on helping the mother to learn to set limits in the play sessions, and recognized the difficulties she may have if she attempted to alter her parenting style abruptly in daily life.

MOVING FROM FEELINGS TO TEACHING

It is also often important that leaders return to didactics during GFT after exploring parents' feelings. When setting the meeting's pace and having to return to teaching, leaders need to do this without any parents feeling rejected. Co-leaders may be able to more easily recognize and process such emotional moments with a parent, then help leaders in the teacher's role to resume their task.

ILLUSTRATIVE EXAMPLE

This example occurred during the leader's feedback to a father after his first practice play session with his 7-year-old son, Jeb. The father, Howard, objected to having to allow Jeb to lead the way.

Howard: I don't see what would be wrong with my giving Jeb a few ideas about doing things he would have liked. Instead, he just went around playing a little with this, and a little with that, and didn't really play with anything meaningfully. How will that help him work through his problems? Isn't that what this play is supposed to do?

Leader: That seemed like a really nothing session to you. You wanted Jeb to take an interest in something, really get involved.

Howard: Yes, if this is going to help him with his problems, he's going to have to play out something. You said play sessions would help him with his troubling feelings.

Leader: It doesn't seem to you like that can happen, if he isn't more involved.

Howard: No!

Leader: You would like to see some evidence of him expressing his feelings.

Howard: Yes. There is no time to waste because Jeb's in trouble at school because of his behavior.

Leader: You need to see some promise that he can play meaningfully and play through his problems.

Howard: Well, isn't that why we're all here?

Leader: Right now, it's hard for you to see how change can ever happen.

Howard: Well, maybe later, but how much later? We don't have years, you know.

Leader: You can imagine change, possibly, in the future. But how far in the future?

Howard: Yes, that is it.

Leader: It would help you a lot if you knew that things would turn out all right, and not take too long to do so.

Howard: Yes.

Leader: The session tonight was hard for you. It didn't look like Jeb would become involved. He probably will, and will need to do so to experience change. I would like to pass on to you that many children start out play sessions in a bland way, as we have seen with Jeb. That is how they "warm up" to the really different experience they are having. Then, in a session or two, they are really involved… perhaps with toys and games, perhaps with imaginative play—playing out fantasies of good and bad. Children play so many different ways when we let them direct themselves. It generally turns out in our experience that the things children do without our direction are their way of dealing with things they need to, to feel better and to behave better.

I would like to suggest that you give Jeb a few more sessions, before you conclude that he cannot play meaningfully. When they are held at home, it may be easier for him. Then we all might be able to see that what he is playing is related to his emotional needs. He could possibly want to play with superheroes. He did look at them during his play tonight. Remember, we said earlier that the content of play sessions is not as important as how the children feel or perceive them. It is this perception, and their feelings, that drive their behavior.

Does this sound encouraging?

Howard: Well, I guess I have no choice, really. And it does make sense. I always feel that Jeb's mother won't allow Jeb to express himself.

Leader: I am glad that you are willing to go on. I believe you will be glad, too, in due time.

Comments on this example and timing considerations

The leader spent several minutes on this father's issue; first, with his feelings, and then with instruction that the leader judged as beneficial for both the father and the group as a whole. However, the leader chose not to pick up the father's reference to the mother. This may be a very important family dynamic, but right at that moment the father and the group needed to move on. If the father still wanted to focus on the mother in the group, this could be discussed later, after the group's play sessions were well established. Important family issues can generally be depended upon to be brought up again, and are likely to not go unattended. In the meantime, if the leader had responded to the father's comment about the mother, this may have taken a lot of the group's time to deal with an issue that was not timely in relation to the training phase of GFT.

The time set aside for training is precious and critical. When therapists are lured into other issues, attention to the needs of the whole group's agenda is neglected. If the father-mother-child relationship becomes more pressing to this father, and time needed for group work does not permit in-depth attention, the mother and perhaps her husband could be offered time to meet with one of the GFT leaders, or another available therapist, to deal with the issue outside the group.

Supportive research

At a more abstract level, there is research to support the value of dealing empathically with parents' feelings when conducting GFT, as Eardley's (1978) study demonstrated (see Chapter 1). The leader's tactic of shifting focus from learning to reflecting parents' feelings at key points is further reinforced by the theory and research on attachment-based exploratory interest sharing. (See Heard & Lake [1997], Jaeger & Ryan [2011] and Ryan [2004] for fuller accounts.) Following this theory's explanation, if people have strong negative feelings, they activate their care-seeking system or defensive system. People cannot then explore new ideas and share the interests of their peers, until their own needs are met sufficiently. Therefore, the immediate goal for GFT leaders when parents voice strong feelings becomes a caregiving one, helping parents to process their strong feelings and to feel understood and cared for. After this acknowledgement, parents are then better able to adopt a non-defended position, which in turn enables them to have their minds free for further learning.

Time management and discussion of parents' feelings

Because there is so much for parents to learn and leaders to teach, it is sometimes easy for leaders to focus too much on trying to help parents grasp all the information required for learning to conduct play sessions. For this reason, many of this book's examples concentrate on focusing on parents' feelings. However, it is also important that leaders do not spend too much time dwelling on one or more parents' feelings, as mentioned earlier. At times, and for some leaders, the therapist part of themselves can over-focus on parents' underlying emotional issues that may arise as they struggle to master the skills of conducting play sessions. These feelings issues should routinely be dealt with empathically by the leaders for a short time; lengthy individual emotional problems should not become part of the group agenda. Indeed many parents, given the opportunity and an accepting emotional climate, will at some point want to engage in time-consuming personal problem solving in GFT that is only tangentially related to their parent-child relationships. While psychological theorists may argue that any internal conflict might be relevant to parent-child relationships, the primary agenda for GFT is based on the power of the parent-child play relationship. Therefore, time spent in the group that diverts from that agenda, and closely related issues, can reduce the power of the GFT method.

Balancing GFT tasks with two leaders

Balancing these two basic leadership tasks of empathic support and instruction, and their subcomponents, can be more easily done by two leaders, so that neither component is relatively neglected. With two leaders, it is possible for one leader always to take a "feelings" role and the other leader to take a "teaching" role. However in our experience, it is much more effective to have both leaders take both roles, taking turns with one another in teaching and responding to parents' feelings. One leader can present the instructional points and the other leader can respond to the parents' reactions to this information. Because it is vital for leaders to empathize and understand where parents are at an emotional level at all times, it is also important that, as one leader presents didactic material, the other leader helps by monitoring parents' feelings and addressing them where needed during the presentation. These roles can be reversed in some meetings, so that each leader can become (or remain) proficient in both components of the process. This way of responding is beneficial for parents, but also entails close coordination between the two leaders.

An alternative method for two leaders to complement each other is to share both tasks for different portions of each group meeting. For example, one leader might conduct play demos with children and lead the related discussions, and the other leader may lead the skills training segment. Alternatively, the discussion of the home play sessions and accompanying feedback can be shared, with one leader focusing, for example, on one parent and the other on the next. Moving back and forth from one leader to the other for different components can be done smoothly and naturally, just as a single leader would move back and forth between feelings and instruction responses. This sharing of roles by two leaders helps parents not to identify one leader with only one component; parents will not as easily believe that one leader is concerned only with their feelings and the other with teaching. This modeling to parents of empathic understanding and skills teaching by leaders also helps parents integrate both facets of the program into their individual play sessions with their own children.

Whatever sharing scheme is used by co-leaders, it is important that the leaders alternate in their particular functions from meeting to meeting. Of course, either leader should be free to pitch in to assist the other leader if the latter is experiencing some difficulty in making an instructional point, or in following the feelings of a parent. This is unlikely to be needed often, but should be planned for in advance so that the leader who needs a hand does not feel upstaged or give the appearance of being upstaged to the parents. Nor should it appear that the helping leader is being intrusive. To avoid these problems, we suggest that co-leaders work out a statement to use, which invites the other leader to join in, for example, *"I'm wondering if…(other leader's name) might be able to put it a bit better."* If the first leader is having trouble, but does not invite in the co-leader, the second leader could say, *"I'd like to add something here that might be helpful."*

Another important advantage of two leaders, in addition to those already outlined, is during demos. When one leader is demonstrating a play session to the group, the other leader can be quietly labeling the play therapist's behaviors as these are demonstrated, as we discuss more fully in a later chapter. This "in progress" labeling can be very helpful in parents' acquisition of appropriate play session behaviors and skills because it is done in "real time," rather than after the events occurred.

Overall, leaders need to remember that modeling of acceptance, showing understanding and other therapeutic attitudes, are basic leadership functions. It is critical that leaders use the same skills themselves that parents are learning. By using this GFT approach, leaders create an atmosphere of continual acceptance of each parent, which has repeatedly been shown to provide a highly successful learning environment for programs with a therapeutic component. The wide range of leadership skills needed by leaders in GFT was discussed in this chapter. In the following chapters we detail the 20-week program from start to finish, after exploring the rationales for the skills taught in GFT in the next chapter.

CHAPTER 4

The Main Skills Parents Learn in GFT

The last chapter gave leaders general guidelines for conducting the GFT program, including helping parents with skills learning. This chapter sets out the CCPT practice skills and rationales leaders need in order to conduct demos and help parents conduct play sessions with their children. Familiarity with all of the skills set out here is essential for leaders from the outset. They are needed in order to set up the program, to answer parents' questions with confidence, to think beforehand about teaching CCPT skills to parents, and to help parents anticipate what is to come in the program. Leaders must be proficient in using CCPT skills in child therapy practice before conducting GFT.

The main play therapy skills for GFT

Play session skills in GFT are derived from Axline's (1947) seminal summary of eight principles on which non-directive play therapy/CCPT is based. These eight basic principles lay out the foundation for the skills play therapists use in CCPT (Guerney L., 2003). In GFT, these same skills are taught to parents, who are trained to conduct CCPT sessions with their own children. These principles are as follows:

- Trusting and accepting relationships are developed by adults with children in one-to-one play sessions.

- Children, rather than adults, choose the issues, the focus and the pace of their play, activities, and interactions in play sessions.

- Empathy with children, expressed by reflecting children's feelings and thoughts in a sensitive manner, is essential.

- Therapeutic limits that "anchor" children's play sessions in reality are needed, in order to engender children's sense of emotional safety (Wilson & Ryan, 2005).

Outcome studies show that the completely integrated set of skills used in CCPT and FT play sessions are effective in bringing about change in children (see Chapter 1).

However, there is as yet not enough process research available to indicate whether one skill is more important than another in helping children therapeutically (Ryan & Edge, 2012). Therefore, the complete set of CCPT skills must be integrated and applied in actual practice for meaningful and effective play sessions. It is important for leaders to remember, and to remind parents in turn, that all the skills taught to parents go together as a system. These skills are separated out for teaching purposes only. After they are learned separately during the training phase of GFT, parents integrate their skills into a whole by practicing all the skills in a mock play session, before they conduct their first practice play sessions with their children.

There are several different ways that trainers and authors set out CCPT play skills (e.g. Bratton *et al.*, 2006; Cochran, Nordling, & Cochran, 2010; Landreth, 2012; VanFleet, Sywulak, & Sniscak, 2010; Wilson & Ryan, 2005). This chapter and the rest of this book follow the way skills are set out in the Parents' Training Manual for Play Sessions in Appendix 15, which is given out to parents at the end of the first meeting.

A summary of the main skills taught to parents

The Parents' Training Manual sets out the four most important skills that parents need to learn for play sessions. They are as follows:

- Focusing on children's feelings and actions.

- Following children's lead.

- Structuring play sessions.

- Limiting children's behavior.

These four skills are now briefly described.

Skill 1: focusing on children's feelings and actions. This skill is essential to the success of parents' play sessions. Parents are helped to track their children's conversations and actions in a non-intrusive way, and to recognize and make empathic responses to their children's feelings. In this way, children feel both valued and understood at a deeper emotional level, which in turn increases parents' and children's attachments to one another. How to respond to children's questions, commands, and requests in a child-centered manner are included in training parents in this skill.

Skill 2: following children's lead. This skill involves training parents to fully attend to their children during play sessions, and to participate in play sessions, either through actions or words, at their children's request. Responding to imaginative play, including role-play, is included in this skill, as is responding to children in child-led conversations.

Skill 3: structuring play sessions. This skill helps children know what to expect in play sessions with their parents. It includes introductory and closing statements for the play sessions that are given by parents to their children.

Skill 4: limiting children's behavior. Parents are helped to assert their own authority effectively by learning how to set limits behaviorally, how to select the important limits to adhere to in play sessions, and how to manage their own emotions in ways that do not create or maintain conflict-laden responses.

The order of teaching the main skills

As we already discussed in the last chapter on running successful groups, leaders need to help parents learn these major skills in the most accessible way, using shared examples from demos during early meetings, and concentrating on one skill at a time. The following chapters discuss the usual order in which the skills are taught in the GFT program. Empathic responding, or "showing understanding" is taught first, since this skill is the cornerstone of child-centered practice and one that, once taken on board, helps parents make sense of the rest of the skills. Equally, it is important to wait to teach the skill of limit setting until the other three skills are understood. Effective and attuned limit setting is dependent upon the mastery of the first three skills. When parents have reached the last stage of the program, and are beginning to generalize play session skills over to parenting in their daily lives, it is again important for leaders to start with applications of empathic responding and understanding children's underlying needs, before limit setting is addressed.

The next sections set out each of the four skills, including their sub-skills, in more detail, along with several concrete examples. Rationales are included in each section because throughout the program leaders should be prepared to provide parents with the general reasons why they need to learn and practice these skills.

Skill 1: focusing on children's feelings and actions— empathy, empathic responding and tracking

The reasons for using empathy are examined first, followed by a discussion of tracking, a skill practiced alongside empathy.

Empathy and empathic responses

Empathy is a key therapeutic skill, and central to practicing CCPT for both play therapists and parents. One of the main tasks for parents in GFT is to learn to express empathy—that is, to learn to understand and, where appropriate, accurately reflect feelings back to their children during play sessions. Using this skill in play sessions has important functions in that it enables:

- children to feel more accepted, and to become more securely attached to their parents

- parents to understand and accept their children more fully

- children, when their feelings are accepted, to in turn understand, accept, and cope with their own feelings and those of others.

Parents learn to identify what feelings their children are expressing both verbally and non-verbally through actions and facial expression. Ways for leaders to help parents master this skill are discussed in the next chapters on skills training. Here we set out additional reasons for parents to show empathy towards their children in play sessions.

More rationales for empathy and empathic responding

These additional rationales are as follows:

- In play sessions, parents are trying to see the world from their children's point of view. This includes what children are feeling and thinking.

- Feelings do not usually disappear, if they are not acknowledged. Instead, they tend to become fixed and strengthen.

- Not acknowledging feelings can short-circuit coping processes, leading to feelings of irritability and discontent in children. Research shows that continued use of non-coping responses can lead to a variety of problems in children (e.g. psychosomatic problems, escalation of anger and aggression). (See, for example, Wenar & Kerig, 2006.)

- Empathic responding enables children to become more confident in themselves; they understand their feelings, label them, and learn to cope with them. For example, a child waking up from a nightmare and talking about it with an empathic adult who does not try to minimize the experience (e.g. *"That dream was scary."* and not *"Forget about it. It's not real."*) is usually enabled to return to sleep.

- Acknowledging children's feelings leads to clearer and more confident communication between children and parents. Children learn appropriate "feelings" words and expressions. When children verbalize their feelings, they do not have to use inappropriate behavior to express them (e.g. they can verbally communicate that they are angry, rather than having temper tantrums).

- Acknowledging children's feelings tends to facilitate, rather than interfere with, what parents expect of their children.

- When children accept and communicate their own feelings clearly, they also learn to respect and listen more to their parents' and siblings' feelings and ideas.

- Parents are not placing value judgments on children's feelings during play sessions. They are allowing children the freedom of exploring their feelings and making value judgments for themselves. *When parents accept their children's feelings, it does not necessarily imply agreement.* Parents frequently worry that accepting their children's feelings will make the children believe that they agree with them. For example, a child says, *"I am going to hit Bugles (the dog) with a stick because he tore up my comic book."* If the parent responds, *"You're really angry with Bugles,"* this acceptance in no way suggests that the parent is in agreement with the child hitting Bugles with the stick. It simply acknowledges the child's feeling; it does not endorse the desired action.

- Accepting feelings does not imply that these feelings are either "good" or "bad."

- Another point that must be stressed with parents is that the acceptance of feelings does not lead automatically to outcomes that are consistent with those feelings. In other words, feelings do not determine outcomes; they are simply a critical factor involved in outcomes. This rationale usually becomes more important at the generalization phase of GFT, where more complex situations arise in daily life.

The uses of tracking

During GFT, parents learn to show their children that they are attentive and interested in what they are doing, and accepting of them. A basic skill learned by parents in order to demonstrate this is called "tracking." Parents learn to keep focused on their children in both verbal and non-verbal ways. When practiced on a verbal level, tracking sometimes is referred to as restating the contents of what a child is doing. How to train parents in this skill is examined in the next chapter. The rationales for learning this skill are given next.

Rationales for tracking

- Children are able to attend to their own actions, thoughts, and feelings more easily when an interested second party helps them focus their attention on themselves and their activities.

- Tracking is part of the larger goal of making sure that children know that adults are interested in what they are doing and accepting of it.

- An older study in CCPT found that, even with very experienced play therapists, tracking what children were doing was a major part of their job. Sixty percent of their comments were related to the behavior they observed in the children during play therapy sessions (Landesberg & Snyder, 1946).

- "Pure" listening in an attentive manner (i.e. non-verbal tracking) can be more appropriate sometimes during play sessions than verbally tracking activities. When children are not verbal and, for example, involved in a silent activity such as building a bridge or drawing at an easel, tracking responses should be minimized. Too much verbalizing in relation to children's activity is very "heavy" and should be avoided because it can be overwhelming to most children, and can become intrusive.

- By listening and accepting an activity, parents can convey to children their trust that the children can work out their own solutions. And solutions thought through by children for themselves often have a more powerful, personal, and educational impact than outside, imposed solutions.

Leaders also should be aware that tracking alone, without empathy, is insufficient for therapeutic purposes. For example, a parent saying to a child in a play session who is looking very pleased with himself, *"You are turning the truck upside down,"* is tracking an action, but not reflecting a feeling. A fuller empathic response is: *"You are really enjoying turning the truck upside down."* This latter statement is more therapeutic because it includes both tracking and empathic responding.

Skill 2: following children's lead

In GFT, parents are trained to fully attend to their children during play sessions and to participate in play sessions, either through actions or words, at their children's invitation. By following their children's lead, parents create a child-led atmosphere, within the well-defined structure and limits of play sessions. Children in turn feel accepted and emotionally secure. During skills training, leaders help parents avoid asking questions of their children, and refrain from praising them or suggesting activities to them during play sessions. Yet all of these responses, which are avoided in play sessions, serve important functions in daily life, where parents have the role of stimulating their children, managing their behavior, and educating them.

In play sessions, parents learn to accept their children and reflect their feelings and actions, rather than actively directing their thoughts and behaviors. They are responders to their children in play sessions. Parents do not express their opinions and share their thoughts with their children.

Opportunities for parents to express their own feelings

Parents process their reactions during group meetings, which provides the opportunity to release any feelings they may have about their inability to express themselves in their play sessions. For example, a parent, Laura, confessed to the group after her practice play session that she had wished during the session that her child had not wanted her to sit and hold a pile of bricks that he kept adding onto for her to hold. She would have much rather been involved in the ramp he was building. The leader was able to empathize with Laura's feelings in turn, as well as pointing out to the group that she had managed to prioritize her child's activity, thus practicing the skill of following her child's lead.

Level of involvement of parents in their children's play

As this example of Laura shows, leaders help parents learn that children direct their own imaginative play, conversations, and activities during play sessions, and parents follow their lead. But unlike Laura's example, parents are commonly involved in play sessions in more active ways. The three types of involvement that children tend to request of adults are:

- *As witness:* parents observe, track activities, and make empathic comments about what their children are doing.

- *As co-player:* children request that their parent join in their craft work (e.g. building a model), physical activities (e.g. throwing a ball), their play with toys (e.g. racing cars), or playing games (e.g. card games or other formal or informal, rule-based games).

- *In role-play:* children direct their parents to play out an assigned role. Children may assign their parents to be anything from a household member to a circus acrobat.

When children, either actively or implicitly, place their parents in the role of witness to their activities, parents show they remain interested in what their children are doing and feeling during play sessions by tracking their children's actions and empathizing with their feelings. Parents' main role as witness is to maintain an open and interested attitude, letting their children develop their own way of experiencing their play. Some parents need help in realizing that this more passive role is as important to their children as the more active roles of being a co-player and taking part in role-plays.

Rationales for children deciding on parents' level of involvement

- Children are most able to play spontaneously and relax when they know there is no pressure on them to perform in a certain way. By allowing children to set the pace for how they want their parents to be involved, there is no pressure for children to fulfill their parents' expectations.

- Parents want children to be both independent within their capabilities and to be able to ask for help when needed. These attitudes lead to positive relationships with parents, and with adults more generally. A sign of children's social and emotional well-being and attachment security is to be able to move back and forth easily between these two positions (O'Sullivan & Ryan, 2009).

- Research has found that children need their parents to be emotionally available, not simply physically present, even though the parents may not be directly involved in their children's activity. Play sessions are designed for children to feel more emotionally connected and relaxed in their parents' presence, and they begin to realize that their parents are fully emotionally available to them.

- Experiencing hesitation and indecision is often a necessary step in children finding their own means of self-expression and in accessing stored memories. Children's natural tendency is to be active and engaged in events, but sometimes emotional issues may hinder their natural spontaneity. Active empathy by parents, the basic skill discussed first, is needed, rather than parents attempting to suggest activities to them.

Children's requests

Three areas that parents often need additional skills training and rationales for when learning CCPT skills are when their children ask for practical assistance, ask them to participate in an activity, such as making something or playing a game, and ask them to participate in imaginative play. Each of these areas is now discussed in turn.

WHEN CHILDREN ASK FOR PRACTICAL ASSISTANCE

Children are not pressured to perform in certain ways during play sessions, except for adhering to basic limits to their behavior. Therefore, play sessions are not for teaching children how to be independent and how to do things, or for parents to show their children that they themselves are skilled and capable adults. During special play sessions, children can decide how they want to approach things, what they are capable of doing, and how much help they want. Parents learn to focus on their children's feelings; leaders help parents acknowledge these feelings first, before taking any action or making other verbal responses.

PARENTS WORRYING ABOUT IMMATURE BEHAVIOR

Some parents worry that, if they accede to their children's requests for practical assistance, they will return to earlier behaviors that are not appropriate for their ages and abilities. There are several rationales leaders may consider using when addressing parents' concerns over their children's immature behavior during play sessions. These include the following:

- Attachment theory and research show that adults as well as children sometimes want to be looked after by others who are emotionally important to them, even when they are capable of being independent.

- Children have a basic drive towards autonomy and self-fulfillment. They need to learn about what they can manage and what they cannot, and they need space and time to assimilate this. This space should be one where they do not have to perform optimally, where they can try things out for themselves. Child development commonly entails relatively rapid transition from one level of independence to the next. "Breathing space" in order to assimilate these developmental tasks can be one purpose of play sessions for children.

- Some children have particular issues that they revisit in their play from their earlier childhood. Children may use play sessions with their parents, who are giving them full attention and accepting their expressions, to work on some things from the past that may be difficult or troubling.

ILLUSTRATIVE EXAMPLE

This example is of a leader helping a parent to accept their child's immature behavior during a play session:

Peter is the stepfather of 8-year-old Jack. Peter has just conducted his second practice play session with Jack during a meeting, and he has now been asked by the supervising leader what was difficult for him.

Peter: *Well it really tried my patience, with Jack asking me three times to tie his shoelaces.*

Leader: *You did what he asked, but you didn't feel accepting inside.*

Peter: *I had to hold myself in. I wanted to say, "You know you can do that yourself, just like you've been doing the last two years!"*

Leader: *So you felt annoyed about it, but tried to follow his lead. That took a lot of control, to keep your feelings to yourself. You deserve credit for that... It would be helpful to reflect Jack's feelings in that situation, too. What do you think he might have been feeling?*

Peter: *It was hard for me to deal with my own feelings, never mind what he felt!*

Leader: *You felt on the spot in the play session, and didn't have enough time to think about what you felt, and how Jack may have felt.*

Peter: *Well, I sure know that he didn't feel the same as I felt!*

Leader: *Harder to recognize what he felt, but you know it wasn't the same.*

Peter: *I wonder if he wanted to boss me around... No, he didn't seem too bothered about that. I don't think he was feeling that. He just stuck his foot out each time and seemed to accept that I'd help him. I know those laces of his are a pain, they keep coming undone.*

Leader: *So he may be tired of tying them, and wanted your help.*

Peter: Yes, that's what it seemed to be.

Jack's mother: I liked seeing you do that for him. It reminded me of when he was little.

Peter: He did seem sort of young today. I guess I never saw him when he was really little, like you did.

Leader: You seem to be losing your impatience as we talk about it together, Peter. I think it was a really good illustration of how children sometimes show younger behavior or behavior they haven't had a chance to show earlier in their lives so easily. I wonder if Jack was acting younger with you because he wants to build up some experiences where you help him, like you might have done if you had been around when he was younger.

Peter: I like that idea, to let him choose in the play sessions how young he wants to be. But I sure don't want him to be a baby all the time at home, and especially when we're out.

Leader: We'll look at how all these play skills are transferable to home much later in the program. Remember we said that for now, try to do the same things that you usually do at home, and concentrate on learning how to do play sessions here. And also remember that children do in general have a strong drive towards greater independence, like we've seen Jack have at times during his play sessions.

This example shows how the leader first empathized fully with the stepfather's feelings, then helped him to explore the reasons for Jack's requests, and finally drew on the rationales given earlier to help both Peter and the group to understand and accept children's immature behavior more fully.

WHEN PARENTS ARE OVER-INVOLVED IN THEIR CHILDREN'S ACTIVITIES

Another attitude encountered by leaders in GFT is parents who are overly involved and controlling of their children's activities, thoughts, and feelings. Some parents may not allow their children to try out things or to fail in activities. These parents seem to have developed an overly protective attitude, which may stem from anxiety and/or from past traumatic experiences, either to their children or themselves. Other times, parents' anxiety may manifest itself by attempting to block out their children's negative responses, as the example of Mary Jane and her adopted daughter in the last chapter demonstrated.

Leaders may apply some of the rationales given earlier for following a child's lead with parents who become very anxious when their control is relaxed over their children. For example, leaders may state that children naturally strive for self-actualization and independence, and that they need to make mistakes themselves at times in order to learn. In addition, it will be important in some cases to help parents realize and adjust to the relative robustness of their children's capacity to absorb frustrations and negative feelings, given the supportive and child-centered atmosphere of play sessions. (See an extended discussion on issues of autonomy versus shame and doubt, and initiative versus guilt, applied to non-directive play therapy in Wilson & Ryan, 2005, Ch.3). Leaders need to be particularly sensitive to parents' own emotional reactions in emotion-laden circumstances, and to show empathy for these parents' feelings, as the earlier example of Peter illustrates. Occasionally, when parents' attitudes are extreme and reflect more serious personal issues, it is important for leaders to address these concerns outside of group meetings, as discussed in the previous chapter.

A REQUEST FOR CO-PLAYING: WHEN CHILDREN ASK PARENTS TO PARTICIPATE IN CRAFTS AND GAMES

When children choose to involve themselves in more structured activities during play sessions, such as craft making or playing a game with set rules, it can be difficult for some parents to allow their children to lead. Again, some of the same issues discussed earlier about immature behavior are relevant. Parents may not want their children to fail in an activity, and may want to protect them from feelings of frustration, lack of confidence in themselves, and feelings of worthlessness. Leaders can usefully discuss with these parents the importance of children learning to manage feelings of disappointment, anger, resentment, and inadequacy during game playing and in daily life. Play sessions are protected environments in which children can experience these emotions at a level that they can manage. Leaders can point out that parents responding acceptingly and with empathy can be extremely helpful for children in processing such feelings.

Leaders also may wish to say to parents that in daily life children do need to learn that games—a metaphor for life to some extent—have set rules, and that when playing with others they share a common set of rules. Because parents are well aware of the importance of playing games fairly and cooperatively in real life, they may have some negative feelings about their children playing by their own, arbitrary rules, if this occurs in play sessions. Leaders should help parents express such reactions during group meetings. Leaders also can helpfully point out that, while parents are giving up their opportunity for teaching their children the proper ways to play games and do crafts in play sessions, they are also spared the responsibility for seeing that rules and instructions are followed correctly.

Leaders may need to help parents accept that some children quickly learn they can change rules in their favor, or falsely declare that they are winners, during play sessions. These children often seem to need to experience a victory in order to feel superior. Frequently such children have few successes in life: it is other children who do the winning, or they lack control over their lives in other important ways. They wisely realize that, in the rarefied atmosphere of play sessions, they are able to experience feelings of triumph, real or not. During discussion of these issues with parents, leaders may find it appropriate to share their knowledge of children who were proud of false accomplishments in play therapy sessions, who then, in the last phases of successful play therapy, followed the rules of games appropriately. Play sessions apparently worked their magic to help these children adapt to socially accepted behavior without adult direction. At later stages in the GFT program, leaders sometimes refer to this change in children's behavior as one sign of successful completion of therapy—many children, apparently as a result of gains in emotional maturity and ego strength, begin to allow adults to win games in play sessions.

WHEN CHILDREN ASK PARENTS TO PARTICIPATE IN ROLE-PLAY

Play sessions are set up to foster imaginative play, allowing children to use materials such as sand, water, dressing-up clothes, and family or superhero figures, to name several types of toys, in ways that they choose in their play sessions. Imaginative play has a strong natural, therapeutic quality; children are able to express a wide range of personal feelings in this type of play. Imaginative play in childhood has similarities to both nocturnal dreaming and daydreaming in adults. Children freely let themselves enter a "not real" world and are thus able to problem solve and assimilate personal experiences in creative ways (Wilson & Ryan, 2005).

When children play imaginatively, there are usually two different types of play they ask their parents to be involved in. They may choose to play imaginatively with toys, natural materials (e.g. sand, water, stones, shells), and real-life objects (e.g. a flashlight) with their parents, or they may use some of these materials to involve their parents in role-playing, another type of imaginative play. When following their children's lead during role-plays, parents may find it easier to participate in their assigned role if they keep in mind that in role-plays children are the producers, directors, and stars of the situations they create for their role-plays (Cochran, Nordling, & Cochran, 2010).

Some important areas for leaders to consider in responding to parents' queries about their children's imaginative play are as follows:

- Children generally know the difference between their fantasy play and reality during their preschool years.

- Mentally and chronologically younger children, and children who have not mentally assimilated traumatic experiences they have had, seem to have more vivid images on which they base their imaginative play. If children are extremely immersed in their imaginative play, leaders need to help parents respond appropriately based on their own play therapy experience. If a role-play dictated by a child becomes too distressful to a parent, or to the children themselves, generally leaders recommend that the role-play be restructured to reduce the emotional level. For example, if a child wanted the parent to slice him up with a plastic knife, and was very specific about the detail, restructuring so that an anxious parent could be less vigorous may be required. Or even redirecting the child to some other form of "surgery" that would be less stressful may be needed. However, in our experience, children rarely take parents beyond what they sense would be very difficult for their parents to tolerate.

- Younger children are less able to take the perspective of the other person playing with them. Therefore, parents have the advantage over play therapists in knowing their children well, being able to anticipate their communication more readily, and therefore following their leads appropriately in play.

- Children during play sessions may express themselves in fantasy by antisocial means, because they realize that their play does not have real-life consequences. Sometimes children's imaginative play can be highly aggressive, with killing and mayhem being played out. This does not mean that these children will carry out these actions in real life as parents sometimes fear. Imaginative play permits these expressions of victimization, control, anger, and destruction in a safe environment.

Skill 3: structuring play sessions

Leaders help parents learn to structure play sessions for their children and to understand the rationales for learning this skill in play sessions.

The underlying value of structuring

An important part of parents structuring play sessions for their children occurs in the sessions' introductory message. The opening statement for play sessions sets out the nature of the sessions, that they are child led. This statement is: *"[Name of child], this is a very special room [time, place, depending on the space parents use]. You can do ALMOST anything you want*. If you cannot do something, I will tell you."* (**This statement may include the optional statement: "You may say anything you want in here."*)

The closing statement, after two time warnings (i.e. five minutes and one minute), is: "Our time is up for today. It's time to leave now." The closing statement and warnings are intended to help children know how much time they have left, and when the session will be over. Other structuring statements may be needed, during children's ongoing participation in their play sessions, discussed further as follows.

Rationales for structuring play sessions for children

The main rationale for using structuring statements in play sessions is that children can play best when they feel relaxed and know what to expect in a new situation. Based on attachment theory and research, children can explore their environments most easily when they are not emotionally defended and anxious (Wilson & Ryan, 2005). In general, structuring statements help children when situations are unclear to them, and when they want things that are different from what other people want (e.g. they may want to continue to play after the end of the play session). These structuring messages give children a good chance of success in the new situation of play sessions.

Parents are urged to keep to the formulas for the beginning and ending messages during play sessions. The rationale for parents' keeping the messages the same each play session is that the messages reinforce for children that everything is the same from one play session to the next. Later, once home play sessions are well established, structuring statements can be abbreviated for most children and become markers for children to continue to view the play sessions as separate from their daily lives at home.

Leaders may need to help parents think about the individual differences among their children when presenting these concepts on structuring, giving examples and/or drawing out participants' examples of how some children need more help with transitions and new events than other children do. It may also be important for leaders to make the following points:

- All children, in order to develop properly, need to try out new behavior and explore their environment. Play sessions are intended to help children relax and explore their feelings, thoughts, and relationships.

- Parents can help their children be successful in play sessions by planning ahead and taking their children's viewpoint about what they need to know in this new situation.

- Structuring by parents in play sessions can make it possible for children to succeed and feel good about themselves, especially when they may have impulses that are more difficult for them to control (e.g. wanting to continue with the play session).

Uses of more general structuring comments in play sessions

More general comments include statements such as *"In here it's what you choose"* or *"You can decide in here."* Parents make these more general structuring comments when it seems important for their children to have the introductory message reaffirmed. For instance, such a comment may be made when children look at their parents to see if they have permission to do something.

ILLUSTRATIVE EXAMPLE

Bobby, a withdrawn and timid 7-year-old, is playing with farm animals, fences, and farm buildings while his mother watches him.

> Bobby: *I'm not sure which animals go with which buildings. Where should I put them?* (He turns to his mother and looks questioningly.)
>
> Mom: *You'd like to be sure that you do it right. In these special playtimes there is no right or wrong about things you are doing. Whatever way you want to make it will be okay.*
>
> Bobby: *Yeah, but I don't want to put them in the wrong places.*
>
> Mom: *You want to be sure that the animals go where they belong. You are hoping that I can tell you.*
>
> Bobby: *Yes.*
>
> Mom: (smiles at him) *You can choose in here.* (Bobby goes ahead and arranges them to suit himself and seems satisfied.)

When Bobby's mother mentioned afterwards during the group meeting how difficult this had been for her during the play session, she also recognized that Bobby was able to move forward in his play without the help from her that he originally thought he needed. The leader, after empathizing with the mother's feelings, pointed out that this kind of independent action from Bobby will in time increase his confidence in his own decision making. The leader then reinforced for both the mother and the group how confident and skilled in her answers Bobby's mother seemed, despite her inner reservations.

Leaders help parents make these appropriate structuring comments when their children seem to be seeking a reaffirmation of the rules of the sessions. It also may be useful for leaders to point out to parents that by using the phrase "in here" during these general structuring comments, parents are automatically saying that these play sessions are "special" and unlike daily life. This clarification may counteract some parents' fear that permissiveness in play sessions will lead their children to out-of-control and demanding behavior in daily life.

Skill 4: limiting children's behavior

In GFT, parents learn how to set limits behaviorally and how to select the suitable limits in play sessions based on their children's emotional and developmental needs. As a result, parents learn to manage their own and their children's emotions in ways that reduce conflict-laden responses, and promote more secure attachments. Limits are defined as rules or guidelines for behavior which are enforced by imposing consequences when the limit is broken (Guerney L., 2013) There has been frequent discussion of limits and permissiveness in the CCPT literature, including the ways in which permissiveness is conveyed to children in order for them to feel able to express feelings and thoughts that may be inappropriate in other contexts. Wilson & Ryan (2005) point out that setting boundaries for children's behavior during play sessions offers them both a sense of security and the potential for particular therapeutic experiences (e.g. developing self-control, developing imaginary solutions).

Rationales for limit setting

On a pragmatic level, limits such as keeping messy play to an area that can be cleaned easily, and safety limits, such as not allowing a child to deliberately hit his head against a wall, are necessary both to protect children and to allow both therapists and parents to carry out CCPT effectively. Leaders who are experienced play therapists help parents to set these practical limits during their play sessions, while maintaining a generally permissive attitude.

On an emotional level, limits convey to children that their parents are maintaining or clearly establishing their adult roles and responsibilities during play sessions. Parents are taught to empathize with their children's desire to engage in behaviors that are limited (e.g. dumping a lot of water, or throwing a block at their parent), while enforcing necessary restrictions to some behaviors. It follows that *empathy* is an important part of effective limit setting. When adults set appropriate limits consistently and appropriately with empathy, this engenders emotional security in children (O'Sullivan & Ryan, 2009). Limits also allow children to gain mastery over their feelings in the following way: strong, easily remembered feelings often arise when children want something that is not allowed. Therefore, they are more able to become consciously aware of these feelings during limit setting. Parents, by recognizing and accepting these feelings in their children, rather than ignoring or trying to alter these feelings, do not limit their children's feelings. They limit only their behavior.

In GFT, parents are trained to decide on essential rules before beginning play sessions with their children. They learn to state these rules clearly and with authority in child-accessible language, and to reflect children's feelings first, where possible, before imposing the rule. Consequences are not to be given in the first statement of the rule for two reasons. Stating a consequence at the same time as the rule takes away the power of the rule itself. It may also imply that children will not listen or comply with the rule without a following consequence.

Play session rule setting counters the common practice of parents saying at home, "*If you don't stop doing that, I'm going to punish you*" or "*If you keep jumping on that bed, you're going to have to go to your room and stay there.*" By tacking on the consequence in the same statement as the desired limit on the behavior, parents weaken the limit, and almost make it a choice between choosing a rule and choosing a consequence (e.g. a parent says, "*If you don't take out the garbage, I'll cut your allowance*" and the child says, "*OK, I don't care about the allowance that much.*") For FT, in contrast, parents give a consequence to their children in play sessions only when the limit is broken a second time (with the exception of rules that for safety reasons demand immediate compliance). This therapeutic rule setting gives children the opportunity to develop greater self-control and follow the rule before a consequence is imposed.

It is also important for leaders to help parents realize that it is not helpful for children to be told in advance what the few limits are in play sessions. Sometimes parents argue that it would be helpful if their children knew what was against the rules from the start. Parents think their children could then restrain themselves from the beginning. This approach is actually a disadvantage to children for a few reasons. First, while the limits are in fact very few in play sessions, when they are listed, they seem more numerous. Second, a list of rules gives children too many to remember, especially young children. Finally, when rules are listed at the outset of play sessions, some oppositional children deliberately try to break them in order to set up a conflict situation, while timid children become less able to relax and engage in play activities.

Consequences for rule breaking

In CCPT, many play therapists are trained to have a range of consequences for children's non-compliance with rules (e.g. putting a toy away until the next session), with the ultimate consequence, which is rarely imposed, of having to end the session early. GFT recognizes that parents conduct play sessions in their own homes, and not in the more ideal conditions most professional playrooms offer. Therefore, parents need very clear consequences at home, in order to assert their authority when limits are broken more than once. The GFT program teaches parents to set the consequence that the play session ends immediately if children do not adhere to the rule after the second statement of it. There are several reasons for this:

- Parents need to convey an accepting attitude in stating rules and consequences to their children. If parents do not have an immediate way to enforce one of their rules, it is possible that their attitude of acceptance of their children's feelings may be undermined.

- Children need to have a clear demarcation between play sessions' permissiveness and their home life, when sessions occur at home.

- Parents learn the easiest way to enforce all their rules, and do not have to consider alternatives in a stressful situation.

The CCPT literature debates whether it is more beneficial for children to be shown alternatives for unacceptable behavior when rules are broken (e.g. Landreth, 2012) suggesting that cars are for crashing into a cushion, not into the wall) or to leave alternatives to the children themselves (Wilson & Ryan, 2005). In GFT as set out here, parents are taught to set rules without suggesting alternatives. This way of setting limits seems more in keeping with the program's aims of increasing children's self-direction, avoiding suggestions, and following children's lead wherever possible, leaving the reactions and next steps children take after a limit is imposed entirely up to them. Some child centered play therapists (e.g.VanFleet, 2013) both themselves use, and teach parents conducting play sessions to use, an additional statement: "*But you can do almost anything else*" after introducing a limit, to further structure for children what limit setting consists of in play sessions.

It is also important to stress to parents that rules need to be within their children's developmental capacities. Sometimes parents have unrealistic expectations of their children's capacities, and either under- or over-estimate their capabilities. Play sessions offer the ideal environment for parents to learn about their children's needs and the ways in which rules can be set in order to ensure understanding and compliance. Short, simple phrases and vocabulary are usually most effective in emotionally charged situations, even for older children. In addition, for very young, developmentally delayed, or disabled children who have more limited cognitive capacities, they may need to have a rule stated more than twice before consequences are mentioned.

During any discussion of limit setting with parents, it is important for leaders to remember that limit setting and compliance are not the ultimate aims of the program.

As mentioned elsewhere in this book, distressed parents tend to focus on wanting to learn how to ensure their children's compliance with their rules, especially early in the program. It is important for leaders to help parents to learn about and accept their children's feelings and needs, along with ways that structuring can reduce conflict and confusion for children, before helping them to apply limit-setting skills.

In practice play sessions during meetings, parents are helped to practice all of their skills of showing understanding, following their children's lead, structuring, and limit setting. They often relate vivid personal examples of the effectiveness of using all of these skills together, particularly later in the program during home play sessions with their children.

ILLUSTRATIVE EXAMPLE

During his first practice play session, a father, Rory, clearly set the rule for his 6-year-old son, Tom, of keeping the play dough on the mat, but he did not reflect his son's feelings about this rule, even though Tom had looked a bit angry. When Tom did not keep the play dough on the mat the second time, his father set the consequence that the play session would end, if that happened again. But once again Rory did not reflect Tom's feelings of frustration, which this time appeared to be over both the rule and the consequence. During feedback with a leader after the play session, Rory realized that he had not understood or verbalized Tom's feelings, and decided to do so the next time.

During their next practice play session, Tom once again did not keep the play dough on the mat. This time his father set the rule, "*Remember the rule, the play dough stays on the mat*" and added, "*It's hard for you to do.*" Tom turned to his father and softly said, "*It is.*" His father replied: "*It is hard for you.*" For the rest of the play session, Tom seemed to easily keep the play dough on the mat.

During feedback after this play session, Rory told the leader he was amazed that a simple reflection of Tom's feelings actually had the effect of Tom changing his behavior during the play session. The leader empathized with Rory's strong feelings about this change in Tom, and reinforced Rory's skilled use of limit setting, which now included showing understanding of Tom's feelings. The leader also ensured that this experience was an effective learning point for the entire group.

Preliminaries to starting the GFT program, including background information on FT and GFT, intake considerations for GFT, advice to leaders on running successful programs, and the rationales for helping parents learn play session skills, have now been explored. The delivery of the GFT program itself is considered from start to finish in the following chapters.

CHAPTER 5
Starting the GFT Program
Meeting 1

The first meeting is a very important one in setting the tone and pace of the GFT program. This meeting has several important aims for leaders, including beginning to develop group support, and helping parents effectively manage their anxieties over both their group membership and their skills as parents. Participants are given an overview of the content of future meetings and the program as a whole, a review of the effectiveness of FT, and introduced to FT skills on a general level. Part of this introduction to FT skills entails leaders demonstrating a child-centered play session and discussing this demo afterwards with group members. Finally, leaders prepare parents for the next meeting.

Leaders already will have prepared carefully for the first meeting, in order to ensure that it achieves all of its aims, as we discussed earlier. New leaders' preparation before starting should include reading this book in its entirety, then studying carefully and assimilating fully the material for the first few sessions. As stated earlier, attending an intensive, practice-based training course on GFT also is important, in order to practice GFT skills in vitro before running the program for the first time with an experienced co-leader.

Briefer summaries of agendas for each meeting in the program are found in Appendix 13. This appendix lists the aims, pre-meeting tasks, and educational and practical tasks for leaders in a 20-week program. These outlines are intended for use as aides memoire, with leaders bringing a copy of the relevant meeting outline into each meeting for their personal use, adapting them as required to their group's needs.

This chapter starts with suggestions for leaders on creating an informal atmosphere, and establishing consent and confidentiality parameters. The majority of the chapter gives leaders guidance on conducting the first meeting, and includes an illustrative example of a dialogue following the demo at a first meeting between leaders and participants.

Beginning GFT

The first session usually sets the pace and tone for the rest of the meetings. Leaders are much more relaxed, if they know they are well prepared. In this meeting, and the other early meetings, leaders take a much more active role than in later meetings. They are fully responsible for working with individuals to help them establish their group membership. Therefore, GFT leaders should not expect too many contributions from group members at the outset, until parents feel more familiar with what is expected of them and other members. Above all, it is important that leaders set a positive tone and convey to often demoralized parents that participating in the GFT program will have positive results.

Introducing the roles of co-leaders to the group

It also is important for co-leaders to remember that parents are not familiar with both leaders, since each leader conducted the GFT intake process for only half of the participants. Leaders themselves have shared information, and hopefully FPO video contents, with one another beforehand, and therefore are more familiar with all group members. Therefore, it is important to allow adequate time for both leaders to introduce themselves to the entire group at the beginning of the meeting. Leaders also should be mindful that it is very important to divide up their tasks during the first meeting, to ensure that parents have interactions with *both* leaders, and view them as equally responsible for, and able to deal with, all aspects of the group's agenda.

An exception to sharing tasks occurs when one of the leaders is in training with an experienced leader. Introduction of apprentice leaders would go something like the following. More experienced leaders introduce themselves and their responsibilities to group members. Leaders then introduce apprentice leaders and explain what their involvement will be. For example: *"This is Mary Porter, our assistant leader, who will be conducting play sessions, supervising you and sometimes presenting some information and fielding questions. If I should ever need to be absent, Mary will fill in for me."*

Creating an informal atmosphere

Some practical suggestions are given in Appendix 8 that will help make the first session more relaxed for both leaders and parents. These are all simple things, such as using first names, but they serve to create an atmosphere of relaxed, informal acceptance, which is essential to the success of GFT.

Recording group meetings

Leaders who intend to record meetings will already have received written permission from parents during the final intake meeting. Recording GFT meetings helps leaders in several ways. First and foremost, it permits leaders to recall the exact nature of all interchanges. Second, reviewing recordings can help leaders determine what changes may be needed in future sessions, and what has worked effectively. Third, they give leaders ideas about examples to use, and ways to help certain parents learn FT skills more successfully. Finally, they are very useful for general supervision purposes, both to show supervisors what is going well, and, if leaders run into trouble, where help is required.

When turning on videoing equipment during the first meeting, we suggest a low-key approach, which is usually less anxiety provoking for parents (e.g. *"We'll always turn the video on when we start each meeting. This will help us be more effective leaders for you."*). It also is prudent for leaders to have the video recorder already set up before the first meeting begins, and in a prominent place where it can pick up all voices and faces. It is unlikely that anyone will object to the video recording but, if someone does, it is important that leaders reflect their feelings and accept them, then wait for a moment. If one or more parents continue to object, it is crucial that leaders do *not* record the meeting and, instead, unplug the recorder and put it aside. In the first author's experience, the rapport and confidence that leaders gain with the group for listening to parents' strong feelings more than compensate for the lost videos. Finally, where one or two parents object to taping originally, it is usually worth leaders asking at a later meeting whether the objection still holds—it may not, once these parents begin to trust the leaders and group more fully. Alternatively, these parents may not object to a fixed camera focused away from them, so that only their voices are recorded.

It also is very useful for leaders to video all the play sessions with children in the program, including demos and all the practice play sessions with parents during meetings. There are several advantages of recording demos and play sessions. On a practical level, the group may need to watch demos and practice play sessions via video link, if an observation room with one-way mirror is not available. Other reasons for videoing include helping leaders self-supervise their own practice, and helping parents and children become familiar with video recordings during meetings, before they are asked to do recording themselves during their home sessions. Occasionally, leaders may also choose to use video from the meeting's demo or play sessions afterwards, during the meeting's discussion of these experiences with group members.

Addressing group confidentiality issues

Another essential introductory issue is group confidentiality. Again, we suggest leaders themselves treat this issue in a low-key, anxiety-free manner, in order to show parents that this issue, while important, can be handled easily by the group. Leaders may wish to say that all of the parents present want to help their children, and will be talking about their family life during these meetings, as well as learning from each other while they do play sessions with their children. Groups work best when family information is shared with others in the group, and with their partners at home, but not when information from groups is shared with friends and relatives more generally, either in person or less directly in phone calls or texts or on the internet. Parents in the group will feel respected and safe if they know that what they say is private in this way, just as information is kept private as much as possible when therapists themselves work with families. The commonly used group adage that *"What is said or happens in this room stays in this room"* can be stated here.

Depending on the group and on cultural considerations, leaders may decide whether or not to have participants fill in group confidentiality agreements, handed out at the end of the meeting, to be returned by the next meeting. Alternatively, leaders may opt to add a short statement on group confidentiality to the recording consent agreement form signed by parents at their last intake meeting, if required.

Leading introductions by group members

After briefly introducing recording and confidentiality issues, one leader then asks parents to introduce themselves to one another, giving their name, and the names and ages of their children who are participating in GFT. Leaders already emphasized at intake with each family that GFT is a whole family intervention. If there are family members who are not participating, as agreed at intake, participants should be given the option of mentioning these other children and family members, if they wish. The leader also asks group members to include a brief statement of what they wish to accomplish by participating in the GFT program.

Leaders already have important information on personality characteristics of parents attending the group from both general intake information and from their own intake meetings. With this knowledge in mind, leaders may choose to call first on a parent to introduce him/herself who appears confident and talkative enough to set the tone of easy communication within the group. If these qualities are not apparent in participants, then the leader can simply go around the group methodically. This strategy also applies to all the skills training discussed later: a group member who has more ability and confidence can be asked to demonstrate skills in front of the group first. This allows other members to learn vicariously, and often reduces their own performance anxiety.

During introductions, the most important role for leaders is actively helping group members to begin establishing rapport with the leaders and with each other. Leaders should remember to be in control of the timing for these introductions. They should only take a couple of minutes each, and move relatively quickly from one person to the next. Leaders also should aim to proportion the time equally among participants. If leaders fail to draw out all group members relatively equally, this sets an unwanted tone for the group. It may create feelings of inequity among participants, which in turn can result in feelings of disengagement in the group process (and even withdrawal), or competition among group members for leaders' attention. Another task for both leaders during introductions is to form working hypotheses on each individual, and on potential group dynamics. These ideas are crucial for leaders to air with one another during debriefing and planning after the end of the first meeting.

It is common for parents to want to share their distress and negative feelings about their children and their lives generally during these introductions. It is important for group leaders to regulate parents' personal discussions; leaders may need to remind parents tactfully that this is not the place and time for such extended discussions. Parents' need to talk at length is usually less problematic, in the authors' experience, if parents already have had the opportunity to discuss their concerns during their final intake meeting with a leader. As explained in the intake chapter, leaders mentioned to parents during intake that there would not be time for such extended discussions during the group itself.

If group members do mention their struggles, it is important first that leaders show empathy with the feelings being expressed, and, second, to interrupt any parents' extended narratives. It is helpful to remind such parents and the entire group that these feelings are legitimate, and ones that the group itself hopes to address over the course of the program. However, as stated in an earlier chapter, leaders need to help the group stay focused on group goals for the meeting and the program, rather than taking undue time with the personal issues of one or two parents.

Providing an overview of FT

The next task for leaders, after each parent has introduced themselves, their families and their aims for the GFT program, is to briefly review explanations of the effectiveness of FT. Again, these points already were covered by leaders in more depth with each family during the intake meetings.

Leaders' aims for the GFT program

Leaders usually begin this part of the program with a general statement about what they hope the group will accomplish, usually mentioning that one of the main aims of the program is for families to get along better together, and enjoy life together more. Next, leaders mention the skills that will be taught in GFT, which are to allow children to lead the way, to focus on children's feelings and actions, to structure situations so that children know what is expected of them, and to limit children's behavior where needed. We suggest leaders save general explanations of these skills until the discussion of the demo later in the meeting.

Leaders then give an overview of what play sessions with children are and how they are effective. Key points to be made in this teaching are:

1. *You will be learning to conduct play sessions. Play allows children's feelings and thoughts to be expressed easily, and is often better than words.*

2. *Play sessions are not directed to children's symptoms and behaviors; the sessions aim to go below the surface. The play sessions address what drives children's behavior. These underlying issues often are more similar for children than the behaviors themselves that they display. Play sessions therefore are effective for many problems. You can learn a lot about your own children by seeing a variety of behaviors and different children.*

Leaders need to insert an example here to illustrate this teaching point. One example that can be used is that many distressed children feel they are not as appreciated as other children (in the household, in class, etc.). This sense of low self-esteem may result in angry behavior in some children, and withdrawn behavior—or both—in others.

3. *You will be learning how to follow children's lead in play and to show your children that you understand their feelings. You will be giving your children permission, within limits, to concentrate on what is important to the children themselves. (Parents usually need to be reassured that limits will be returned to later.)*

4. *After mastering the skills involved, and children learning to use their play sessions well, your play sessions can become a relaxed, unhurried, and stress free time for you and your children. This is because during these play sessions you will just be concentrating on each of your children alone, and not on all the other million and one things that need to be done at home to be a good parent. Your children will*

see a different side of you, and you are likely to see a different side of your children too. These playtimes aim to increase your positive time together and you have a chance to see one another in a different way.

5. *You have decided [or "You have been asked..."] to attend this GFT program. These groups are very useful for parents and we think they will be for you. Many parents over the years have learned to do these playtimes. There's research to show that many children and their parents benefit from GFT.*

Summarizing the whole program

The next task for leaders is to give parents an overview of the contents of future meetings and the program as a whole. A handout for each parent to follow should be distributed at the beginning of this discussion (see Appendix 12 for a prototype). However, in the authors' experience, the detailed schedule of all the meetings in the program and the Parents' Training Manual works best when distributed at the end of the meeting. The purpose of this part of the meeting is for leaders to clarify and review what happens in the program in general terms, previewing contents of all of the arranged meetings in the program. Each stage of the program is referred to briefly and parents' learning tasks should be alluded to throughout this brief discussion.

Once again it is important for leaders to move the discussion along, and not spend too much time on this, but it *is* important for leaders to empathize with the feelings parents may express in relation to their own role in the program. We suggest that leaders skim past the information on the demo phase of the program, noting for parents that there will be further discussion of the demos before the end of the meeting.

The following brief points about parents' learning during the program are important for leaders to include and paraphrase themselves in this overview:

1. *One of us leaders will demonstrate a play session during the meeting with a familiar child who is not participating in this group [or leaders can use a video; see options later].*

2. *Over the next several meetings, demonstrations—we will call them "demos" for short—will be done by leaders with each child in the program for all of you to watch. The demos will be no more than 15 minutes each.*

3. *These demos by leaders are done to help parents learn the skills for play sessions. After the demos, held at the beginning of each meeting, parents concentrate on learning these skills. We will use discussions, role-plays and direct practicing for this training.*

4. *After we have done all of the demos in the first several weeks, and helped you practice play skills, then each parent will conduct two short sessions of 10–15 minutes with each of their children who are fully participating in the program. We leaders and group members will be quietly watching and learning, without interfering.*

5. *Further skills training will be given at each meeting during this part of the program. The skills practice prepares you for playing with your own children. Nobody*

expects that you will get everything right at your first few attempts. We know that it is a learning process that takes time.

6. *After you are skilled enough, home sessions will start. These home play sessions will be twice as long as the ones we have in the group; they will be 30 minutes long with each child who is participating in the program every week.*

7. *When home play sessions are going along well, we will then turn to transferring some of the skills you have learned in play sessions to your daily family life.*

We advise that leaders make light of generalization to daily life here. Leaders do not want to overwhelm parents, and transferring skills can sound forbidding to many of them. (When parents have the necessary skills, generalization seems quite natural to them.) It is essential for leaders to keep in mind during this discussion that their job is to remove doubts about participation, to show participants that the leaders are practical and supportive, and to maintain hopefulness. It often is more difficult for parents to feel curiosity and optimism at the beginning of the program. This is when parents most often feel defeated about their problems with their children. The general attitudes for leaders to convey are *"We will work it out"* and *"We empathize with your concerns."* Conveying these messages in varying words, and as often as needed, keeps the group interested, and some reluctant parents may even become eager to continue.

Introduction to the parents' role in the program

Leaders can paraphrase the following essential points, either during the previous discussion, or over the next few meetings, as appropriate:

1. *We will help all of you learn to do play sessions, and it will be a journey together. There is no hidden agenda. We are not trying to manipulate you into changing the way you operate at home. Your children and your family are your domain.*

2. *Many of you will feel challenged at the beginning because play sessions are different from what parents do in daily life. But we will make sure that we train you to carry out these special play sessions. We will train you in an easy way, and have you practice the skills you need in the group first, before you do play sessions with your children.*

3. *We strongly urge you to maintain the status quo at home during the learning phase of this program, and not try to change the way you do things at home for now. This bigger change will come later, after you have learned to do play sessions. Your main job in the program right now is to learn the skills you need to carry out play sessions.*

Demonstration of a play session

The purpose of this part of the meeting is to show parents as soon as possible how client-centered play sessions are conducted. There are two reasons for introducing the demo early in the first meeting. First, it is an effective way to begin teaching basic skills and stimulating group discussion. And, second, if leaders keep the participants' focus on the play therapist conducting the demo, it shifts parents away from their own anxieties about skills learning more readily.

Leaders decide before the first meeting which of the following options is feasible for them and their group. These options are:

Option 1: give a live demonstration with a child who is brought to the group for this purpose.

Option 2: show a video of one of the leaders conducting a play session.

Option 3: use a commercial video of a CCPT session.

Demo options and some considerations for leaders

Leaders ask the parents to do the following while watching the demo: *"You will look at what I am (or 'the therapist is') doing because that's what you'll be doing with your own children later. After the session, we will talk about it together."*

Leaders should remember that, because parents' anxieties are high at this point in their training, it is important that the demo is one in which no serious emotional issues are raised by the child with the play therapist, and that the demo is in no way emotionally distressing to view for parents. And since leaders want to encourage parents to do play sessions, the demo needs to be interesting and engaging, in addition to clearly showing the play therapist talking and demonstrating CCPT skills. The three demo options are laid out in detail next.

OPTION 1: LIVE DEMONSTRATION

Live demos are the most interesting for the group to watch, and the easiest for them to engage in emotionally. This type of demo quickly establishes a leader's credibility for the group, given that the leader is competent in conducting CCPT. We recommend, if this option is chosen, that the leader have their live play demo with a familiar child, in order to ensure that the play session is interesting and informative for the group. The leader will be able to predetermine that the demo will not be either distressing to the child to take part in, or too taxing for the leader to conduct. Given that it is a live demo, it is useful for the leader to add beforehand for parents: *"I may not be perfect. Where it's relevant, I'll tell you where I slipped up, so that you won't be steered off course in your own learning."* This statement allows for the unexpected. While a minor mistake is not useful or relevant to discuss with the group, a major mistake should be addressed by leaders in a low-key way during the discussion following the demo.

Leaders may wish to obtain written permission from parents and verbal or written permission from any children who participate in a live demo, after leaders have given the family an explanation of the purpose of GFT and the role of the demo in the program. Leaders also need to consider whether parents in the group would feel uncomfortable with a family outside the group knowing their identities and the purpose of the group. This consideration may be especially pertinent within small communities, or when groups contain well-known participants. (The likelihood of parents in the group being identified by the family is remote when a one-way mirror or video link is used.) If there are any doubts about confidentiality, we suggest that a video may be preferable over a live demo. Leaders should avoid using their own children for these demos. All children can respond unpredictably when they are being observed, and preserving harmonious and low-anxiety relationships is important in professionals', as well as clients' families. Finally, we suggest that leaders try to use the same kinds of toys and materials in their demos that parents will be asked to provide for their own home play sessions later in the program. A more detailed discussion of the equipment parents collect for their home sessions is given to parents later in the program.

OPTION 2: DEMO USING A LEADER'S PERSONAL VIDEO

If the video option is chosen, we suggest that it is most effective for leaders to make their own recording of a play session to show to the group, after getting all the necessary permissions from a family, rather than using a commercial video. When parents see their own leaders on video with a child, it increases participants' rapport with their leaders. Leaders need to make a 15–20 minute video of a demo play session with a clinically neutral, familiar child (e.g. a neighbor's child, a young relative, or a friend's child who does not have emotional difficulties). It is important that leaders show videos that demonstrate their CCPT skills practiced competently overall, in order to establish credibility as leaders for their group. It is most useful if all of the four main skills taught to parents are shown in the demo video. Similar to live demos, minor mistakes should be ignored during discussion after the video; mentioning minor mistakes may distract parents from learning about the main skills shown. But leaders should avoid showing parents a video of a play session with major mistakes (e.g. not setting a necessary limit), so that parents do not become confused.

OPTION 3: USING A COMMERCIAL VIDEO

Using a commercial video is a third and less desirable option in our opinion. A commercial video can be used if a live or personal video demo by one of the group leaders simply is not feasible. The commercial video example again should be 15–20 minutes long, show a client-centered, non-directive play therapist playing with a child who is not displaying emotional problems, and demonstrate the main skills parents will be learning. (See Appendix 1 for suggestions.)

Group discussion of the demo

The last task for leaders before the meeting's midway break is to lead a discussion of the demo with parents. Leaders start with general questions, to help participants get into their first group discussion with one another. These questions, and the attitudes leaders display during this discussion, tap into both the therapeutic and educational functions of GFT, which parents experience for the first time here. We suggest the following questions:

1. *What were your reactions to the demo?*

This is the most important question to begin with, in order to have participants concentrate on their own feelings and thoughts within the group. The other two questions may follow in any order.

  2. *Did you notice anything about the therapist's behavior that was different from how adults usually respond to children during play (e.g. no questions, no praising, no suggestions)?*

This is a more factual question that is important to ask. It shows participants that their cognitive abilities are used in GFT to learn new skills. (It also is the point in the discussion where a leader can point out a major mistake in the live demo, if this has occurred.)

  3. *What are your concerns and feelings about play sessions with your own children?*

This question is very important to ask. It is essential at this point in the group process to pull out the main doubts parents may have about themselves, their children, the method to be taught to them, the capacities of the leaders to help them, fears about group criticism, and other issues of concern. If these reactions are not addressed directly and managed effectively by leaders immediately, parents' doubts can either lead to participants deciding not to return next time, or simmer as an undercurrent during subsequent interactions. Leaders need to be certain they provide empathic responses when addressing these issues. In our experience, empathy alone may be sufficient in response to these issues, since such concerns by parents are often feelings based. Information can follow empathy, if the issue requires it.

   For example, a question couched in cognitive terms by a parent can require an empathic response first:

> *Parent: What would you call that behavior in the video? My child also spends a lot of time classifying toys. Would that be compulsive?*
>
> *Leader: Your child's behavior may be a worry to you.*
>
> *Parent: Yes, it is. Do you think it's compulsive?*
>
> *Leader: Whether a behavior can be considered compulsive or not is not important in this approach. What is important is responding appropriately to the child's behavior in the session. We try to address the behaviors and what is going on for the child, and think about underlying causes later if it seems necessary. I can assure you, though, that should we observe any behavior that needs attention beyond what the healing power of the play session can provide, we would tell you. We would help you figure out how to deal with it.*

Illustrative example of a group discussion following a demo

This example illustrates a dialogue between leaders and parents after parents watched their first demo. The live play session was conducted by Leader 2 with a 6-year-old boy who had already been a volunteer for a play therapy training workshop.

SUMMARY OF THE DEMO

Kevin came into the playroom eagerly and clearly enjoyed investigating the toys. He settled upon playing with the water in the play sink. He poured water on the plastic puppets, but did not play with them as puppets. He used a teapot, which he really seemed to like, and asked the therapist if he could take it home with him. The therapist set the limit about toys staying in the playroom. Some water spilled on the floor, which did not bother Kevin or the therapist.

This demo was only 15 minutes and, at the five-minute warning, Kevin was annoyed that he had not had time to play with other toys. He complained about having to leave, and started to play with the bop bag. He wanted to stay longer. The therapist reflected his desire to stay, and his annoyance with the short time. He poked at the bop bag a few times but, when reminded by the therapist that he really had to leave, he left with no further comment.

GENERAL COMMENTS ON THIS DEMO

The child in this live demo of a play session had the appropriate level of involvement in his play for a first meeting. It provided the group with a first exposure to a play session that was active, but simple and easy to conduct. In the short play session, Kevin was very appropriate for his age in his activities, and in the amount of talking that he did. It is worth noting that he did not play with the puppets as puppets, but seemed to include them as props in his water play. His need for two limits gave the therapist an opportunity to illustrate limit setting—one regarding leaving toys in the playroom, and the second to remind him that his time was up. He responded well to both, giving the parents who observed an opportunity to see that firm, simple limits can be enough.

GROUP DIALOGUE FOLLOWING THE DEMO

> *Leader 1: Well, you have now seen an example of the kind of play sessions we've been talking about. I am wondering what you are thinking and feeling about it?*
>
> *Mary [parent]: I thought it was interesting—different from what I thought it would be.*
>
> *Leader 1: You had some other ideas about what it would be like... Any other reactions to what you just saw?*
>
> *George [parent] (talking to Leader 2): I noticed that you simply commented on his picking up toys, and when he played with the water, you didn't encourage or discourage him. I would have wanted him to play with the puppets, instead of just pouring water over them.*
>
> *David [parent]: Would it have been wrong to start playing with the puppets with him? He held them up to you a couple of times before he wet them.*
>
> *Leader 2: This seems like a natural thing to do for both of you. For everyday play, that would be OK. In these play sessions, which are intended to be therapeutic, we do not enter children's play unless invited. This is what all of you will be learning to do. An important feature that makes this play therapeutic is that the*

children become the leaders of the play session activities, and are not directed by grown-ups, as would be the case most of the time in real life. If children ask adults to play, say if Kevin had handed the puppet to me, then I would have done so, under his direction. Pulling on their own impulses and resources is one of the things that help children learn about themselves and how to control themselves.

George: Sure sounds farfetched. Can a child like our little Lena [4 years old] possibly do that, without our telling her how?

Leader 1 (responding to George): It seems kind of unreal. We do need to teach children in real life how to do and say certain things. But the inner life of children is not something you can really teach. You will learn that this non-directed play allows children to free themselves from real-world demands, and express their own inner thoughts, feelings, and conflicts.

George: I can't disagree with what you are saying, but I will need more convincing, I think. Maybe if we see more children playing with you.

Leader 2: More play sessions may be more convincing. But you need more examples of this to be sure about it. We will be doing a lot more sessions to demonstrate this.

Leader 1: Getting back to Kevin—did you notice anything else that was different from what you usually do? Did anyone else have any reactions?

Sarah [parent]: Yes, I was kind of expecting him to go on a bit about having to leave the toys at the end of the session. I must say that I was impressed that Kevin did not question your answer about not taking home the teapot. It was clear that he wanted it. Also, that he wanted to stay longer.

Leader 1: That was better than you thought it might be. It was a pleasure for you to see such cooperation. It seemed to you that he wanted to stay longer, since the session was very short. In play sessions there are limits on time and behaviors— never on feelings. We believe that it is in the blend of freedom and needing to conform to limits that children develop necessary controls. The free expression in play sessions helps them get out feelings that need to be expressed. The limits help children put controls on expression. Because there is so much freedom in play sessions, children generally rein themselves in on those occasions when requested to do so. When possible, we try to state limits in a positive way. For example, "Keep the sand in the sandbox" instead of saying "Don't throw the sand on the floor."

Mary: That's really different from the way I tell my own kids what they can and can't do at home. It must be hard to get the hang of that.

Leader 1: It seems hard for you to think about doing it this way. We do leave learning limit setting until other skills are learned, but we always help you learn all these CCPT skills in ways that are not too difficult. And of course, no one learns right away how to do something very different. All parents need to practice these skills. We'll work on these in our group meetings, including practicing these skills *in pairs, so you'll be competent in these skills, and feel more confident, before you start doing play sessions with your children.*

This dialogue illustrates the usefulness of the shared experience of a demo to stimulate parents' interest in play sessions and compare what they saw with their own lives. The dialogue also illustrates a few parents' reservations about learning to conduct play sessions themselves, and shows how important it is that this demo is a positive one. Parents' reactions were sought by the leaders and their feelings accepted. Several important teaching points emerged during this discussion, and leaders gave parents brief information, as the need arose, on the structure of the program during skills learning.

Other teaching points needing to emerge during discussions

If possible, leaders should allow teaching points to emerge from the group discussion, but first they need to make certain they have elicited parents' reactions to the demo. During further discussion, leaders should remember to always prioritize responding to any parents' comments that are relevant to the demo, while minimizing parents' comments and questions that are unrelated—leaders always need to keep mindful of the time.

In our experience, the following teaching points often emerge spontaneously during the discussion of the first demo, and need to be picked up and underlined by leaders. If they do not arise spontaneously, leaders should themselves find opportunities to introduce these points, either during this meeting's discussion or over the next few meetings.

1. *In the demo, the therapist showed interest in everything the child was doing and playing with. The therapist commented on what was happening several times and included children's feelings.*

Leaders should point out that this is a skill parents will learn to do, and link this comment to the point that research on play therapy shows that this skill seems to be part of what works well for children, with predictable results.

2. *The therapist didn't ask the child questions or praise the child during the special play session.*

If this comment does not emerge spontaneously, leaders should invite parents to notice. Leaders can then explain to parents that this was deliberate on the therapist's part. Leaders may wish to paraphrase the following explanations:

- *Questions are not asked because these play sessions are children's own time to express themselves. If they have to stop and think in order to answer our adult questions, it takes away from children's time and changes their focus onto us.*

- *We don't praise in the play sessions because we don't want children to try to please us and win our approval. If children focus on doing well to get praise, there is a good chance that they will not get down to the root of their problems in play sessions, which at times might not be praiseworthy. That doesn't mean that praise isn't a good thing! So don't stop what you're doing in real life. We all feel better when people who are important to us think we've done well. The play sessions are exceptions.*

- *Play sessions are child directed, and therefore the views of the adult present are excluded. This allows children to try out behaviors that may not be approved, but are essential to children overcoming their problems.*

If play demo examples have not arisen spontaneously during the first few meetings, leaders may wish to use the following type of example for illustration:

Since the rules allow children to say anything they wish (if this option is taken), some children will use words that are normally forbidden outside their play session. This defiance of convention, for the short time it generally lasts, permits children to see if parents have different rules for play sessions or not. It also allows children to express anger and/or other negative emotions that can assist in their healing process. Children feel especially accepted when parents can permit this deviation from the norm.

3. *This is a family program, so all important family members are encouraged to participate in it.*

Whether arising spontaneously, or introduced by leaders, this is the point at which leaders are advised to make another plea for parents, who at intake chose not to be engaged in GFT, to become members of the group and attend the second meeting. Leaders can point out that *"This program is intended to improve parent-child relationships, so if one parent is not as involved with their children, taking part in this program could provide a unique and promising opportunity for this to change."* Leaders also should try to include other children and teens in the family, mentioning that all the children in the family get great benefits from participating in their own play sessions with their parents. (While leaders already decided on the maximum number of children for play sessions in their designated groups after the intake meetings, some groups may be able to absorb one or two more children with subclinical issues from families who are participating, if parents decide early in the program that these children would benefit from the program.) Leaders should add:

We will include toddlers and teens after you move into home play sessions. Any of you who think there may be special issues about who should participate in your family can talk briefly at the end of the meeting to either of us, or you can arrange to talk it over more on the telephone with one of us before the next meeting.

4. *We leaders are not making promises that each child will be helped the same way in this program, because each child is unique. But typically children are helped, and this program has been run often with parents who all report that there were some positive changes their children made. And often parents say there were big changes, with their children becoming much more lovable and capable. Also, when measures of change are used for evaluating programs, they show meaningful changes in children's behavior. (After making this point, it is timely for leaders to briefly mention the means of evaluation their group will use at the end of the program.)*

5. *This kind of playing together builds better relationships. You will feel better about yourselves and so will your children.*

Midway break

The tendency of new GFT leaders is to allow the discussion of the demo to run on past break time. However, as we discuss elsewhere, breaks have the dual purpose of allowing parents "time out" as well as allowing them an opportunity for informal interactions. Keeping to break times also establishes that leaders are able to structure meetings effectively, thus giving parents a model for keeping to consistent time limits during their own tasks and attendance on the program. The break should follow the discussion of the demo, and occur before leaders formally introduce the four main play skills parents will learn in the program. Midway breaks are well placed approximately halfway through each meeting.

The second half of the meeting

Overview of the four basic CCPT skills

After the break, leaders should briefly summarize the four skills parents are taught during the program. Similar to other educational tasks in GFT, simple, jargon-free explanations should be used. It is helpful for leaders to acknowledge that this is a review, and that the general idea of FT already was covered during intake meetings. (This statement is to acknowledge that some parents may well remember what the skills are.)

It is important for leaders to ensure that a clear link is made between each of these four skills and the contents of the demo parents saw before the midway break. (When leaders use videos, these examples can be prepared beforehand.) Leaders should remember that the demo is the experience they and the participants have in common at this early point in the program. The demo provides concrete examples of child-centered play skills. Using these examples serves to enhance skills learning for parents, giving them experiential memories on which to tie new concepts. Ideally participants themselves give examples for each of the four skills covered in the handout. For instance:

> Leader: Skill 2, following children's lead, was already noticed by Mary [a parent]. She pointed out in our discussion before the midway break that in the demo the therapist, Judy, got up and moved over to where Julian was playing in the sand, after he told Judy that the soldiers in the sand were getting buried by a sandstorm and wanted her to see it. Does anyone else have an example from the demo? (If not, leaders should provide one of their own.)

Introduction to the toys used

Leaders also may choose to mention in general terms the toys that will be used, saying that there will be a range of toys used in play sessions to allow children to play out different feelings. We suggest explaining briefly to parents that the toys allow children to play out positive feelings, like taking care of others, negative feelings like aggressive feelings, more mature and immature feelings, and also feelings of achievement or not being able to do things, like getting a lid to fit on a bottle. Also toys are there that can be used by both boys and girls, not just by one gender.

Leaders should be aware that when this topic is introduced, parents may want to go into detail about the types of toys to be used. We suggest leaders say that there will be a full discussion of the toys to be used later on. The leaders also need to caution parents *not* to go out and purchase extra toys now: *"We will talk about what is needed later on."*

Sometimes discussing the use of certain toys arouses strong feelings in parents. Gender-specific toys may be difficult for a few parents to accept for both boys' and girls' play. And objections to aggressive toys in the playroom also can be raised by parents here. It is important that leaders deal with any potentially emotive issues briefly, being mindful of the time constraints they have, by empathizing with parents' feelings in the first instance, before providing more factual information (e.g. aggressive toys—guns, foam bats, etc.— are in the playroom to give the message that negative feelings are OK, and dolls are there to give the message that younger, softer feelings are acceptable). Leaders also should add that parents have to be able to manage the feelings they have about the toys in the room too. We suggest leaders say:

> We will discuss any uneasiness you have about toys, if this issue arises again for you during the next few meetings. At any rate, we will return to it before you start doing your home sessions. We'll work something out together if you still have concerns.

Managing parents' anxieties on being observed

Another crucial area for leaders to address, if it arises here or, less commonly, later in the program, is any anxiety parents may express about being watched. Leaders should take time to empathize with parents' anxiety about being exposed to scrutiny. They also may try to engender a more positive attitude towards being observed. Perhaps a leader might say in a light-hearted way, *"We haven't lost a parent yet!"*, if the discussion seems to be turning negative in tone.

If one or two parents strenuously insist that they or their children will not allow these observations, we suggest that leaders first acknowledge these parents' strong feelings and then say that they will come back to these issues later. It is important for leaders to say that they will work something out with these parents that take account of these feelings, if they still feel the same way in a few weeks' time. If parents state that one of their children will object to being watched by strangers, leaders can suggest that this child (if a sibling) wait until another sibling has a turn first (and wait until other demos have been conducted). If this strategy is not feasible, leaders may suggest that parents bring their child in early for a meeting. The demo can be videotaped beforehand and then shown to the group afterwards. (This is also a possible, last-ditch solution if a parent objects to being watched by the group during practice play sessions. See Chapter 10.)

Some other parents may state that they will have logistic problems with home sessions. For example, they may say they do not see any way to conduct home play sessions, given their home environment. Again, leaders should state that this can be worked out later. Leaders may want to add:

> We always find a solution, once we come to doing the home sessions and get our heads together about this. In the meeting before you start your home sessions, we will spend time looking at all the issues you may have.

Technical and practical issues

Preparing parents for the next steps in the program

Leaders need to allocate time towards the end of the meeting to discuss with parents the demos that begin the following week with their children. Leaders have two or three demos each meeting, depending on the size of the group and the number of siblings. We suggest leaders make the following teaching points:

1. *There will be two or three demos each meeting that we will work out before we end today. One of us leaders will play with each of your children, and all of you parents will watch without talking among yourselves. For families with more than one child, we will do demos with all the siblings, one after another, at the same meeting.*

Leaders ideally should aim for no more than two demos conducted per meeting, but numbers may dictate three per meeting.

2. *These demos will be done with one child to one adult, just like your own play sessions will be.*

3. *Just like you did during the demo today, you will watch what leaders are doing because that's what you'll be doing when you play with your own children later. We'll watch all the demos for the meeting, and then talk about them together, after all of them are finished for that day.*

The most practical reason for doing all the demos before discussion is that children are waiting for their turn to play. Leaders do not want to test their patience too much, since it could affect the quality of their play session.

Leaders also should take note that it is much more economical, from a time standpoint, if all demos are conducted during a meeting before having a discussion. It sometimes is tempting to talk about each demo as soon as it has ended. People do seem to remember demo details better. However, experience by many leaders has shown that the change of set, from observing to discussion, requires more time:

> Leader: You'll be watching your own children and we're sure you'll be very interested in what they do. It will be interesting for you as parents to see how your children will react. This is something new for your children and you.
>
> Your children may behave perfectly, or do things you wish they hadn't done. Children react differently in different situations and with different people. So don't be surprised if your child shows you a new side. That may be because they are on their best behavior, but it's also because the atmosphere of these special play sessions allows children to express different aspects of themselves.
>
> Please do not prime your children to behave in a certain way. It is most useful for parents to see one another's children just as they are on the day. We also know that each parent realizes that they will only be seeing a small part of what each child is like. Whether it's more positive or more negative will depend on what each child is feeling at the moment.
>
> After the demos, we'll talk with each parent a bit about how it's the same or different from at home, and then talk about what we can all learn from each demo.

The children who have done the demo with the leaders will be the focus for our discussion. Other parents will have their turns talking about their own children week by week, until each child is discussed.

You will find that, by watching one another's children in the demos, you will not only understand children in general better, but that you will develop a better understanding of your own children. Plus it's always very interesting to see how other children react to the demos.

We'll work out the demo schedule together before we leave, as we said. We will be starting on time for each meeting, so that the children don't have to wait too long for their turns. That's also why we will be having all the demos at the beginning of the meeting.

You need to be early when your children are taking part in a meeting's demos. You will need to settle your children into childcare before the meeting starts (NB: leaders give information on childcare facilities here), rather than bringing them directly to our meeting. One of us leaders will be there to collect the children one by one, bring them along for their play sessions, and then return them afterwards.

Preparing children for the demo session

Leaders explain to parents:

> *Your children will need to be prepared for the demos they do during meetings. They will need to know who will be looking after them. We'll arrange this childcare next.*

Ideally, parents have one or more options to choose from for their children's care during meetings. These options include the following:

- The therapy providers have a room for the children to play in while the meeting is on, attended by a childcare person paid by the agency.

- Parents bring their own familiar childcare person to stay with their children in the childcare room for the entire meeting.

- Parents arrange with either their own familiar childcare person, or another adult they designate (e.g. grandmother), to take the children home after they have done their demos. These children do not wait during the entire meeting.

> *Leader: You will need to tell your children, and we'll repeat it when we collect them to come with us, that they will take part in a short playtime. You should explain that this playtime with leaders is to help parents learn to have the same kind of playtimes with their own children.*

At this point in the discussion, leaders should hand out a copy of Appendix 14 on preparing children for demos and practice play sessions, as well as a copy of the children's leaflet (Appendix 10), and then review them with parents.

Preparing parents for the next meeting

THE AGENDA FOR THE SECOND MEETING

Leaders prepare parents for the agenda for the next meeting, by stating:

> *Next time we'll watch these demos, talk together about them, and then have a midway break. We'll come back together again after the break to begin learning play therapy skills together. Remember that you will be using these skills when you do play sessions.*

WORKING OUT THE DEMO SCHEDULE

At this point, leaders inform parents of the following:

> *We will be doing demos with your children over the next several meetings, as you know from the schedule. The demos will be done with each of the children who are fully participating in the program. If you have more than one child participating fully, bringing all of the children in your family in on one date would be best.*
>
> *These demos will start within five minutes of the start time for the meeting. As we said earlier, it is very important that we start on time.*

SUGGESTIONS FOR SELECTION OF DEMO CHILDREN

We advise that leaders pick what appear to be the easiest children first for demos. These selection decisions should be based on their interactions with families during the intake meetings. This strategy is recommended first of all to ensure that parents in the group are not overwhelmed by extreme behavior. Sometimes the most difficult children are eagerly volunteered by their parents! These children may provide demos that are too atypical for good teaching. If parents have early exposure to more typical sessions, they are not as likely to be put off by atypical sessions. Another reason for this strategy is to ensure that leaders are not overwhelmed themselves by difficult and unexpected behavior from children during early demos. This is important because it is essential that leaders show their credibility as child-centered play therapists during these early demos. Play sessions that "go bad" in some way for leaders can potentially undermine the entire program. Parents, as a result of serious difficulties by leaders during demos, may feel that play sessions produce nothing worthwhile.

Leaders also should make certain that the most reliable parents have their children selected first in the program, so that there are no unexpected absences and the program can be assured of starting on time. After using their clinical judgment on these dimensions of reliability and children that are easier to play with, leaders should make up their own tentative schedule for the order in which children will have their turn for demos. Leaders also should make parents aware that leaders' decisions on the order of demos are tentative and that changes are likely to be made along the way to accommodate children's and their parents' family situations and learning needs.

Once leaders decide with parents on the order of children for demos, we recommend that they take out the additional insurance of sending an email and/or making a telephone call the day before these early demos, to remind parents to bring their children, until parents get used to this routine. Before any meeting with demos and practice play sessions ends, the names of the children scheduled for the next week should be reviewed. This is in case a parent suddenly realizes that the time is now inappropriate; another child can then be placed on the schedule for a demo during the next meeting.

Ending the first meeting

At the end of the meeting, leaders aim to engender hopefulness and interest in the next meeting with parents. Leaders may choose to paraphrase the following statements for themselves:

> We have covered a few points about the play sessions this time. I think we could all see that the child in the demo you watched enjoyed playing, as do most children. So next week we will see how a few of your children react to being played with by us leaders. We leaders will take turns playing while you watch. George and Diane are scheduled to bring Lena, and Mary and Sam are scheduled to bring John and Larry. We will all be very interested in what happens, and believe that the children will enjoy themselves. We are off to a good start and are looking forward to seeing everyone next week.

Group leaders also distribute the Parents' Training Manual for Play Sessions (Appendix 15) at the close of the meeting, along with the schedule of dates and times for all meetings. The Training Manual is easy to read and engaging for parents, and in our experience helps motivate parents to attend and participate fully in the program. Parents should be told that this Manual is to be read during the week, before the next meeting, to prepare themselves for the leaders' demos with the children that they will see. It is important that parents *bring their Manuals* along with them to each meeting. They also are asked to enter all the meeting dates and times into their phones, diaries or calendars, so that they are certain to attend all of them. Finally, there is a general goodbye and encouragement by leaders for parents to be certain to attend next week.

The next chapter continues with the second meeting in the 20-week GFT program.

CHAPTER 6
Starting Play Demonstrations and Skills Learning
Meeting 2

This chapter and the next two chapters consider Meetings 2–4 in the 20-week GFT program. This chapter discusses demos in detail and gives an extended example of a group discussion following the demos, when skills training is introduced. The next chapter explores ways to directly teach the FT skills that have been modeled in the demos, giving illustrative examples and suggested exercises.

In these three meetings, leaders aim to show parents the skills they need for special play sessions, to motivate parents to continue participating in the program by reminding them of the end goals, and to have shared examples from demos for use when directly training parents in CCPT skills. Other aims are to foster parents' interest in conducting play sessions with their children at home as a next step, to help parents view their children in more objective terms during demos, and to build positive group support.

Skills training during these three meetings is a step-by-step process, gradually evolving into helping parents use all of the FT skills together during their "mock" play sessions, held during Meeting 5. A "mock" session is a mini-play session with a leader playing the role of a child, to give parents the experience of selecting appropriate FT responses. This is a rehearsal for parents' play sessions with their own children, starting the following week.

The second meeting

Meeting 2 begins with two or three demos by leaders with children in the program. Most of the group time following the demos is taken up with processing what happened in this meeting's demos. Leaders then use demo examples to illustrate the skills that parents are being taught. As parents begin to master child-centered skills during these early meetings, there is more skills training, and less emphasis on what leaders did during demos.

Conducting demos

THE UNIQUE CHARACTER OF DEMOS

Parents commonly are intensely interested in seeing how their children respond in a play session. After observing demos, the group then shares a common experience that can be discussed and referred to later, as mentioned earlier. The demos are rich experiences for participants because each demo is in "real time" and therefore shows the challenges, complexities, and rewards very directly of play sessions with the children in the program. Conducting demos with each of the children involved in the program is intended to maximize parents' interest in and knowledge of their children's reactions to this new situation. In addition, it reinforces parents' knowledge of each other's children; this familiarity helps when parents are discussing their children in future group sessions. Leaders also have a better picture of each child involved in the group, making it easier for them to provide meaningful feedback to parents when it is their turn to play with their respective children.

PRACTICAL DETAILS

Leaders already have decided the allocation of children between themselves for demos during the meeting. One leader starts the demos with the children, each demo followed immediately by the next one, with a maximum of three demos per meeting. While each demo takes 15 minutes, leaders should remember that on average each demo will take 20 minutes, by the time a child is collected and returned to the childcare room by one leader, while the second leader tidies the demo room. Leaders should note that it is important that they collect children for the demos themselves, and that they are experienced in helping children relax and anticipate their playtime, in order for this transition between rooms to be easy for the children to accomplish.

Parents already were forewarned by leaders during the first meeting that the first demo would start within five minutes of the start time of the second meeting, and we suggest not waiting for latecomers. Keeping to the group start time minimizes waiting times for the children and discourages parents from getting into discussions with one another that are very difficult to terminate quickly.

Leaders need to remind parents again at the beginning of the meeting that demos should not be interrupted by either leaders or parents. The only exception, which is very rare indeed, is when a leader decides to end a demo abruptly because a child is extremely distressed or aggressive, which in turn distresses parents. It is rare that a young child may wish to leave, or an older child may receive a consequence and is required to leave. In the authors' experience, children nearly always are able to participate in most of the demo and feel contained by the filial therapists.

Sotto voce comments by leaders during demos

Ideally, a one-way screen or video link is available for parent observation of the demos from another room. When this separation of rooms is possible, the co-leader who is not conducting the demo is able to remain with observing parents and make very brief, unobtrusive, and quiet comments from time to time, while they are all observing the demos together. Leaders' comments should be limited to giving a label to an observed skill, or answering a quick and easy parent question. For example, if a child during a demo hides something out of the therapist's view, and one or two parents become concerned about how the therapist will manage this, the leader can mention that the therapist conducting the demo probably will try to reflect what the child is feeling. Some other examples that can arise during demos are:

1. Katie, 5 years old, moves rapidly over to the doll's house during the first part of her demo. The leader/therapist states: *"You are going over there quickly."* The leader behind the one-way screen whispers briefly to the parents: *"We call this 'tracking' what the child does."*

2. During her demo, 10-year-old Gemma is trying to make a cube shape out of stiff paper and wrinkles her nose as she squeezes out the glue. The leader/therapist says, *"Gemma, you don't like that glue."* The co-leader behind the screen whispers to the parents, *"Showing understanding of Gemma's feelings here."*

Less simple questions from parents or discussions about more complex behaviors should be postponed until after the observation. The leader may make the following statement: *"The answer will take too long. We'll talk about it in our meeting."* In general, there are a few caveats for leaders when making *sotto voce* comments during demos:

- Dialogues and discussions with group members are not appropriate and can be disrespectful to the child, parents, and the therapist in the demo, as well as modeling inappropriate behavior for group members during demos.

- A leader commenting on many things that are happening can be both distracting and overwhelming for observing parents.

- It is vital that no diagnostic comments (e.g. labelling a behavior as obsessive) are made by the observing leader. These comments are very out of place because they may seriously undermine all the group members' confidence, which may be at a low ebb at the beginning of the program. Diagnostic comments set the leader up as the "expert" and "critic" and could possibly interfere with parents feeling that they can use the skills in a comparable way.

Issues for the leader conducting the demo

CCPT has some variation in the way it is practiced. For example, we referred earlier to differences over giving alternatives to children during limit setting, and Wilson & Ryan (2005) argue for the importance of verbal as well as non-verbal congruence in CCPT. However, in the GFT program detailed here, we follow Louise Guerney's method of training that in her experience is the most straightforward way of teaching parents FT skills, without the CCPT variations used by other authors. Since leaders are modeling the CCPT skills to be taught to parents in the GFT program, it is important for consistency that they closely adhere to the ways CCPT skills are set out in this book in their demos and skills training.

Another practice situation that leaders conducting demos need to manage for parents' benefit is when leaders make mistakes during a demo. We already discussed this briefly in the last chapter. With minor mistakes, particularly if these are not noticed by observing parents, the leader has to decide whether it is useful to mention them or not. Some minor mistakes can be a source of much more concern for leaders than for parents, particularly if leaders tend to have perfectionist tendencies. In these cases, shortcomings are perhaps not useful to point out (e.g. finding *exactly* the right word for an expressed feeling, when an adequate one was used), nor are other minor mistakes, if they do not recur. Should such a minor mistake be noticed by a parent, the leader can manage this easily by pointing out that, even though the leader is an experienced play therapist, sometimes a minor mistake is made. Leaders can add that parents, when learning these skills, will naturally make some of these kinds of errors themselves. For example, one addition of a question, or use of a questioning tone, can be overlooked, but repeated use of questions must be avoided in demos. An occasional slip does not destroy the model, but a minor mistake that is repeated can undermine it. Therefore in our opinion, this type of mistake should be mentioned when it happens more than once, and an acceptable substitute offered.

If a leader makes a major error during a demo—for example, not setting a limit when one is required—leaders already have prepared parents for this eventuality in the first meeting. In these cases, it is important for the leader to be transparent, pointing out the mistake and correcting it in the discussion of the demo. But it is not useful to the group for the leader to engage in unnecessary self-recriminations or self-doubt. If these feelings do arise for a leader, the co-leader is in an ideal position to help the leader who has made the mistake. The co-leader is able to monitor whether the other leader needs support or time to regroup. Where needed, the co-leader can take over the discussion from the first leader and help group members to use this mistake to further their skills learning. Overall, leaders need accepting and transparent attitudes towards their own and the parents' mistakes in GFT, rather than a critical, including self-critical, attitude. These positive attitudes are very important for leaders to model in the group, particularly during early meetings before group support has been established.

Discussion of demos

The discussion following the two or three demos consists of, first, the parents sharing their reactions to seeing their children in the demo; and second, discussing the therapist's interactions with the children.

The parents' reactions to the demo

Leaders first give the parent(s) a chance to give their reactions to observing their child during the demo. It is very important that the leaders and all the other group members are respectful and attentive when parents share their feelings about their child's behavior. One typical reaction parents may voice during demo discussions is that they were surprised that their child was so well behaved. Other parents may have different reactions, perhaps expressing surprise that their child was so nervous, or so immature. Leaders should use these reactions to point out that play sessions are new and different for children, as well as for their parents. It is often timely for leaders to add that other parents may be curious as to how their children will react during their demos. An example of a possible discussion of a parent's reaction to their child's behavior during an early demo is given next.

ILLUSTRATIVE EXAMPLE

Mother: Matthew was unbelievably good during that demo! I can't believe that he simply stopped throwing that ball against the mirror when you asked him to! And he went like a lamb when the time was up. All the other parents will wonder what we're complaining about with him.

Leader: You are really surprised that Matthew was so well behaved. You think that this wasn't a real example of what he's like. It looked too easy to you.

Mother: Yes, it certainly did!

Leader: Children do react differently in different situations, and I expect other parents will be interested to see how their children will react when it's their turn. Of course Matthew may have been on his best behavior, with everyone watching.

Mother: Maybe... I didn't know he could do it!

Leader: You're amazed that he was so well behaved. Part of the reason may be because of the play session itself, where children "lead the way". Children are more inclined than usual to listen during play sessions when they're told something for that reason. Matthew certainly seemed to! We'll talk next, after our midway break, about what the leader was doing while Matthew played. Is there anything else, Steve [Matthew's dad], that you noticed about Matthew's behavior you wanted to mention?

COMMENTS ON THIS EXAMPLE

This example shows how the leader led the feedback during this early stage in the program. The leader gave precedence to empathizing with the mother's emotional reaction to the demo with her son, then brought in two teaching points, and referred to other parents in the feedback in order to motivate them to have their children take part in play demos. It also is important for group leaders to actively include the second parent in the feedback, as the leader demonstrated in this case for Matthew's father.

Demos in relation to midway breaks

Two, rather than three, demos are preferable for the second meeting, where possible. In Meeting 2, leaders should aim to have the break after all the demos and the initial discussion of the demos eliciting the parents' reactions to their children are finished. Parents may want to air their reactions to their children taking part in the demos with one another informally during the break. This airing often serves to build group support among them. However, it is always important that the group leaders already have set up a positive approach within the group, where children and parents do not feel criticized; otherwise this informal discussion can be inhibiting and perhaps divisive. For this reason, the leaders should ensure that the break occurs *after* they lead the initial feedback with the parents in early group meetings.

Discussion of the leaders' interactions during the demos

After the parents give their reactions to the demos and have a midway break, leaders move the discussion forward to address the therapist's behavior and what group members noticed. There is not much time during this second meeting, when CCPT skills are at the beginning stage of being modeled, for the leaders to find time to teach these skills directly to parents.

It is important for leaders to start as they plan to continue—they need frequently to provide examples of what skills and attitudes they are referring to during these early discussions, and not rely too much on verbally describing these skills. Examples always go a long way towards engaging and motivating parents. Examples used judiciously by leaders also help parents to observe the demos and their own children's reactions to them (and to events at home) more carefully.

Important emotional issues are often raised directly by parents in these early discussions, as the earlier example of Matthew shows. Another common issue raised by parents in early demos is that their child seemed to have permission to do *anything* during the demo. When this occurs, leaders should first of all empathize with these parents' feelings (e.g. *"That annoyed you,"* or *"That worried you…'* or *"It's not like at home."*). After this acknowledgement, leaders then need to bring the discussion back to the parents' task of learning the new skills involved in play sessions, mentioning both the more permissive attitude during sessions, the reason(s) for this (see Chapter 3), and the judicious use of the limit-setting skill alongside the other skills.

An example of such a discussion is given next to illustrate these points and show the teaching opportunities that arose spontaneously for leaders in this particular group. It also shows the ways in which discussion is shared between the two leaders, and ways in which parents can be included in this discussion. The ways that leaders manage their practical tasks at the end of the second meeting also are illustrated. These tasks include briefly discussing the agreed demo arrangements for the third meeting, and preparing parents for beginning to practice skills themselves during the next meeting.

Extended example of a second meeting's group discussion

The discussion here followed parents watching two demonstrations of play sessions by each of the two leaders. The children were two brothers, Ray and Connor (aged 9 and 10); neither the boys nor their parents, Jessie and Greg, had ever had any involvement in play sessions prior to these demonstrations.

PRELIMINARY COMMENTS

We remind readers here that the purpose of the demos is for the parents to observe what the therapists do during a play session, so that they will learn to model their responses after the therapists' when they play with their children. While the behavior of the children is secondary to trying to learn the responses of the play therapists, parents are drawn to thoughts of the way their children are behaving. Leaders need to accept that interest, but deal with it as minimally as possible in order to focus on parents learning the responses of the therapists.

GROUP DISCUSSION EXAMPLE

Leader 1: When Ray wanted to build that tower, I commented about how pleased he was that he could do it. The focus was on his feelings. I said, "You're really happy that you know how to do that."

Hannah [parent]: Would you ever tell him how you felt about it? Like, "I'm proud of you," or something like that?

Leader 1: Those would be very natural and good responses in real-life situations. But in the play session, it's the child's feelings that are the only focus. How you feel about it is not part of this model. Your time to talk about your feelings is in our meetings together.

Tom [parent]: After watching the play demos that you did tonight, I think I can play the way you did.

Leader 2: That is good to hear. I am sure you can, too. We are sure that you all will.

Jessie [Ray's and Connor's Mom]: I seem to remember your telling us before that the first thing you might see in play sessions is aggression. I didn't really see aggression tonight. I saw Ray playing with a gun, but it was just play, not aggressive.

Leader 1: So you're wondering whether this is the kind of aggression we were talking about. You are right. Just playing with a gun, not using it in an aggressive way would not really be called aggression in the way we were talking about, although it is a toy that would typically be thought of as an aggressive toy. Aggression, where a child tries to shoot the gun at a therapist, or aim at some other object, would be what is classified as aggression.

Children usually get into more open expression after the first demo. But aggressive behavior can actually start any time. You will notice as you observe more play demos that they will all be different. While certain patterns are seen frequently, there is no single pattern that typically occurs. After a period of active aggression during play sessions, children very often engage in behavior in which they seem to be seeking nurturance. They seem to need to be nurtured and act much more immature than they are in real life. This seems to come after aggression with most children because, we figure, it is more difficult for children to accept their feelings of immaturity that can come out when they feel free to express them in play sessions, than it is to accept their feelings of aggression.

In our society, children are very much encouraged to act grown-up, and being aggressive from time to time, unless it is extreme, is not as punishable in most cases as not acting their age. That is, it is safer to express aggression than to act immature. That comes second. But nobody knows why this is for sure.

Leader 2: For example, one of your children might ask for help taking off the play dough lids, something that they have done themselves lots of other times.

Tom: What would you do if a child asked you for help?

Leader 2: We would show we understand their feelings and provide the help. This is because we would assume that the request was made as an expression of this need for nurturance and reliving a more immature phase of life. Going through that phase is part of the healing process of play therapy. It allows children to move on to the phase of mastery, where they have worked out these immature feelings and aggressive feelings and have become more mature emotionally and behaviorally.

Kate [parent]: I really don't know why you have such resistance to answering questions in the play sessions.

Leader 2: It seems a little strange to you to take such a hard stand on questions.

Kate: Yes, if children ask questions, they want answers.

Leader 2: You want to help children that way. First I'd like to say that it's not as absolute as it might seem that you don't answer questions. There are some questions that can be answered, and we'll give you examples, but this is only after first commenting on the child's feelings that are behind the questions. In play sessions we first address intent before dealing with content.

There can be questions where simple information during a demo is requested that is relevant to the situation. Some examples might be: "Is my grandma waiting for me?", in which case the play therapist would say, "You're concerned about where she is." Or "You want to be sure she's waiting." Then add the simple information that she is waiting in the childcare room.

Leader 1: Another example might be, "How much time do we have left today to play?" Since I don't know whether this child is eager to leave or, more likely, the child wants to be sure he or she has time to finish a project, I might simply say, "You want to know how much more time you have left." Or, if I know what the child's intent is, I might say, "You want to be sure you have enough time to complete that building you're making." Then, I would provide the information, "Ten minutes."

A final example of providing simple information would be for a child, who cannot read yet, asking what something written on a package says. The child's question is: "What does this say?" The adult playing with the child would say: "You'd like to know what it says on that package." Then the adult provides the answer, "Soap."

Leader 2: Simple information does not disrupt the flow of play sessions, or the child's thinking. It really enables the child to continue the session. The kinds of questions that we do not answer in the session are ones that are not information, but instead would limit a child's play and choices if they are answered. For example, if a child said, "How should I color this?" and the adult said, "Make it blue and red and gray," this would be taking away the child's decision-making power. Remember that play sessions are intended to enhance children's ability to make their own decisions.

Leader 1: Or a child may ask, "What shall I do now? Tell me what to do." In this case, the adult would address only the child's feelings, and not provide an answer. The adult would say something like, "You really don't know what to do now. You're not sure there's anything to do. You'd like me to tell you what to do." Let's do a simple role-play for you. (One leader takes the child's role and the other is in the therapist's role.)

"Child" [Leader 2]: Yes, tell me what to do (in a nasty tone).

"Therapist" [Leader 1]: You don't like it if I don't do what you say. (Aside to group: Notice that here I focused on the feelings that are underneath this "child" pushing her point.)

"Child": Yes, tell me what to do!

"Therapist": In here, this is your time to decide what to do. If you don't know what to do, that's OK. You don't have to do anything, if you don't want to. This is your time. You decide everything in here, unless it's against the rules. ("Child" moves on to something else.)

Leader 1 (to group): In this case, we're not providing answers because we want to be sure that children understand that the rights and responsibility for the play session are theirs.

Leader 2: When parents play, they are spared a lot of personal questions that children tend to ask professional therapists such as "Are you married, where do you live, do you have children?" However, sometimes children may ask questions that have nothing to do with the play session that parents should not answer with content. For example, "Can we go to the mall tonight after we are finished here?" or "Are we really going to go on vacation this year, or are we going to skip it like last year?"

These questions are not ones that are relevant to the play session, and again require the adult to deal only with the child's intention and put a limit on these being discussed in the playroom. The parent would say, "You really want to go to the mall after we finish playing. You're hoping I'll say yes. That's something we talk about outside the playroom."

Leader 1: We find that the hardest questions for parents to resist when they are trying to stay in the model are educational questions. These are the kinds of questions that we all like our children to ask and it's part of our parenting role to provide useful information. Examples are: a child might ask about why the sky is blue, where does electricity come from, or questions about nature. These are again questions that can be answered at home when the child sees fit to bring them up there. In this case, during play sessions, show understanding of the child's interest, such as, "You're interested in electricity and would like to know how it works. We can talk about it after the play session, and look it up."

Tom: I have a tendency to enjoy answering Jerry's questions, and I find I tend to get into a lot of detail, far more than he wants. I find that I like that role of knowing the answers, and letting him know about that.

Hannah: Sometimes children will keep asking more and more questions, if you answer, and I think they like to be in control. They are the center of attention and they've got your attention while they can keep thinking of questions.

Leader 1: It sounds like you have found that, on some occasions, children's questions have other purposes and rewards than information, which is what we have found in the play sessions. We have found that, except for the kinds of simple information questions that we told you about first, like "What time is it?", children typically do not insist on answers beyond two or three statements from the adult. They move on to other things when they see that the ball is in their court, and that things are left to them.

There is the occasional child who is annoyed on a long-term basis about questions not being answered. It's the job of the adult to address that with the child at whatever length is necessary to help the child work out feelings about that. Getting into "You're angry, you're frustrated, you're annoyed with me" and so on until the problem is resolved. Should this happen to any of you, we will help you work that out. We'll give you the words to get over that hump with your child. However, you should know that this problem is rare, and most children learn to appreciate that they are not dependent on parents' answers and directions in the play sessions.

Betty: I noticed that you did not ask any questions of the boys. I would have wanted to ask Connor why he was keeping such close track of the score when he was shooting the darts.

Leader 1: You are curious, and you would like to satisfy that curiosity. In the play sessions, the adult does not ask questions, even when bursting with curiosity about what children's motives might be, or what outside information they might be alluding to. The play session is strictly in control of the child, and is dealing with just the here and now. Not interrupting children's train of thought is important. Asking him about who somebody is that he might be referring to in the play session is not something that you do. This is hard on parents and therapists, since we tend to be very curious about people mentioned and reasons behind things children do. We need to remember that, in the play sessions, it's the expression of feeling that we emphasize and feelings do not need to be justified or tied in with reality. Some anxious parents will ask unnecessary questions, or ask for unnecessary direction from their children, such as "Do you want me to catch the ball?", when their child is obviously intending to throw it to their parent.

Kate: I think that's going to be pretty hard. I just naturally want to know what my son is thinking when he tells me things. I want to know more about it.

Leader 2: This is not an easy thing to learn—how to do the play sessions so that you give your children the opportunities that they need to work out problems. It requires restraint sometimes, which is hard to do. It is also important to remember not to quiz children about their play after their sessions. However, you will find that there is a payoff for all your hard work. And don't forget, we will try to help you through these struggles.

Greg [Ray and Connor's father]: I noticed that Connor didn't really play with you. He was doing his own thing, and you were making comments to him about it, which he agreed with. But, he wasn't really playing with you. When I play with Connor at home, we really do things together. We wrestle, or we play some game, like checkers. So isn't that part of this? Playing together?

Leader 1: Yes, it's a part of it, if a child chooses it. How much and what kinds of wrestling you do is up to you and the leader to work out together. Some parents would not care to wrestle at all. Others would wrestle up to a certain point. We would talk about that with you. Remember we do have limits, and we want to make sure that something as physical as wrestling would not get into limit issues. So, we would want to be sure in advance that you and your child would be clear about the boundaries around it.

Some children play alone and want the adult to be a witness or observer to what they do, to make comments and appreciate their play. Others want to involve the adult in a very full way, and give them a role, such as "You be the policeman and I'll be the robber" kind of thing. I would say that most children tend to do several kinds of play in their sessions. Parallel play and role-playing and game playing... various kinds of competitions can happen. They change from session to session and within a session; they can do all of those kinds of things. We will help you learn how to handle these different kinds of playing...role-playing, competitions, and game playing. The easiest thing for the adult is to be an observer or witness where your only responsibility is to make empathic and tracking responses, showing that you are accepting and understanding what your child is doing and saying.

Leader 2: Looks like our time is just about up for tonight. We will need three children to play next week for demos. Andrew, Jessica, and Morris are scheduled to play—I hope there are not any problems with that? Each of us [leaders] will play with one of them for 15 minutes while you observe, as we did tonight. We will discuss what you saw us doing afterwards.

After we've discussed the sessions, we will add a new piece to our time together and that will be to practice one of the responses that you see the leaders making. We will practice empathic responding, also called reflecting feelings or showing understanding. This is where you try to make statements that show understanding of the feelings the child is expressing while playing. It's in your Parent's Training Manual. This skill goes with the other ones we will be practicing later, as you saw us leaders doing in play demos. But it's easier to learn the skills separately to start with. We will do some practice play among ourselves later in the meeting, so that you can learn to use that skill when you play with your children. Thank you all for coming. I think that we are going to have a wonderful group, and we're off to a very good start.

(Leader 1 joins in this positive statement and the goodbyes.)

GENERAL COMMENTS ON THIS EXAMPLE

In this discussion during a second meeting, both leaders made significant contributions to the exchanges with the parents. Who made what comments were not planned in advance, although Leader 1 was the more experienced leader and Leader 2 was less experienced. In instances where the leaders are not equally experienced, the more experienced leader generally takes more responsibility and contributes more.

Exchanges with the parents by leaders focused almost exclusively on the demonstrations parents observed and their spontaneous questions and thoughts afterwards. However, leaders also took the opportunity to talk about the progression of stages in children's play during a series of play sessions. This information was intended to help orient parents to the play content they will observe during future play sessions. The leaders also prepared parents for the next meeting, when parents will be introduced to practicing the first skill that they will need to master in order to conduct play sessions themselves.

The leaders made use of the learning opportunity provided to discuss how questions are dealt with in play sessions. They reinforced one of the positive functions of being a parent, the educative function, and acknowledged that some parents find it very difficult to refrain from trying to educate their children during play sessions, many times because they value the competence and sense of self-worth that are byproducts for their children of mastering skills and knowledge. Leaders reminded parents that this function is very necessary and very much appreciated in daily life, but that it is not the main purpose of play sessions. Leaders informed parents that in play sessions they follow their children's lead, and therefore help their children to explore, consolidate, and discover new learning for themselves. Parents facilitate rather than direct this process.

Leaders' reactions to the second meeting

In the last example, the parents seemed amenable to learning new skills and listened attentively to the leaders' comments, along with sharing their doubts and questions within the group. However, parents in other groups may not be as engaged and non-defensive as these parents were. Leaders sometimes become disheartened with such parents after Meeting 2, thinking that some have a long way to go before accepting and implementing child-centered play skills. If these feelings arise, leaders may wish to remind themselves that Meeting 2 is at the very beginning of parents' training. When leaders keep to the agendas suggested here, the GFT program allows considerable time for leaders to give parents examples of the skills they used in demos, along with ample time for parents to practice learning these skills.

As mentioned in Chapter 3, there is a usual order for teaching the main child-centered skills in GFT and the next chapter presents this blueprint. However, as we explained earlier, it also is important for leaders to keep in mind that groups have their own unique shared experiences and distinctive composition. Therefore sometimes during demos, when parents observe a skill being used by leaders, this experience may capture and focus the entire group's attention spontaneously on that particular skill, making it the optimal time for *that* group to learn a new skill. We urge GFT leaders to use these fortuitous moments fully to motivate parents' skills learning, rather than waiting until the usual time in the program.

CHAPTER 7
Continuing Demonstrations and Skills Practice
Meeting 3

This chapter and the next explore ways for leaders to build on parents' learning from the demos in the second meeting, and help parents practice for themselves the main FT skills observed in the demos. The chapter concentrates on teaching empathic responding, giving illustrative examples and suggested exercises. It also discusses general issues involved in group skills training.

The third meeting

In the third meeting, leaders should aim to more formally introduce and have parents practice the first of the CCPT skills, empathic responding. However, as we have mentioned already and discuss more later, some flexibility in the order of training may be needed in early meetings.

During the third week, parents in the group are more settled in the routine for meetings of demos and skills development, after seeing it in action during the previous week. Meeting 3 follows the same format as Meeting 2, with demos first, then a brief discussion of parents' reactions to their children's demos, followed by the break and discussion of the skills leaders displayed in the demos. The main difference from the second meeting is that in Meetings 3 and 4 somewhat less time is given to discussing the leaders' responses during the meeting's demos. Instead, approximately 25 minutes is scheduled for directly teaching skills to parents in Meeting 3, and slightly more time in Meeting 4. Leaders' aims for skills training in this part of the program are to convince parents of the usefulness of the skills they are learning, and to ensure parents know how to use these skills on a basic level. Introducing early skills learning and practicing skills, along with the issues that arise during this early skills training, are discussed next.

General comments for leaders on Meetings 3 and 4

Even though parents now are more familiar with the format of early meetings, leaders still have to schedule in and deal with all the questions and comments individual parents make about their children when they see them during the demos at the beginning of each meeting. Issues continue to arise for each family as their children play, such as *"Why did my child do that?"* Leaders should not assume during later demos that parents are familiar with the underlying emotional issues of their children in play sessions simply because, in general, they are by now familiar with the demos and how they work. Parents seem to generate their own questions as they directly watch their children play, and always need time to process their responses afterwards in the group.

Meetings 3 and 4 are very important in fostering and maintaining group cohesion, as well as fitting in all the demos and skills training. Leaders should aim to have each part of these early meetings flow from one another as seamlessly as possible. They need to balance parents' concerns with the timing constraints inherent in the meeting, and help parents realize that leaders are flexible and empathic to their concerns, as well as focused on training.

FLEXIBILITY OF APPROACH IN EARLY MEETINGS

Early meetings can be a challenge for leaders; they need to be flexible about scheduling demos, teaching parents the basic skills, and adapting to circumstances that arise in particular groups. For example, leaders may have planned for three demos in one of their early meetings, with two siblings from one family. But at the last minute, when it is too late to slot in another family's children to focus on, the two siblings are unable to attend. These gaps need to be put to good use by leaders to work on skills training and other extras that are scheduled for future meetings in the program.

This need for adaptability, as we have explained already, requires leaders to be very mindful of the overall program goals and the program's training requirements, rather than being prepared only for the next few meetings. However, keeping to the progression from one stage in the program to the next also is essential for leaders to maintain. Therefore the pacing of each of these early meetings is very important for groups, especially for those with the maximum number of children.

GROUPS WITH LARGE NUMBERS

When leaders have nine or ten children to fit into demos, timing is particularly tight. Leaders have to be very much on top of the time, and be certain that major points are covered, while postponing parental concerns that are not so critical. Leaders need to keep track of these parental concerns for later discussion, and convey to parents: *"That's something we will need to deal with. However, tonight, we need to..."*

Another suggestion when the meeting's agenda is long (e.g. three demos, parental feedback from four parents, three discussions of demos, and some skills practice) is to consider shortening the demos to ten minutes per child, while still ensuring that sibling groups are scheduled in the same meeting. A possible secondary effect of such a tight agenda may be that the meeting ends approximately ten minutes late. (This time adjustment, of course, needs to be negotiated with group members during the previous meeting.)

FLEXIBILITY IN TEACHING SKILLS

Leaders also may find that they need to spend a little less time on skills practice during one of the early meetings of GFT, if, for example, the demos have run on too long, or the discussion has become too complex. A particular group may become highly involved in the demos and learn a great deal from them, with the result that formal skills training becomes less of a focus during that meeting. Other times, however, leaders can cover a large amount in skills training.

As already mentioned, the order of teaching skills suggested here also may vary sometimes. It is very much in keeping with the spirit of GFT to come back after very emotionally engaging demos and adjust the training to where parents' experiences and motivation strongly lie. For example, where the demos for Meeting 3 turn out to be dominated by allowing children to lead, leaders need to discuss and practice that skill in more depth with the group, because the training is timely, even though their planned focus was empathy. When such adjustments are made, leaders should inform parents that empathy and acceptance in the play sessions are primary, but sometimes, because of the children's activity in demos, the group needs to learn first about a different skill and then return to empathy in the next session. (Leaders should remind themselves in these exceptional cases that parents will not have any difficulty with this order of teaching, since they do not have experience of any other approach. It is the leaders themselves who must adapt to this change.) Leaders also should be aware that they need to pace the skills training throughout Meetings 2–4, in order not to cram too much of the formal skills training and practice into Meeting 4.

Beginning skills training

It is essential during early skills training that the leaders' approach is somewhat light hearted, low key and humorous, especially for parents who experience performance anxiety. Parents' anxiety about their competence also may lead them to engage in more animated conversation and information gathering or giving in order to postpone practice, as discussed earlier in the book. If this occurs, leaders need to take the initiative and move into skills practice, explaining that questions and information giving will be addressed another time. However, leaders also should remember not to get too intent on skills teaching and ignore parents' indications that they are dealing with their own emotional responses to events. In the latter circumstance, leaders' main role is to empathize with and understand these feelings. When leaders respond empathically to parents in GFT, as stated earlier, parents usually are released from troubling feelings and able to return to learning. We remind leaders that it also is important after responding empathically to a parent that leaders return to teaching the group, and do not get sidetracked into a one-to-one discussion.

Leaders may need to stress that learning the main therapeutic skills in early meetings serves parents well throughout the program. Leaders can encourage parents, if the same skills teaching issue arises several times during early meetings, that learning these skills takes time and that this is the beginning of a process of learning. Leaders also can remind parents that many issues will be looked at later, as parents become more familiar with these skills and ready to start home sessions.

Materials for leaders to supply for practice exercises

Leaders provide packets with small toys for parents to use for skills training; one packet for every two parents suffices. Each packet should be filled with small items (e.g. blocks, paper for drawing, crayons or colored pencils, cars, a deck of playing cards, necklaces, soldiers). These toys make it a little more realistic for parents to practice in role-play style the skills they need to learn, such as setting limits or playing the role of a racing car driver. Keeping these bags ready for handing out each week at the start of skills practice lightens the work of leaders and involves minimal expense, particularly when these toys are rounded up from leaders' practice settings.

Each week leaders can include 3 × 5 cards in the toy packet with play scenarios as suggestions for parents to develop during their practice. For example, a card might say:

> Here are two scenarios you can develop in your play. Please choose one of the following, or do one of your own: "Cars in a traffic jam and an accident" or "Fixing and eating dinner, with someone coming late for dinner."

Leaders can use this opportunity to remind parents that they will be collecting their own toys soon for play sessions at home and that a list of toys and ample time to discuss details of these toys further will be provided in a later meeting, along with a recommended list of materials.

Introducing the skills

One leader introduces Meeting 3's skills training on empathic responding, which includes "showing understanding," and "tracking." Leaders already discussed some of the rationales for these skills during the first two meetings where opportune moments arose, and used relevant rationales. When helping parents practice any of the main four skills, leaders need to start with the basics within each skill and then build on parents' learning towards more advanced skills development. Leaders also need to preview for parents the other skills they will be learning; however, it is not useful to do this in too much detail during the early part of the program.

Leaders may wish to introduce skills practice by reminding parents that the core skills will be integrated into a whole package for them after each skill is learned separately. This will happen as part of a "mock" play session with a leader pretending to be a child. Mock sessions are scheduled for the meeting before any parents begin conducting practice play sessions with their children.

We suggest leaders introduce the skill of empathic responding by paraphrasing the following:

The skills we will be learning now help children to know that their parents are showing understanding of them, and taking their point of view. Children can then figure out their own feelings better. This helps children feel emotionally safer and more secure. This is similar to what you already tried to do with your children as babies: you tried to follow their leads in what interested them, showed you understood their basic feelings verbally and non-verbally, and gave them periods of close and sensitive attention. You will be building on these things and learning two main skills. We will be practicing "tracking," which is making brief comments on what your children are doing, so that they know you are with them and not ignoring them. This skill of tracking is practiced along with the other skill of "responding to children's feelings." Sometimes the skill of tracking is referred to as "restating the content of what children are doing." In the first part of your training in tracking, you will be asked to say what you think are the most important things that are happening in the play, just as you saw us [leaders] doing during demos.

At this point, leaders should try to draw out parents on what they saw in the demos so far, and help them come up with a couple of examples of tracking responses that leaders have made. Leaders may have to give clues to help the group remember and relate the demos to this skill, if this new concept proves difficult for parents to pick out. For example, one child may have zeroed in on the sand during a demo. The leader can help the group recall what was said during the demo. For example, *"Do you remember when Aaron ran over to the sand? He seemed so eager and the leader said, 'You're really hurrying over to that sand!'"* Or a leader may give another example of a child who played for a long time with the baby doll, feeding and dressing it:

> *Do you remember when Beth played with the baby doll for such a long time? She wasn't saying much, and neither did I [the leader]. Beth knew that I was still interested when she heard me say after a while, "You're making sure that doll is wrapped up warmly."*

Leaders using this kind of example of a quiet child also may point out that it usually takes parents a while to know when to comment verbally and when to focus on their children without saying anything. Leaders may wish to add: *"Children are not used to parents tracking what they are doing, so it sometimes takes both children and parents a little while to get used to this skill."*

We advise leaders to spend only a short time on teaching the tracking skill and then quickly move on to teaching parents how to "show understanding." Leaders should point out how important it is for parents to learn and practice what feelings children have underneath what they are doing. If the leaders used the last example of Beth, they could say:

> *For Beth, she seemed to be feeling very loving towards the baby doll she was caring for. Her feeling of love for the baby seemed important for me [the leader] to mention during the demo. Maybe you remember what I said.*

(Again, leaders may need to provide clues, if parents find this recall difficult.)

> *Remember that showing understanding goes below the action—what children are doing—and identifies the feelings beneath the action. An example of tracking is:*

"You are rocking the baby." The response getting at the child's feeling is: *"You are enjoying rocking the baby."*

Exercise 1A: large group exercise on empathic responding

Once the skills themselves are introduced, leaders first practice very basic feelings and actions with everyone in the large group. One of the leaders enacts brief play examples in the role of a "child," and the other leader prompts for answers (or one leader does both tasks). The leader as "child" should use normal play sequences, playing out a child without emotional problems who is playing alone. Leaders should have a readily accessible stock of normal play scenarios to draw from. These normal play sequences are designed, as stated earlier, to reassure parents that their own play sessions will be manageable, and to allow them to concentrate on their skills learning, rather than risk their becoming engrossed in the play itself. It also is essential that the leader as "child" act out feelings very clearly, with definite facial expressions and actions. During these role-plays, the leader as "child" gives pregnant pauses and parents are asked to give feedback on the feelings and actions being displayed, as illustrated next.

ILLUSTRATIVE EXAMPLE: CONDUCTING THE FIRST PART OF EXERCISE 1A

> *Leader 1: We want you to watch me play as a child—that may be the most challenging part of this exercise—to imagine me as a child!*
>
> The leader plays out a child who tries a few times to hitch a trailer onto the cab of a truck, and then pauses.
>
> *Leader 2: What tracking response can you make there?*
>
> After this question is answered successfully, Leader 1, as "child," starts shaking the trailer, saying crossly "That dumb trailer," along with showing frustration facially.
>
> *Leader 2: What would you say now? What is the "child" feeling?*
>
> Leader 2 might want to suggest alternatives here and have the group choose the right answer (e.g. *Is the child feeling calm, sad, or annoyed?*), if they seem stuck.
>
> Next, the leader as "child" plays out trying and succeeding in getting building blocks to stand up in a tower. The other leader asks the parents, *"What is he doing? What do you say now? What is the feeling?"*

Some groups that seem unable to respond easily on this feeling level to these uncomplicated exercises may need to get in touch with their own feelings before moving on to children's feelings. If necessary, leaders should talk about simple things in daily life that generate feelings in people (e.g. *"You were overcharged at the store. How do you feel?"*). The leader can practice this scenario in front of the whole group with one of the parents, asking this parent to briefly describe how they are feeling in this situation, with the leader reflecting their feelings.

After the parents become more successful in recognizing feelings and tracking responses in very basic examples, a leader then plays out a scenario showing several feelings in sequence. The leader should ask parents to call out, during (deliberate) pauses in the play, the "child's" feelings and the tracking comments they would make. Sometimes in this exercise on sequencing of empathic responses, parents have trouble going beyond their first response and get stuck on the second and third feelings. In nearly every group, someone says, *"I can respond to the first feeling easily enough, but after that I'm at a loss."* Therefore, extending the role-playing through several exchanges is recommended in order to extend the parents' response repertoires, as the next example shows.

ILLUSTRATIVE EXAMPLE: CONDUCTING THE LATTER PART OF EXERCISE 1A

> *Leader: You need to call out the feelings I am showing when I have a long pause. You can call out a tracking response a few times too. Don't worry! I'll be an easy child to read, with clear feelings. After we do this together, both of us leaders will show you what we want you to do in pairs.*

The leader then plays out, with pregnant pauses, a child, say, who, playing a ring toss game on his own, displays a range of feelings as the game progresses (e.g. excitement, persistence, frustration, success, and boredom), and who then goes on to play with the cars, lining them up on the floor before having them crash into one another.

Exercise 1B: the first role-play exercise

After leaders help parents successfully respond to tracking and empathic feeling responses during a longer play sequence, leaders then model the next exercise. In this exercise, parents are asked to split into pairs, with one parent taking the role of the child and the other giving tracking and empathic responses to the "child's" play. In their demonstration of this exercise, one leader takes the child's role and the other takes the parent's role. For large groups, leaders may choose to divide the group into two subgroups with one leader each. In such subgroups, each leader should select the most relaxed parent to pair up with for this demonstration of skills, assigning the parent the child's role, and suggest one or two play sequences to this parent. This help enables the parent to more easily and quickly adopt a child's role. Single leaders also need to adopt this approach for their whole group. Leaders need to ensure that there is enough time to complete this paired exercise and discussion before the end of the meeting.

PRACTICING IN PAIRS: WHY IT IS HELPFUL

We suggest leaders do not spend time discussing the skills they modeled, and instead quickly move the parents on to their own practice in pairs. Not only is learning facilitated by this opportunity to act and react in this skill modality, but practicing in pairs minimizes embarrassment and awkwardness that might occur in the larger group. Everyone in the group is occupied with trying this new behavior, and they are not being observed by the entire group. Working together in pairs to master a skill also seems to serve as a rapid "group consolidator," allowing parents to show support of one another's successes and understanding of one another's failures during feedback on the exercises afterwards in the large group. This enables parents to become more adept at role-playing as a technique, and to gain practice in specific skills.

PRACTICING IN PAIRS: HOW IT IS DONE

Leaders should explain to parents that role-plays are intended to be easy to do, not a major crisis in the making! Parents are asked to pair up with the person sitting next to them for this exercise. (Leaders should use a threesome, if there is an uneven number in the group.) If these two parents are members of a couple, leaders suggest that they should pair up with someone else. Becoming familiar with other group members besides the ones they already know can help promote group cohesiveness. However, when a pair has finished the task to their satisfaction, they frequently start extraneous conversations that are pleasant, but not a good use of group time. When leaders discover that most pairs are beginning to converse, they should direct group members to reverse roles, take on another exercise, or reassemble if the task is completed. Leaders also need to mention to parents that they will be circulating around the pairs to see how their practice is going. A suggested introduction to this exercise is:

> You have now seen us do the kind of practice we are asking you to do together in pairs. We want one of you to take the child's role for five minutes—we'll give you suggestions for a few play sequences in a minute, or you can do your own easy ones—and the other person will show understanding by reflecting the feelings of this "child" and tracking some of what they are doing. We'll then have you reverse roles and play again. We'll walk around to keep track of how things are going for you. After that, we'll all come back together and talk about it.

Leaders ask parents when they are playing the child's role to play a child they are very familiar with, but not a child who is out of control or unable to play. If these suggestions are not concrete enough for some parents, then leaders may recommend that they play "a happy child getting into their playing" or suggest to parents that they may want to use something easy they saw one of the children doing in the demos and act that out themselves. The suggestions included in the packets of toys for play scenarios also may be helpful for some parents, if they do not have any ideas themselves.

WHEN TO BEGIN WITH THE LARGE GROUP OPTION

When the group splits up into pairs easily and readily begins role-playing, leaders monitor how each pair is doing unobtrusively. However, if the group seems very hesitant to pair up and take on the assigned roles in this first exercise, there is another recommended option. Leaders can suggest that one of them will role-play with a parent in front of the whole group first, and follow the same approach outlined earlier for split and single-leader groups. After this large group exercise, the leader first asks the parent who participated how that felt, and then very briefly discusses examples of reflecting feelings and tracking from this exercise, before moving on to the paired exercise for all group members. Again, leaders have to ensure that there is enough time before the end of the meeting to give all the parents time to practice this skill in pairs and discuss the exercise afterwards.

PROMPTING DURING ROLE-PLAY EXERCISES

Parents practice in pairs while leaders circulate singly among the pairs in an unobtrusive way—it is not a time for leaders to talk to one another—showing parents that they are available to pairs for consulting. If leaders need to help pairs, they should aim to work with each set of role-players long enough to provide positive reinforcement and corrective feedback. However, inexperienced leaders may not realize that sometimes adults feel more comfortable talking about what they are supposed to do, rather than enacting their role-plays. In these cases, it is important that leaders do not engage the parents in extended discussions, but instead refocus the pair onto continuing their skills practice. We recommend leaders circulate around and sit with each pair. Sometimes whispering suggestions to the pair during their role-play is useful; however, leaders need to remember not to interrupt too much.

DISCUSSION AFTER THE EXERCISE

After the practice in pairs, one of the leaders begins the discussion of this exercise with participants. The leader first asks parents, *"How did that practice go for you?"*, drawing out a range of parents' feelings, and trying to include more reserved parents in this discussion. Some of the usual feelings parents state are that it was *"hard to do," "unnatural," "easy to understand some of the feelings but not others," "hard to find the right words for the feelings,"* and *"interesting to try."* After leaders make empathic responses to parents' comments, and remind them of the rationales for the skills where appropriate, leaders may wish to point out that this task is demanding because parents were attending to both the content of what was being played out and the underlying feelings, just like they will be doing in their children's play sessions.

Leaders should then concentrate on successful responses. They first ask parents what they thought went well, if this has not already emerged in the discussion. If parents are reluctant or unable to respond, leaders are able to point out successful responses they witnessed during their circulation around the pairs during the exercise. Leaders should aim to end the exercise on a positive note. As mentioned earlier, adult learners can be highly self-critical when learning new skills, forgetting that adulthood does not confer special, superhuman powers of learning! Leaders often need to help parents to look at positive responses, while remaining empathic towards them in their struggles.

Other issues related to early skills training

USING ROLE-PLAY JUDICIOUSLY

When leaders introduce role-play to parents, they may need to give several suggestions to them of how to play the child's role, since this role is outside of their normal adult experience. In addition, it is important for leaders not to overload participants at this early stage in the program, and to remember that parents will want a very brief trial, rather than a lengthy role-play, for their first exercise. Therefore, leaders need to be casual about the first exercises, and not overwhelm parents with too many toys or instructions.

While role-play is probably the best single device for demonstrating and practicing skills in GFT, we remind readers that it can be overdone. Leaders should encourage, rather than force, parents to role-play, if they are not ready for it, or if they are reluctant to take part in a demonstration in front of the group. Also, it should not be overused because it can become tiresome quickly, especially when parents are not skilled at it, and when there are only a limited number of roles to be played. This is why short role-plays are suggested during early skills training in GFT.

Refining empathic responses by parents

Leaders actively help parents make clear "feelings statements," such as *"You like that"* and *"You're angry about that."* Leaders should not expect parents to have verbal responses that are perfect during early role-plays. For these early stages in learning empathic reflecting, leaders need to settle for less, and ensure that parents learn to have the basics of empathy, before refinements are made. For example, leaders should not exaggerate the importance of the quality of the wording of parents' reflective responses during early skills training. Leaders may accept at this point that a parent reflects *"You don't know if you feel you can get the right answer"* instead of *"You're afraid you will fail."*

With minor errors, such as tacking on a question at the end of an empathic statement (e.g. *"isn't it?"*), or using *"You feel"* prior to addressing a relevant feeling, parents should be gently reminded these are not preferred. Leaders can say:

> You really accurately reflected his feeling. Next time, just leave off the question at the end. Remember that we specialize in making statements in the play sessions. If you are really so uncertain of the feeling that you thought you should reflect, it may be better not to say it at all, and maybe make a tracking comment, than to suggest that the "child" should be agreeing or disagreeing with you.

Reinforcing parents' efforts

Leaders reinforce any or all steps in the right direction. Shaping to reach the ideal responses will follow, once basics have been fully demonstrated. Leaders may wish to adopt the teaching rule: *"Strive to get appropriate responses in the beginning, then guide parents to more refined and totally accurate reflections of deepest feelings in the later stages."* In general, leaders should try to eliminate undesirable responses in the early stages of training in as many ways as possible, without undermining parents' confidence in their ability to learn new skills. Correction on the part of leaders is particularly important when parents reflect feelings that are not capturing deeper feelings. For example, some parents can overuse the phrase *"You like/don't like that"* with their children. Helping parents to widen the range of feelings they observe and reflect is very important for leaders to do in these cases, while maintaining parents' morale. By asking for possible feeling words in examples given during large group exercises, especially when more than one parent has this difficulty, leaders deflect from any implied criticism of individual parents. It is worth underlining here that leaders also must always work actively against any parental responses during GFT that potentially insult, belittle, or criticize their own and others' children, and children in general.

Overall, we suggest that leaders avoid "don't do" statements, and give positively worded alternatives instead to what was said. Positive teaching is much more effective in the authors' experience. At this early stage, it is vital that leaders set the tone for the group of being accepting and not overly demanding of results from skills training, to counteract the tendency already discussed of adults' tendency to be unduly self-critical. Leaders may suggest that parents might want to work on being kind to themselves and not too demanding of their need to "get it right." The leaders need to show by example that the group is intended to be a place to practice and learn, not a place to receive a mark or grade.

Leaders may want to explain to the group that it is difficult for everyone to keep new skills in mind at the beginning and to inhibit their usual responses. We often find it useful to remind parents what struggles they had mastering other skills in their lives when they first started, such as riding a two-wheel bike, roller skating, or learning to play the piano. Leaders may wish to remind parents:

> Skills learning requires that you first go through the steps to master what is required, and then have a considerable time, in most cases, to actually put this understanding into action. Usually many practices are required before being able to exercise the skill smoothly.

Helping a parent who is emotionally burdened during skills training

Sometimes starting to practice therapeutic skills during GFT can trigger traumatic memories and emotional distress in parents unexpectedly. An example of a parent who has serious difficulty accepting the value of empathic responding is the following.

> Mary: I have a lot of trouble talking about the feelings that a child is supposed to be having. I was taught by my own mom and dad that what I felt was not important. Doing what we were supposed to do, regardless of how we felt, was the most important thing. I can understand what you are suggesting, but I am having a lot of trouble really acting on it. My own life has always been "duty above everything else."

> Leader 1: In your own life you were taught that there is no room for feelings to get in the way of what you're supposed to do. It is hard for you to let go of that when you're practicing playing with Jimmy [her son]. Not just because of the habit of thinking that way, but because you wonder if it's really right to focus so much on feelings.

> Mary: Yes, I am afraid that I will make Jimmy think that feelings are more important than doing the right thing.

The leaders continued to respond with empathy to Mary. However, she then began talking about her own childhood, and how not doing what she was supposed to do resulted in severe punishment. It was clear to the leaders at this point that Mary was burdened with more than just new didactic information that she had to process. Both leaders sensed that there was a great deal of past material for her to deal with, before she could apply new learning to play sessions effectively. They therefore suggested that they arrange a time to talk further with Mary after the meeting. The leader then returned to the teaching on empathic responding for the group, and suggested that Mary may need to observe, rather than participate in, any further role-plays during the meeting. During their discussion afterwards with Mary, who remained very distraught, the leaders suggested that seeing another therapist outside of GFT would be helpful.

Empathy in relation to teaching on other facets of CCPT

Leaders should remember that, once parents understand the basic concepts involved in empathy, other issues become more meaningful to discuss and practice as they arise in future demos and practice play sessions. Therefore it is important that parents are taught first, if at all possible, to concentrate on what their children are feeling and how to show understanding of these feelings. For instance, in the extended example of Meeting 2's group discussion in the last chapter, leaders taught parents to find the underlying emotional needs being conveyed within questions during play sessions, and to use empathy first, instead of simply answering children's questions factually. However, even though several points about asking questions may have been made in an early meeting by leaders, often it is only when parents practice the skill of showing understanding themselves that they begin to be able to think deeply about and apply these principles. Parents' insights may occur after demos and during skills training, but it usually arises during their practice play sessions and the discussions that follow.

This chapter set out teaching the essential skill of "showing understanding." The next chapter discusses the remainder of the CCPT skills taught to parents, before they undertake a mock play session with leaders in which they apply all the skills together, as needed.

CHAPTER 8

Continuing Demonstrations and Skills Practice

Meeting 4

This chapter concentrates on parents' skills learning in the fourth meeting. The second, third and fourth basic skills—following children's lead during play sessions, structuring, and limit setting, respectively—are introduced and actively practiced by parents. Meeting 4 also prepares parents for their mock sessions during the next meeting in the program. In the first part of Meeting 4, leaders finish conducting the remainder of the demos with children in the program, followed by discussion of the demos, as discussed in the previous two chapters. Skills training is the main aim in the second part of Meeting 4 after the break, for approximately 45 minutes; a briefer time is allocated for discussing the demos than in previous meetings.

The examples and discussions in this chapter also show that from Meeting 4 onwards, and occasionally by Meeting 3, leaders address particular issues parents begin to raise about their children, their worries about them, and their own parenting responses, in addition to carrying out their main task of skills learning.

Skills training: following children's lead

Children generally request parents to witness or participate in their play. First, leaders provide the rationales (see Chapter 4) for parents learning to follow their children's lead in play sessions (e.g. children work on their emotional issues themselves and become more able to master them). Then leaders ask parents to give shared examples from demos that showed this skill in action, just as they did for the skill of empathic understanding during the previous meeting. Leaders again may have to give clues to help the group remember and relate the demos to this skill, if this new concept proves difficult for parents to pick out. Leaders should emphasize that children either tell their parents, or give other obvious non-verbal clues, whether they want parents to witness or to take part in their play. Leaders may wish to give their own examples from real life and from demos of how children are able to play spontaneously and relax when they know there is no pressure either to perform in a certain way or to include others in their play.

Leaders should remind parents that, if children want their parents to act as witnesses to their play or activities, parents actively use the skills they practiced during Meeting 3, those of tracking their children's activities and making comments that show they understand their children's feelings. This is a prime place for leaders to review the empathic skill, if this has not already been done during the discussion of the meeting's demos. Leaders can ask parents to pick out a few examples from Meeting 4 demos where leaders showed understanding of children's feelings and tracked them. After this brief review, leaders should then turn to the main ways that parents take part in activities with their children during play sessions and follow their lead. These include giving practical assistance, participating in an activity (e.g. making something, playing a game), and being involved in imaginative play, all under the direction (specific or implied) of their children.

Exercise 2A: following children's lead

As stated earlier, leaders most usefully start this exercise by drawing out parents' examples from demos of leaders following their children's leads. However, if these examples are not forthcoming, or if the group seems to need more specific training in this skill, leaders may wish to use their own examples or make use of some of the brief examples that follow. The first example concerns responding when practical assistance is requested by children. The negative and positive examples here can be given, and leaders can then ask which choice actually follows the child's lead.

EXERCISE 2A1: PRACTICAL ASSISTANCE AND FOLLOWING CHILDREN'S LEAD

The leader can introduce this in the following way:

> We've already said that play sessions are not a time to teach your children how to be independent, and how to do things. And it's not a time to have your children see what skilled and capable adults you are yourselves! During these sessions your children can decide what they are capable of doing, or how much they want help right now (even for things they are capable of doing themselves). Remember, you are already learning to focus on your children's feelings. These feelings are important to respond to first. I'll give you two examples and you can tell me, when I'm finished, which one is the response to use during play sessions.

> (Negative illustration:)

> Mandy [8 years old]: Daddy, I want you to put the doll's clothes away.

> Dad: You can do that for yourself, Mary.

> Mandy: I don't want to do it right now.

> Dad: Come on, Mandy, just do it.

Mandy: It's hard to put them away.

Dad: It's not. I'll show you how to do it the easy way.

(Positive illustration:)

Mandy [8 years old]: Daddy, I want you to put the doll's clothes away.

Dad: You want me to help you (focusing on Mandy's feelings).

Mandy: I don't want to do it right now.

Dad: You can do it, but right now you want me to help.

(Dad then puts them away as requested.)

Leader: Which Dad followed Mandy's lead? What feelings did he reflect?

If parents question why the father in the positive illustration put the clothes away, leaders may add that everybody feels like Mandy sometimes, that it's just so nice to be taken care of, and not have to work at it yourself all the time. The other rationale leaders may offer is that children tend to have a drive towards autonomy and self-fulfillment. In general, people *don't* like to have everything done for them, but children are learning all the time about what they can manage, and what they can't. They need time to assimilate this knowledge about themselves. They also need some space and time to not have to perform optimally and independently. This may be a good place for leaders to introduce the idea that sometimes children have particular issues that they revisit in their play sessions from their care in earlier childhood, and this can result in wanting to be taken care of in play sessions.

PARENTS' REACTIONS TO CHILDREN'S NEED FOR NURTURANCE

Parents can have difficulties with the ideas mentioned earlier about children showing immature behavior, and with some other rationales set out in Chapter 4. Leaders could mention that CCPT is designed to allow children to make their own corrective moves, to help them attain the level of autonomy that best meets their needs. However, again it is very important for leaders to empathize with parents' negative feelings, and not to try to convince them cognitively, when they have emotional issues. As we discussed in earlier chapters, parents may feel threatened emotionally when their children show immature behavior, fearing their children will remain immature in daily life when this behavior is accepted in play sessions. Other parents may have the opposite difficulty, and insist on doing things for their children that they wish to master for themselves. Leaders need to respond to all these parental feelings with empathy, and often need to acknowledge that CCPT skills feel foreign and puzzling when they are new. Sometimes leaders need to reflect that parents have to trust leaders in a lot of things during their early training, before seeing the effects of play sessions for themselves.

EXERCISE 2A2: PARTICIPATING IN GAMES

Another common occurrence during play sessions is for children to give their own rule variations for standard games. If spontaneous examples have not arisen during demos, leaders may need to use the types of examples offered here to help parents distinguish between directive and non-directive responses when their children play standard games during play sessions.

(Negative illustration:)

Rosie [6 years old]: Let's play Snap.

Mom: Let's sit at this table. Then we'll have room to play.

Mom: You're having me turn up lots of cards, and you're waiting with your fish. You know how to play Snap. You have to turn one up the same time, and let go of your fish. (Rosie ignores Mom.)

Rosie: I got it!! Snap!! I won!!

Mom: You didn't win. You cheated!

(Positive illustration:)

Rosie [6 years old]: Let's play Snap.

Mom: You want me to sit here. You're having me turn up lots of cards, and you're waiting with your fish...waiting to find one of my fish.

Rosie: I got it!! Snap!! I won!!

Mom: You're excited!! You won! It's the way you like to play Snap in our play sessions.

Leader: Which Mom followed the child's lead? What feelings did she reflect?

DISCUSSION OF FOLLOWING CHILDREN'S LEAD IN GAME PLAYING

Game playing can arouse strong feelings in parents, as well as in their children.

Leaders should aim to give parents developmental information where needed, and always empathize with parents' reactions. For example, leaders can point out that in play sessions children can choose to *try out* how to take part in games. Leaders may also acknowledge that parents want to teach their children to play games by the rules because this is the way they want them to operate in real life. Leaders need to remind parents that in play sessions children lead the way and often make themselves winners by deliberately violating the rules, or giving themselves an advantage. Play sessions permit children opportunities to shed responsibility for playing games by the usual rules. Leaders can briefly explain that children often use play sessions to learn to cope with issues such as cooperation, jealousy, achievement, and power, all of which are steps in learning to deal with failure, as well as success. They may allow themselves temporarily to experience the pleasure of winning, even though they realize that they violated rules to do so. Often it is too painful emotionally for these children to lose, and in play sessions they are spared that pain. This counter-experience can, in time, help children cope with loss when they cannot win. Parents therefore accept their children's need to win, rightly or wrongly, in their play sessions.

Leaders should add that this assumes that a child has reached the stage developmentally to know how to play games. Preschoolers may not have any real understanding of a game, so that when they play it their own way it may be out of ignorance, rather than respite from the constriction of rules. However, the purpose of play sessions is not to teach the rules, unless children specifically ask their parents for rule clarification.

Some difficult feelings parents have about following their children's lead in games are as follows:

- My child will never have any friends, if he cheats in games.

- My child will never learn the right way to do things.

- My child will get confused.

- My child will always expect to win.

- My child is getting spoiled by me.

Leaders need to acknowledge these feelings, if they arise, and that it is hard for parents to give up some of their goals for their children in play sessions. Leaders should agree that parents do need to teach their children how to get along with other people, and how to manage losing games outside the play session. In addition, it is helpful for parents to hear from leaders that this need to win is commonly a phase in play therapy, and rarely generalizes to outside the play sessions. Children are generally able to distinguish situations where they know that they are not leading the way.

ILLUSTRATIVE EXAMPLE

The following is a dialogue leaders had with a parent who was distressed about her daughter's cheating during an early practice play session. The mother, Beth, has already realized that her play session responses are not the same as the ones she makes in her daily life:

> *Beth: I have always believed for myself, and taught my children, that cheating in games was a very bad thing. It really is hard for me not to try to get Sally to play by the rules in the play session. I just have to grit my teeth not to correct her. When she is delighted that she has won by cheating, I can't bring myself to reflect that delight. I guess I should, if I am really showing I understand her feelings.*

> *Leader 1: It just grates on your nerves to have to watch her do things that go against your principles.*

> *Beth: Yes!! I'm worried too that if she gets away with it in the session with me, that she'll think that it's OK to do anything to have the pleasure of winning, anytime with anybody. I really don't want her to be a "cheater."*

> *Leader 1: It's hard for you to believe that Sally won't think that the new play session rules that she set up for herself to win will not be carried over to real life.*

> *Leader 2 (having the role of commenting didactically): That is the way learning frequently takes place, with children trying something out in one place and, when it works, trying it someplace else. However, I can assure you that feedback given*

to Sally in the real world will make her realize, probably sooner than later, that people outside of play sessions will not show the same acceptance.

Does Sally play games with her brother, Mike? You probably know that he would "tell on her," or tell her off for not playing by real-life rules. However, I am guessing that Sally already knows the difference between her play session ways of doing things and the outside world. Most children learn the distinction after only two or three sessions, if not immediately. You are free to remind them, if they try to play by play session rules outside, that "Now, we are outside and do not play by play session rules." If children object and say, "Why not? It's more fun!" parents can say, "What you do in play sessions ends when they end. Rules outside stay the same."

Beth: I'll try to think about what Sally does as special to the play session, and just continue to keep to what I think is important at home.

Leader 1: You'll try your best. We'll come back to this later in the program, when we think about daily life, after Sally has had a lot more play sessions. We'll see where she is then.

This dialogue, as well as illustrating how leaders can respond to parents' worries about following their children's lead in games, also shows how parents are given developmental and play therapy information and helped to keep their focus on learning to conduct play sessions, rather than generalizing their emerging, less practiced, skills too early to daily life. In addition, the example shows that briefer conversations about following children's lead are usually appropriate to introduce the skill to parents in the early meetings, but, when either a demo by a leader or a parent's early practice play session brings this issue out more vividly, it is important that leaders respond more fully to these teaching opportunities. Finally, the example illustrates again the value of dividing up the tasks between the two leaders.

EXERCISE 2A3: PARTICIPATING IN ACTIVITIES

We next turn to examples leaders can use, if demo examples are not available, for helping parents learn how to follow their children's lead in activities at their children's request.

Leader: In these next two examples, a child wants his parent to draw a park scene while he works on cutting out what they have already done.

(Negative illustration:)

Pete (looking at what he is cutting out): Mom, you draw children at the park.

Mom: What park should it be?

Pete (not looking up): Our park.

Mom (pausing): Should I put a boy like you in the park?

Pete (gets involved in Mom's drawing): Put the boy there, and put his friend on the swings...

(Positive illustration:)

Pete (looking at what he is cutting out): *Mom, you draw children at the park.*

Mom (drawing what has been asked): *You want me to do that.*

Pete: *That's good [the swings] but I don't want that boy there.*

Mom (pausing): *I did it wrong. You don't like that.*

Pete: *Start again.*

Leader: *Which mom followed the child's lead? What feelings did she reflect?*

If parents do not make the point themselves during feedback, leaders should point out that the parent in the first case influenced Pete to lose interest in what he was planning, and become involved in her drawing instead. Leaders can point out that parents can shift the focus of playtimes for their children, like the first mother did, even though they have the best possible intentions.

EXERCISE 2A4: FOLLOWING THE CHILD'S LEAD IN IMAGINATIVE PLAY

We now turn to examples leaders can use, if demo examples are insufficient, for helping parents learn how to follow their children's lead in imaginative play.

Leader: *In these next two examples, a child wants her dad to take the part of the monster in her story. Her story is about a princess who is frightened of being eaten.*

(Negative illustration:)

Jane (wearing a crown): *Dad, I'm the princess and you're the monster—wear that scary mask. You try to eat me up!*

Dad: *I don't want to eat you up. I think I'll be a nice monster, and wear that hat instead.*

Jane: *You be the monster and try to run after me.*

Dad (laughing): *OK, I'm the cookie monster and you're my cookie!*

(Positive illustration:)

Jane (wearing a crown): *Dad, I'm the princess and you're the monster—wear that scary mask. You try to eat me up!*

Dad: *You want me to scare you! I'll be a scary monster coming to get you! (Dad puts on the mask.)*

Jane: *You try to run after me now.*

Dad (laughing): *OK, Grrrr...here I come, princess!*

Leader: *Which dad followed the child's lead? What feelings did he reflect?*

DISCUSSION OF PARENTS' PARTICIPATING IN IMAGINATIVE PLAY

Leaders should point out, if parents themselves do not, that the second example showed how the father followed his child's lead, taking on the role assigned and responding to clues about how to play the part. Leaders can add that parents should try to match the emotional tone, in this case the excitement of the girl, when they respond in role, but not to overplay it too much. This is in order to allow the children to identify the part, along with the feelings that are to be expressed, as well as having the main feelings themselves. It works well, leaders can note, if parents act out their roles more playfully by using different voices and sounds, as the dad in the example did by saying "Grrrr" and talking as the monster. It may also be important for the group to have a discussion about how the dad in the negative example tried to protect his daughter from the aggressive play, perhaps because he did not like to be placed in this role, even in play. Leaders should discuss how pretend play can be powerful emotionally, and it is important for parents to notice when they think their children do seem overwhelmed by their fantasy play. However, in general, children do not need this amount of protection by their parents.

Exercise 2B: following children's lead

After using the earlier large group examples to introduce the skill of following the child's lead, leaders then model the next, paired exercise for parents. Leaders use their own small toys for this modeling, and parents are given the toy packets created for the parent training for their practice in pairs afterwards. Cards are placed in each packet with at least four play scenarios. These are suggestions for parents to develop, if they choose, in the paired "follow the lead," "structuring," and "limit setting" exercises to follow.

In this exercise, one parent in the pair again takes the "child" role, and the other takes the "parent" role and follows the "child's" lead. If time permits, it is useful to have pairs practice making responses when witnessing the "child" playing on their own first, then have the "parent" follow the "child's" lead during the "parent's" involvement in the "child's" activity. (If there are time constraints, the most important one is the latter.) Parents are asked to build on their previous learning, and give empathic responses (e.g. reflections and tracking comments) to the "child's" feelings. Again, leaders should not spend time discussing the skills they model. The group needs to move on to their own practice in pairs, with leaders circulating around the pairs to see how they are going. Parents again need a reminder, when they are playing the child's role, to play a child that they are very familiar with, but not a child who is out of control or unable to play.

A suggested introduction to this exercise is:

> You have now seen the kind of practice we are asking you to do together in pairs. We want one of you to take the child's role for five minutes—we again have given you suggestions for a few play sequences, or you can do your own easy ones— and the other person will follow the "child's" lead and witness the child playing on their own, or involved in an activity chosen by the "child." You will also need to use the skills of showing understanding by reflecting the feelings of this "child" and tracking some of what they are doing. We'll then have you reverse roles and play

again. We'll be circulating as usual to see how you are doing and help you, if you need it. After that, we'll all come back together and talk about it.

DISCUSSION AFTER "FOLLOWING THE LEAD" ROLE-PLAY

One of the leaders begins discussing this exercise by asking parents, *"How did that go for you?"*, drawing out a range of feelings, and trying to include more reserved parents in this discussion. Some of the feelings mentioned by parents are similar to the ones they had in Meeting 3 after the role-play on empathic responding (e.g. *"hard to do, unnatural, easy to understand some of the feelings but not others, hard to find the right words"*). Often parents mention that it was difficult to inhibit their usual responses such as praising, educating, directing, and to stay with following the lead.

Again, leaders should be vigilant of parents who seem to find skills learning difficult because of underlying emotional issues that appear to block their learning. In addition, as well as empathizing with parents' feelings, leaders should tie parents' answers into the skills being taught, and remember to vary their words as they reflect and instruct parents, in order to avoid sounding too repetitious.

AN EXAMPLE OF A PARENT QUESTIONING THE SKILL
OF FOLLOWING CHILDREN'S LEAD

Background: the parent in the "child" role has said to their partner in the "parent" role that the "parent" needs to scrap their drawing and start again. The "parent" brought this issue back to the large group discussion after the role-play.

> *Hazel [the parent]: I really don't get it. Why should I start my drawing again? That's wasting paper.*

> *Leader: It's difficult for you to do this. You don't like it. You'd usually help your child to not waste things. Remember we're trying to learn how to show children that they can lead the way. Following children isn't something that goes with our feelings always. When it bothers your feelings too much, we want you to talk about it here with us, just as you're doing now. But in the play session, try to follow your child as best you can. We'll be teaching you about limits later. You can remind me then to talk about what limits you need.*

After parents' responses to the exercise are acknowledged empathically and leaders have reminded parents of the rationales for the skills where appropriate, leaders should concentrate on examples of successful responses during this exercise. They ask parents what they thought went well, if this has not already emerged in the discussion. If parents are reluctant or unable to respond, leaders point out successful responses they witnessed during their circulation around the pairs during the exercise, and end the discussion on a positive note.

Skills training: structuring

The next main skill to introduce to parents is structuring. The most immediate skill for parents to learn is the structuring message given to children at the beginning and end of their play sessions. Parents already have seen this skill in practice during the demos.

When introducing this skill, leaders should explain the meaning of structuring, which is simply that it involves explaining a situation so that people understand what the situation is, and what to expect of it. An example that may be useful to parents of physical structuring is teachers showing children where to put their coats when they start a new school, and an example of verbal structuring is teachers telling them to go to the toilet and wash their hands before recess. The main rationale for clear and consistent structuring statements at the beginning and the end of play sessions is that they help children know what to expect in play sessions, because they have not experienced them before. Leaders may want to make a general remark about how all of us, young and old, feel better and more relaxed when we know what something is about. (Leaders may choose to make a light-hearted remark that this is what most parents want too, when they start something new, like this group, for example).

Leaders need to remind parents that structuring play sessions is especially important when they are carried out at home. Children need a clear message that play sessions are not the same as daily family life. Parents need to give clear and brief messages, so that children easily understand. Leaders then have parents turn to their Parents' Training Manual and read out the introductory statement—*"[Name of child], this is a very special room [time, place, depending on the space you are using]. You can do ALMOST anything you want.** *If you cannot do something, I will tell you."* (*This statement may include the optional statement: *"You may say anything you want in here."*) —followed by the ending statement: *"[Name of child], our time is up for today. It's time to leave now."* In addition, five-minute and one-minute warnings are always given in a low key as children play, so that they will know how much time they have left (e.g. *"[Name of child], we have (five, then one) minute(s) more to play today."* These are reminders that the play session will end soon, and that children are free to carry on with their activities until the end.

Parents are advised to say the beginning and ending statements in a matter-of-fact, authoritative manner. Structuring statements are intended to convey to children that their parents are in charge of the start of the session, the rules during the session, and the ending. With both the beginning and ending statements, leaders should point out that, just as they saw leaders do during demos, parents should stand up for the beginning and ending statements, to give authority to what they say.

A few children may be unsure of themselves and their parents' reactions in their early play sessions, despite their parents' introductory statement. They may need to have the permissive part of the introductory statement repeated. For example, if children repeatedly ask permission to engage in activities, or seem hesitant in other ways, parents may need to respond with structuring statements during the play session, such as *"In here, it can be any way you want it to be"* and *"Remember, you can do almost anything you want in here."* Finally, leaders prepare parents for the actions they should take, as outlined in the Parents' Training Manual, if their children resist ending.

Next, leaders suggest that parents practice the phrases, voice tone and actions involved in structuring play sessions (i.e. introduction, ending, and one in-session structuring comment) with a partner. Parents are asked to read the statements from their Manual if necessary, and memorize them by the next meeting. After this very brief practice, the group is asked to reconvene for limit-setting training.

Skills training: limit setting

Leaders should note that the preferred order for skills teaching is teaching limit setting last. However, as mentioned already, if this topic arises from observing one or more of the demos, then it is important for leaders to consider limit-setting training for that particular group then and there. In the authors' experience, this happens during early demos more often than not, so leaders need to be prepared.

Leaders introduce the limit-setting skill by pointing out to parents that they will be using this skill themselves, as they have seen leaders do during demos. The success they observed in limit setting by leaders should help parents recognize that the authority in play sessions rests with the adults. This motivates parents to feel that they can maintain this authority themselves. Leaders start by asking parents to give examples of how leaders handled certain situations when their rules were challenged during demos. In some groups, leaders may again have to give clues to parents in order to elicit examples. Leaders then remind parents what they read about limit setting in their Manuals, and go through the main rationales and guidelines for limit setting.

The following points are important to underline:

- One of the main rationales for limit setting in play sessions is that it is the parent's job to make certain that everyone and the equipment are safe.

- It is important during play sessions that rules are narrowed down and only important rules are given to children, so that they can play more freely than in other settings.

- Children are taught the rules for play sessions as the need arises.

- Children are able to choose for themselves to either break the limit and accept the consequences, or not break the limit.

- The consequence of not obeying a parent's rule, after reminders, is that the play session has to finish then and there.

- This way of setting rules helps children to make choices about their behavior, and develops their self-direction and self-control.

- When parents show understanding of their children's feelings while setting limits, children feel more accepted. This usually takes the steam out of their strong, negative feelings.

- When parents carry through with consequences in a calm way, their children recognize that consequences are not merely angry responses from their parents, but rather a result of their failure to follow the rules.

Parents' emotional reactions to this preliminary information on limits should be acknowledged and empathized with by leaders. But it also is important to move this skills training forward, in order to practice all the limit-setting steps during this meeting. Next, leaders need to go through the steps used in setting limits for play sessions in the Parents' Training Manual. The three steps are read through, with examples to illustrate each step, as illustrated here:

Illustration of teaching limit-setting steps

Leader: Step 1 is to state what your child is feeling and then state the rule when your child is just about to break a rule (or is breaking a rule). For example, "[Child's name], you'd like to throw that ball at the clock. I said I'd let you know if you may not do something. (This sentence may need to be eliminated, if quick action is required!) One thing you may not do is throw the ball at the clock."

For most children most of the time, this clear statement of their feelings and the rule in Step 1 is sufficient for them to inhibit their behavior. Step 2 is taken by you if your child breaks the same rule again in the same play session. You give a warning of the consequence, after restating the rule:

"[Child's name], you are starting to throw the ball at the clock. You want to do that again. Remember I said that you may not throw the ball at the clock. If you do that again, we have to end our playtime for today/tonight."

It is important to remember to reflect your child's feelings each time you set the rule. If your child looks annoyed after you set the rule, you can state: "You're angry about that rule."

Step 3 is required only if your child breaks the rule again. This should not be stated until the moment in which it is readily apparent to the eyes of any observer that the rule is about to be broken, also known as "immediate intent." In the example here, the child winds their arm up and is releasing the ball towards the clock. It is important not to state the limit prior to this point, since children sometimes look as though they are going to do something, and pull back at the last instant in order to get a rise out of an adult. You need to follow through with the consequence once you state the limit and consequence. It is important that you carry out the consequence you gave, even if you have a nagging thought that perhaps it was stated prematurely:

"[Child's name], You want to throw the ball again. Remember I told you that if you throw the ball at the clock again, our playtime ends for today. You did throw it at the clock again, and we have to leave now."

(You then get up and move towards the door. A few parents may have to help their child leave by taking their arm or hand.) We will play again next time.

If your child resists leaving, saying, "I didn't really mean to do it," you as a parent respond empathically. Some examples are: "You don't think you should have to leave early," "You don't like that rule," "You think that's a stupid rule," "You want me to know that you don't like that rule."

But it also is important that you do not develop a conversation about this with your child, and that you do immediately end the play session.

*If your child tries to break the same rule in a later session, you skip Step 1
and go right to Step 2, and then 3. But as your Manual says, very young or
developmentally delayed children may need to hear the rules more times, and if
it is a long time later in play sessions that the rule is broken, you may need to go
through all three steps again with your children.*

Practicing the limit-setting skill

Parents are first asked to practice setting a rule by reading out the three steps to another
parent. Then leaders bring the group back together to think about the important rules that
parents will make for their own practice play sessions during meetings, reminding them
to keep to only the rules that are the most important ones. (Questions parents inevitably
have about home sessions should be postponed until later.) Leaders should be able to
anticipate what essential safety rules are needed for practice play sessions, and help parents
with these fairly quickly. More time is need for discussing their personal limits, such as
tolerance for bad language, the privacy of certain areas of both their children's and their
own bodies, limitations due to parents' physical constraints, and the usual play therapy
limits on mess, leaving the room, etc.

Leaders should mention that there will be further discussion of rules during the
next meeting, in order to prepare parents for beginning practice play sessions with their
children the following week. Returning to a discussion of personal boundaries during the
next meeting is important, because some adaptations may be required to meet the personal
limits of a few parents in their practice play sessions, once they have had time to mull the
rules over during the week between meetings.

Leaders then model a five-minute play session. One leader is the "child" and the
other is the "parent," who uses tracking, empathic reflections, and following the "child's"
lead. The "child" needs to break a particular limit three times while playing, in order
for the leader in the parent's role to accurately demonstrate for the group each of the
three steps in the limit-setting sequence. This limit-setting role-play is interspersed with
normal playing by the "child," while the "parent" follows the "child's" lead and shows
understanding. After their role-play, leaders should reinforce for parents that limit setting
is not rushed in play sessions. Children are given time to learn the rule, think about it, and
think about the consequences, as well as their own feelings about the rule.

Illustration of leaders' role-play of pretending to break a rule

A role-play example for leaders to use or adapt in their training on limit setting is now given.

> *Leader: We will now show you a role-play where the "child" tries to break a rule
> three times while he plays.*

> The leader as a "child" is building a fort industriously, with the "parent" making
> empathic and tracking comments. The "parent" then gives the "child" a five-minute
> warning that the session will end soon. The "child" takes one of the bricks and
> throws it at the "parent's" foot.

"Parent": You're angry with me (reflecting the feeling). (Then the "parent" sets the rule.) *Martin, remember I said I'd let you know if you may not do something. One thing you may not do is throw bricks at me.*

The "child" again throws a brick towards the "parent."

"Parent": Martin, you still want to hit me with the brick. Remember I said that you may not throw the bricks at me. If you do that again, we will finish our playtime for today. (Martin pulls a face.) *You're cross with me for saying that.*

The "child" destroys his half-built fort angrily, with the "parent" reflecting his feelings. Then for the third time, the "child" throws a brick at the "parent."

"Parent": Martin, you're still angry with me. Remember I told you that if you threw the bricks at me again, the playtime ends for today. You did throw one, and we have to leave now. (The "parent" gets up and moves towards the door, guiding the "child" by the arm.) *We will play again next time.*

Limit-setting exercise: parents' role-play

In the authors' experience, parents need more intensive practice on limit setting than the other three basic skills because the steps are more complicated to learn, and can be confusing to them. Two role-play attempts each, rather than one each, is recommended. Leaders may introduce this exercise by stating:

> Now we want you to have five minutes to take turns playing in the roles of "child" and "parent," with the "child" attempting to break the same rule three times. We'll go around and see how you're doing. We'll probably ask you to do this twice each, with a different rule each time, to really get the hang of it.

For this exercise, leaders again need to give out toy packets and suggested play scripts for parents to use, this time for four role-plays, in case parents do not readily think of scripts for themselves. Leaders ask parents to pretend to break the rule, if carrying out the action is not appropriate (e.g. the "child" hits the mirror with a solid object).

Leaders monitor each pair, prompting when needed. Usually the prompting is related to when a step is missed or out of order, the "child's" feeling is missed or the "parent" jumps to consequences too soon. Leaders often need to remind parents to slow down, and to play in other ways too, and not just break a limit. This slowing down is in order to help the person in the parent's role have time to remember the three steps needed in limit setting—sometimes parents need to refer to their written "script" during the role-play. It also helps parents have additional practice on empathy and following children's lead, along with limit setting.

DISCUSSION OF THE ROLE-PLAYING EXERCISE

Leaders again draw out from participants how the exercise went for them, including what was difficult and what was easier to do. One or two parents may say that following children's lead and showing understanding were easier skills to learn than the new one of limit setting. Leaders may wish to agree that limit setting is complicated to learn, confirming that it is more difficult because it has several steps to it. Leaders usually need to underline that parents should be matter of fact and authoritative when setting limits, rather than too severe or too tentative, but that this attitude is more difficult to achieve when learning a new skill.

Leaders will again see common issues arising in the group and paired exercises. Instead of singling out individuals for correction, we suggest leaders say they noticed the group had a bit of trouble with an issue (e.g. not reflecting a "child's" feelings, giving consequences too soon, a rule not being clearly stated) and that the group as a whole would benefit from doing a bit more on this skill during the next meeting.

Parents also may have several questions about limit setting. Again, it is important for leaders to distinguish whether the issue is a teaching issue or an emotional issue. If the former, it will be beneficial for leaders to model the answer to such a question through a brief role-play. If the latter, the emotional issue needs to be dealt with first. Parents usually find learning limit setting emotionally challenging, and some may then feel defensive, and question either what they are being taught, or the leaders' skills.

For example, a parent may ask: *"Why should I set limits that way? Why not just tell him what he should do?"* Leaders should strive to convey strong empathy for these parents. Empathy may include comments about the parent not thinking this form of limit setting is useful to their child, or allowing skeptical parents to query why limit setting was successful in a demo (e.g. their child's positive response was a fluke when the leaders set limits in this way). These parents usually worry that they will not have the same control with their child in their own play sessions. Other parents may be overly timid and worried about setting limits firmly, or afraid of making mistakes. Again their fears need to be empathized with by the leaders.

Leaders should end this limit-setting discussion on a positive note, saying that the main purpose of these first few weeks of training is to help parents have a general familiarity with all the main skills used in play sessions and that refinements will come with more practice. Leaders should remind parents that they will have more practice next time, before the sessions with their children start. This usually is a natural point, before the meeting ends, to prepare parents for next meeting's mock sessions practice.

Preparing for mock sessions

A full discussion for leaders on conducting mock play sessions during Meeting 5 is contained in the next chapter. We suggest the following statement as a useful way to structure for parents the mock play sessions taking place during the next meeting:

> You have started learning all the main skills involved in play sessions, and as you know, we have finished the demos with your children today. So there will be no children attending our meeting next week. Next time we will ask you to put all these skills together to conduct a "mock" play session. One of the leaders will be a "child" and each parent will have a turn practicing a short play session. The other parents will watch, so that everyone can learn from one another.

> Next week we'll also hand out a list of things to begin collecting for your home play sessions. We do not have time to talk about them right now, but we want you

to look over the list and think about them, but not buy anything yet, so that we can talk about collecting the materials you need before you start home play sessions.

After this preparation for the next stages in the program, leaders need to listen carefully and respond to any concerns that arise, before ending the meeting. These concerns often center on performance anxiety about the mock sessions, which is covered more fully in the next chapter, and worrying about their children's reactions to starting play sessions.

This chapter discussed helping parents learn the remainder of the basic skills needed to conduct practice play sessions with each of their children. The next chapter concentrates on Meeting 5, and ways leaders help parents use mock sessions to consolidate their skills in the meeting immediately before their practice play sessions begin.

CHAPTER 9

Mock Play Sessions
and Preparation for
Practice Play Sessions

Meeting 5

This chapter looks at mock sessions, and other preparations needed by parents, before they start their practice play sessions in the next meeting.

Conducting mock sessions

The first part of Meeting 5, which is devoted to mock play sessions, is a very energizing and somewhat anxiety-provoking time for parents. They are excited to be trying out all the skills they have learned while practicing playing with a "child" (albeit, a pretend one). But parents' anxious feelings also can be elevated, because they are being asked to use their new skills in front of the whole group, which can create performance anxiety in most parents. Another reason parents commonly put themselves under pressure to perform well during mock sessions is because they want to conduct their practice play sessions with their children adequately, when they start the following week.

Mock play sessions aim to consolidate parents' child-centered play skills by having them conduct a shortened practice play session from beginning to end with one of the leaders in the "child" role. With leaders assuming the child role in as realistic a way as possible, parents have opportunities to create responses that are immediate and appropriate to the leads provided by a "child". This enables parents to practice "thinking on their feet," as they will need to do during play sessions with their children. Parents' skills also are honed by watching the other parents' mock sessions with one of the leaders, as they will continue to do for practice play sessions during meetings. Mock play sessions therefore are an important aspect of GFT. They provide a rehearsal for parents before they attempt to play with their own children.

Issues can easily emerge during these mock sessions that may not have been covered in previous meetings. Indeed, leaders should adapt their role-plays as required to ensure that parents have adequate training in how to manage different situations—for example, questions, commands, and requests from their children during practice play sessions. Opportunities for further discussions of parents' personal limits during play sessions also arise. Leaders need to engineer situations when taking the child's role that challenge limits, while being mindful of doing this in ways that are not too anxiety provoking for parents to manage.

Leaders should aim to finish all the mock play sessions before the midway break. In order to speed up the process of mock play sessions in groups with the maximum number of parents, one leader can take half the group to another area, and conduct mock sessions with them. The second leader plays with the other half. Time is considerably reduced, with no loss of quality; however, a suitable second area is necessary, so that the "players" are not getting in each other's way.

Timing the group to finish mock sessions prior to the midway break enables parents to informally debrief themselves, sharing their own reactions and thoughts about their mock sessions, before they come back to the formal debriefing during the second half of the meeting. Parents commonly provide strong support and reassurance to one another during the break, and often express feelings of relief and exuberance after performing in front of the group. This informal process usually increases parents' motivation and strengthens their alliances with one another, which in turn leads to strong feelings of group cohesion after surviving their "baptism by fire." It also seems to begin a pattern of parents joining together and supporting one another for the next stage of the program, when they conduct practice play sessions.

Introducing mock play sessions to parents

Leaders should aim to have a ten-minute mock session with each parent. We recommend that leaders start with five minutes as the minimum for each mock session. If the parent is managing well in the session, the leader can lengthen the mock play session to ten minutes at the most. In our experience, even when more time is possible for mock sessions in small groups, ten minutes is still long enough to stretch parents' skills, without overwhelming them. Parents are told that the mock sessions are done one after the other in the first part of the meeting, and that there is a general discussion and feedback on each of them after everyone has had their turn.

During their mock sessions, parents are asked to say the opening statement, apply all the skills as appropriate, including limits, in-session structuring statements (e.g. *"In here it can be any way you want it to be."*), and the closing statement, in addition to the time warning of five minutes and one minute. Leaders have to remember to prompt parents when the hypothetical five-minute and one-minute time warnings should be given by whispering, since the leader is the one controlling the amount of time for each mock session.

Leaders should explain to parents that since leaders are not real children, no harm can come from any error that might be made. Parents are reminded that leaders are able to manage all the responses parents may give during mock sessions, and repeat the message that everyone learns from one another by observing. Leaders also need to tell parents that they will whisper asides for the five- and one-minute time warnings while they are playing the "child." For particularly nervous groups, leaders may wish to add that they will aid with asides any parent who seems to be stuck, or getting off track (see below).

Leaders continue to use the toys and materials they have been using for the demos with the children in earlier meetings. Parents already are familiar with these things, which usually aids their relaxation. In an earlier chapter, we highly recommended that leaders use the kinds of materials in their demos that are similar to those parents will be asked to provide in home play sessions. These materials should continue to be used for both the mock sessions and parents' practice play sessions during all subsequent meetings. Using similar materials to those that will be provided at home keeps to a minimum any unfavorable comparisons of equipment children may make between play sessions in group meetings, and their home sessions later. Using similar equipment also serves as a ready example of what parents should be aiming for when collecting their own toys and equipment, a topic parents have been told will be discussed in detail at a later meeting.

Prompting parents during practice

Leaders try to ensure that parents have favorable experiences in mock sessions in front of the group, and that the group benefits from observing. Therefore, if a parent is increasingly lost or confused, or overlooking the obvious, during their mock session, the leader should provide asides suggesting a response, or a clue to guide the parent and help shape their response. These asides should be done in a whisper and not too frequently. Leaders need to guard against too much prompting, in order to help parents develop confidence in their own ability to think on their feet, and to not be too heavily reliant on leaders.

The optimal time to provide a prompt is when a parent demonstrates a level of anxiety that is obvious to observers. This timing of a leader's intervention seems to work well, since the authors have never had a parent who could not complete a mock session. If a parent were to become overly distressed trying to complete this task, despite leaders following advice just given, the leader can simply say, *"We can stop now."*

Leaders in the child's role

As implied earlier, leaders choose the kind of child to play, and the play contents for each mock session. Ideally, leaders should try to portray a child somewhat like that of the parent—but a milder version, if the child is challenging. For example, if one of the children is expected to react in a sulky manner, the leader would role-play a sulky child for a few minutes with the parent, before moving on to other kinds of play. If a child questions adults frequently, the leader would be sure to ask a few questions. The mock play session always should include opportunities for parents to set basic limits and to participate in play activities while following the child's lead.

As already mentioned, it is very important that the leader playing the child helps the parent feel successful and competent in their mock play session. In order to make mock sessions more meaningful for parents and easier for leaders, we recommend that each leader have a general idea of the kind of child and the kind of play "script" they might enact beforehand, as part of the preparation for this meeting. This mock session exercise also needs to be interesting for parents to watch and learn from; therefore, leaders should vary their play activities and the kinds of questions, limits, commands, and requests they enact in their child role.

The role of the second leader

We suggest leaders take turns playing the "child's" role during mock sessions to provide as varied an experience for parents as possible. Leaders should plan together beforehand which parents, what types of children, and which play scripts they will take turns enacting during this meeting. It works well when the leader who is observing along with the parents takes notes on the role-play as it occurs. The observing leader should make certain that the parents realize that the note taking is primarily for remembering examples of what happened, and not evaluative in any way. It is then the *observing leader* who leads the discussion after the midway break about what took place in the mock session of the specific parents (s)he observed. The other leader who played the child is free to enter the discussion at any time. Before specific feedback to individual parents, however, leaders facilitate a general discussion with the group on the mock sessions. Some of the specific comments to individual parents may be more appropriate to make within this general discussion, rather than waiting for individual feedback, as our example below shows.

WHEN SINGLE LEADERS CONDUCT MOCK ROLE-PLAYS OR THE GROUP SPLITS

With small, one-leader groups, or with large groups divided into two halves, note-taking is not possible—another reason single-leader groups for large numbers is not recommended. Single leaders must train themselves to remember the contents of the mock play sessions. We suggest single leaders make notes during the midway break to aid recall—leaders will be cheered to know that it is usually surprisingly easy to remember the specifics of several sessions in which they have played the child.

An example of a mock play session

The following example illustrates a mock play session with a father, Steven. This example is followed by information for leaders on leading group discussions, once mock sessions and informal debriefing are completed, using the example of Steven to demonstrate this process. Finally, the way in which specific feedback to Steven was given, and the ways in which skills were then practiced as a group based on Steven's example, are discussed.

PLANNED SCENARIO BY THE LEADER ON TYPE OF
CHILD, PLAY SCRIPT AND LIMIT CHALLENGED

Leader 2 to play the part of a 7-year-old boy who asks questions and mildly challenges rules. The leader plans to engage in a spontaneous game or two with the father and will try to break the rule of not hitting the parent.

Leader 1: Now we'll have Steven take his turn. (Steven gives a sigh and gets up.) I can see this is not something you're looking forward to, Steven. It takes a bit of doing to get up this first time.

Steven: I just think it might be difficult, if you play a child like Harry.

Leader 2: I'll be doing some things like Harry, but nothing that you can't handle. I'll be called John and I'm about Harry's age, about 7. You start now with the introduction to the session.

Steven: John, this is your special playtime. If you can't do something, I'll let you know.

"Child": OK Dad. I'm going to play with these bean bags. You have two and I'll have three.

Steven: You have more than I do.

"Child": Yes, you're bigger than me. Why? Do you think we have to be the same? Can I have three?

Steven: Well, that's how most games are played. But I'll just have two today.

"Child": I'll go first. I get three goes to hit that doll over there... I missed. I missed. Damn, I missed again!

Steven: You did not like that.

"Child": I'm standing closer. But you have to stand back there where I was when it's your turn.

Steven: You're giving me the rules.

"Child": I hit it! I hit it!

Steven (flat tone): You got really close, so you hit it.

"Child": Now you do it. You stand there. Can you hit it from there? No, you stand back further.

Steven: You want it to be hard for me.

"Child": Yes, you're bigger.

(Steven seems to deliberately miss hitting the doll.)

"Child": You missed! Try again and see if you can get it.

Steven: I'll try again.

"Child": This time do it with your eyes closed. (Steven half shuts his eyes.) I think you're cheating. Are you peeking? Turn your back and don't look, then throw.

(Steven does as he is told and misses hitting the doll.)

"Child": I'm going to turn my back now. I hit it! I hit it!

Steven (flat tone): You were standing very close and you hit it.

"Child": Now you stand where the doll is and hold the doll. (Steven moves to where the doll is.)

"Child": I'm going to turn my back and try to hit the doll.

Steven: You can't hit me. I won't play that game.

"Child": Aw, this isn't fun. I'm not going to do this any more. (The "child" throws the bean bags down on the floor angrily…)

Steven: You don't like that.

"Child": No, but I think I'll play with the cars. You have the racing car and I'll have the big truck. See which one can crash into that doll the hardest. You go first. (Steven is given a prompt here by Leader 2 in an aside to give the five-minute warning.)

Steven: John, we have five minutes left today. Now I'll race my car and crash into the doll.

"Child": That wasn't a very hard crash. Now watch me! I'm going back here and crashing it really hard! Watch, watch!!

Steven: You really want me to see that!

"Child": Crash! That was great! (Steven is prompted by Leader 2 to give a one-minute warning here.)

Steven: We have one minute left. It's almost time for you to finish today.

"Child": But I won't have a chance to play with the soldiers. That's not fair.

Steven: We'll have lots more playtimes. Today it's time to finish.

(The "child" leaves, with dragging feet.)

Steven (to Leader 2): How was that?

Leader 2: You did some very good things in the mock session you just had, Steven. We'll talk it all over after the break.

Formal discussion of mock play sessions

After the midway break, there is a general group discussion of mock sessions, followed by more detailed feedback to each parent.

General group discussion

The group discussion of mock sessions begins after parents have had informal conversations during the midway break which, as mentioned earlier, usually have been high spirited after their unique experience. Leaders should remember at the outset of the general discussion to give very generous praise to all the parents for taking part in their mock play sessions, and surviving well. Leaders then ask parents as a group how it went, what was easy and what was more difficult, as they did during earlier skills training. Leaders usually ask the group what they would like more practice on, which may lead to brief, specific feedback for a parent during the general discussion. Some members may be more vocal than others, but it is important that leaders try to be as inclusive as possible. In this special instance, we suggest specifically asking quieter parents if they wish to contribute their reactions and thoughts.

As explained before, some of the detailed feedback to parents by leaders can be fitted into the large group discussion of how the mock sessions went. Using our example here, Steven talked to the group about how difficult it was to let the "child" cheat in the mock session.

> *Leader 2: That was a real struggle for you, Steven.*

> *Steven: It wasn't easy! I was telling Raymond [another father] about how frustrated I was that I had to keep my mouth shut.*

> *Leader 2: It felt like you needed to restrain yourself, not do what you usually do. Did anyone else feel that way? (Other parents volunteered that they felt inhibited and unnatural too.)*

> *Leader 1: It's a part of learning to do something differently that is not easy for a lot of you. While I was watching, Steven, I noticed that in general, even though it felt uncomfortable for you, you did go along with the "child's" play and followed his lead, until a limit was needed.*

> *Steven: I did?*

> *Leader 1 (referring to notes and giving a specific example): Yes, you accepted playing with two balls, instead of three, for example. (Leader 1 also could have chosen the instance of, say, Steven accepting that the "child" stood close to the target. However, one example should suffice in this general discussion.)*

Specific feedback to individual parents

After the general group discussion, leaders turn to each parent individually and have a discussion of their mock play session, taking up issues from their mock sessions that were not discussed in the general group discussion. More detailed feedback is given to each parent, picking out specific things that went well, along with one thing that needs to be worked on, always ending on a positive note (see Chapter 3).

Leaders continually need to be careful to word feedback to the parents about their play session in such a way that any recommendations for change are given in general terms. In the previous example, Leader 1, rather than saying, *"Steven, you had trouble stating the limits to the 'child'"* or *"You forgot some important words in the introduction,"* would, instead of personalizing these comments, say to the large group, *"In a few minutes, let's all go over the steps for limit setting and the introduction again, which are a little hard to get straight."* If a common error was made by all or most of the group members, leaders can say, *"It seems like almost everybody had a little trouble giving the opening statement. Let's go over that again."*

Once again, we highly recommend that leaders attempt to depersonalize skills correction as much as possible, while at the same time provide accurate feedback for each parent. An example of specific feedback to Steven, with Leader 1 taking the main role, is given next.

SPECIFIC FEEDBACK TO A PARENT ABOUT HIS MOCK PLAY SESSION

Leader 1: Steven, you said already that it was difficult for you to accept that the "child" played his own way, rather than the way it's supposed to be. What about the mock session as a whole? How did it go for you?

Steven: I spent so much time thinking about what I should not be doing that I felt like a robot.

Leader 1: Just like some other parents, it was very difficult to stop yourself from your usual responses when you were playing. However you did manage to practice a lot of the skills that you have been learning. Is there anything that you think went quite well for you?

Steven: It's hard to think of anything. I suppose that I did set the limit of not hitting me when it was needed, even though I didn't do it right.

Leader 1: Yes, you really did get the timing right, and the rule itself too, even though you had to think on your feet for this. Again, this is common for parents at this point in the program.

Steven: I think I have it straight now, but I'd like to rehearse again, just like other parents said. I wanted to set limits in more places. I wanted to tell the "child" not to give himself all of the breaks, like standing close so that he could hit the doll.

Leader 1: The play session goes against your belief that rules should be the same for all players. We'll think more about why children give themselves the advantages when they play in their sessions, if this arises later, as I suspect it will. For now, maybe we can think about what feelings the "child" had during this mock session.

Steven: I know I didn't show I understood "his" feelings enough. I got the basics of "You like it" and "You don't like it," but I missed some more.

Leader 1: I thought you managed to say some of the "child's" feelings very effectively. You weren't thrown by hearing "Damn," for example, and got the tone just right there. You stressed that the "child" did not like doing less well than you. I'd be interested in what other feelings, now that you think about it, you would have liked to say.

Steven: Well, I would have liked to say that the "child" was angry with me when I set the limit.

Leader 1: That would have been very appropriate to do. I also thought you might have said something about the "child's" feelings at the end. You said that there will be a lot more playtimes. Maybe you can think how to turn that into a statement about how the "child" was feeling.

Steven: Disappointed. Yes, I could have said that. I try to encourage my children to know what is going to happen next, but I will try to put that to the side, and concentrate on their feelings, especially Harry's.

Leader 1: In general it is important to give structuring information to children. But it did seem to get in the way of showing understanding of the "child's" feelings at the end.

The last thing I wanted to say is that overall I thought you did an excellent job of following the "child's" lead. You were able to let "him" think about what to do next, for example, after you set a limit and "he" gave up the game with the doll. You didn't suggest anything, and just waited for "him." And you didn't change what "he" was thinking by asking questions or telling him to do things.

Steven, you and the other parents need to appreciate what you did NOT say, as well as what you did say. There are so many things that we might feel like saying that would go against the principles of play sessions. For example, "Oh, that's really good. I like what you're doing," or "Why would you do it that way?" It requires control on our parts to inhibit ourselves from saying what comes to us naturally. You're all to be complimented that none of you used these regular conversational comments that we would respond with at other times. That is a major step towards learning the play session talk we are trying to master.

Steven: I'm glad you think so. I'm not quite so sure myself.

Leader 2: It will take a while for you to feel on top of everything. However, you really conducted a nice session. As we said earlier, all of you have made a good start during the mock sessions. Let's turn to the next parent now.

DISCUSSION OF THIS ILLUSTRATION

This example of feedback is intended to illustrate how effective it is when leaders use examples of each parent's behaviors from the mock sessions. It is important to steer the feedback to the one most important issue for parents to improve on, while emphasizing the positive and hopeful elements of their practice, particularly in the final comments. The example also shows how extended discussions of underlying meanings of play sequences are not well placed during this phase in the program; skills training should take precedence. Finally, general comments of benefit to the entire group are important for leaders to make in a timely way during feedback to individual parents, as this example demonstrates.

Skills review based on mock play session feedback

After each parent receives specific feedback on their mock session, leaders rehearse the group as a whole on skills corrections emerging from the feedback, often restating the rationales for developing these skills accurately. For example:

Leader: Let's rehearse the opening statement. Remember it is: "This is your special playtime. In here you can do ALMOST anything you want. I'll let you know if there is something you cannot do."

We already talked about there being no grounds for limit setting unless you include, loudly and clearly, the "ALMOST", along with "anything." Parents often forget the "ALMOST," when they start. But then children may think any restrictions you make are unfair, and challenge them, since they were told they could do "anything." And remember, these statements need to be made in an accepting tone, to help children relax and freely play out issues that are important to them. Let's practice together now.

Preparation for next meeting's practice play sessions

Preparation for individual practice play sessions that begin the next meeting follow on from specific training raised from the contents of mock play sessions. There are a number of issues that come to the fore when parents begin to conduct their practice play sessions with their own children. Some of these will have been covered earlier, and need to be reviewed as they become immediately relevant. Some issues may be new. We discuss several of these issues next.

Additional skills training and issues to address

ADDRESSING GENERAL LIMITS

Leaders are advised to return to discussing the limits parents intend to put in place during their practice play sessions, and remind parents that, in order for children to be clear about their choices, limits must be consistent from the outset. Some parents may have high tolerance in some areas that are not tolerable to other parents. Leaders should make certain that all parents enforce limits that are for safety and protection of property, such as not allowing objects to be thrown at the walls, windows, and mirrors, not allowing tampering with any equipment in the room (e.g. cameras), not allowing children to draw on walls, flooring, and toys, and not allowing children to poke the bop bag with anything that is sharp, or to deliberately break toys. Leaders should then discuss with parents other activities in the playroom that *are* allowed, which they may have noticed during demos, such as allowing messy play in the area of the room set up for this purpose.

Allowing play sessions to be more permissive of mess is an area for leaders to highlight. Usually parents who have an initial emotional reaction against messy play commonly become more tolerant of it in the playroom, if their feelings and underlying worries are acknowledged first. After this acknowledgement, practical solutions are also explored by these parents, other parents or the leaders (e.g. having their child wear play clothes). As part of this discussion on messy play, personal limits of parents may also be touched on. For example, leaders can help parents decide whether they would not be able to tolerate getting messy or wet themselves during play sessions, and suggest that parents who could not manage this may decide to set a limit, if their child were, for example, spraying water at them.

The other important area to have consensus on is child and parent safety, with children not being allowed to hit, kick, hurt, or endanger themselves or their parents in any way. Hanging out of windows and climbing on high furniture, tampering with electric outlets, and hitting the lights with objects are dangerous and prohibited behavior. Other actions that may be unsafe also are prohibited. For example, parents need to set limits, if asked to do something unsafe by their children (e.g. *"You really want me to drink that pretend tea with small beads in it. Remember I said I'd let you know if there was anything you can't do. The rule is that water with small beads doesn't go in our mouths."*).

ADDRESSING PERSONAL LIMITS

In GFT, a personal limit is defined as a limit that is not part of standard play session rules (e.g. throwing objects at the observation mirrors or hitting the parent). They pertain to behavior that is personally intolerable to parents. A rationale for personal limits is that certain child behaviors may create stress or discomfort in parents (similarly to therapists) that may block parents from accepting their children unconditionally, and lead to anxiety in both parents and children during play sessions. Examples of behavior that may be difficult personally for some parents is a child running his finger around the entire hairline of his father, or examining his teeth, or insisting he drink dirty water. Therefore, it is vital that leaders spend time on parents' personal limits before practice play sessions begin.

Typically, parents will have no more than three or four personal limits. If a parent wants to have more personal limits, leaders should try to work with these parents' feelings of discomfort as extensively as seems necessary. In rare cases, time may need to be given outside of group meetings. For example, a leader may offer a parent extra time before or after the group to help the parent feel more comfortable with normal child's play.

PERSONAL, PHYSICAL LIMITATIONS

Parents need to be asked if they have physical limitations that may necessitate setting a rule (e.g. a bad back). Some parents may say that, while they do not have physical limitations, they do not like children to put things near their eyes, or jump onto their backs. Attitudes towards private areas of the body also need to be respected for both children and parents, and would mostly fall under general limits for all parents. However, in a few circumstances there is room for personal interpretation. For instance, mothers who are uneasy about having stethoscopes put on their breasts can make that a personal limit. During such a discussion, and after the importance of the parents' feelings are acknowledged, leaders may agree that a personal limit is required. Then brainstorming with parents on acceptable adaptations is needed. For example, if a mother does not like the stethoscope on her breast, the leader may suggest she say: *"Mary Jane, one thing I cannot let you do is use the stethoscope on my chest; so you may use it on my back."* If her child objects to this adaptation, the parent then reflects her child's feelings: *"You like to do it your way,"* or *"That's not how you wanted to play with me,"* and then restates the limit. Similar to other limit-setting situations, this would count as the first step of limit enforcement. Alternatively, if no adaptations seem appropriate, leaders should guide parents to set limits without suggesting alternatives on behaviors that seem intolerable to them.

"I" STATEMENTS AND GFT

In both play therapy and Filial Therapy practice, adults learn to match their inner with their outer expressions of feelings non-verbally with children in a genuine manner during play sessions. The first author considers that the only place where parents and play therapists should attribute personal feelings verbally to themselves by using "I" statements in their play sessions is when they communicate with children in the exercise of personal limits. The second author has a modified view (see Ryan & Courtney, 2009), arguing that expressing congruence with "I" statements in play therapy and Filial Therapy is an important part of deepening attachment relationships between adults and children. However, GFT as presented in this book follows the first author's practice: during play sessions parents are taught to use "I" statements only for personal limits. Parents are then taught to use "I" statements to express their feelings when they generalize skills to daily life later in the program, once they understand and reflect their children's feelings accurately.

We suggest the following explanations, when leaders help parents learn to use personal limits for their practice play sessions:

- First, as in all limit setting in play sessions, children's desire to do whatever is being limited should be recognized, whenever personal limit setting is not urgent.

- Personal limits should be communicated to children in the form of "I" statements.

- Because parents are taking personal responsibility for imposing the limit, the wording is, "*I can't let you do that*" and parents then provide their reason briefly. (This explanation is needed because a personal limit is coming strictly from parents, and no other solid universal therapeutic rationale lies behind it.)

- In order for children to be clear about their choices, personal limits must be consistent from the outset.

- Leaders may wish to use their own examples or adapt the following ones to their group's needs:

  "Jamie, it's fun for you to run your finger around the edges of my hair. However, I find that it does not feel good to me. I can't let you do that anymore."

  "Billy, you want to feel all my teeth. I don't like people putting their fingers in my mouth. I can't let you do that anymore."

- If children resist parents' personal limits, they should respond empathically to their children's feelings (e.g. *"You don't like me to stop you doing that; you don't see anything wrong with it."*)

- If children continue to insist, parents need to impose Step 2 of the usual limit sequence (e.g. *"George, you don't want to stop doing that, you don't think that's fair, it is now one of the rules of the play session. If it happens again, we will need to end the play session for today."*)

- Children rarely fail to comply at this point, which is similar to other warnings on general limits. Parents should be informed that it is unusual to need to go to enforcing the consequence with personal limits.

ADDITIONAL PERSONAL LIMITS: GUNS AND BAD LANGUAGE

Two other areas that are often very emotive for some parents are using guns in the playroom and using bad language. For example, some parents in Steven's group may not have tolerated the "child" saying "Damn" during their mock session. Leaders, after responding empathically to any parents' strong feelings, should try to help them increase their tolerance of children's aggressive play and uninhibited use of language in play sessions, if possible. Rationales for permissiveness in play sessions may need to be reviewed, once parents' emotional reactions are shown to be acceptable by leaders.

If leaders need to address parents' concerns about children using bad language during play sessions, they may wish to turn to the Parents' Training Manual. The Manual advocates that ideally there would be no limits on what children say in play sessions, including swearing, dirty words, and hostile comments towards parents. However, if any parents are certain that bad language is intolerable, it is important leaders narrow down what phrases are unacceptable to parents, rather than accepting a blanket ban on bad language. Usually there are certain words that are much more unacceptable than others. Leaders can then suggest that parents set a limit on this narrow set of words, if they find this necessary.

This approach is also useful when discussing guns and other aggressive toys for children's use in play sessions. Helping parents to understand and accept their children's aggressive behavior, then narrowing down the one or two materials that are unacceptable to a specific parent is recommended. Leaders can suggest that they will return to parents' concern about guns and bad language when discussing materials and preparing for home play sessions. Lengthy discussion of these topics at this point in the program can override other issues, and should be discouraged. To repeat, parents may need several returns to such topics in order to increase their tolerance of emotive issues in their play sessions.

Overall, leaders aim in this discussion of personal limits to increase parents' tolerance for their children's behavior that is not dangerous or destructive during play sessions, and begin to accept that their children play more fully when rules are kept to a minimum.

Reservations about imaginative play

Parents' reactions to being involved in their children's imaginative play may also come to the fore during their mock sessions. Most parents very much enjoy participating in imaginative play during mock sessions. However, a very small number of parents may raise the concern that imaginative play does not mean anything, and is "boring," or they feel foolish when dressing up and playing a role. Usually it is sufficient for leaders to accept these feelings and acknowledge their concerns at this stage in the program. Commonly, parents who raise this issue early in the program feel that their adult authority is in danger of being undermined, or worry about the reactions of other group members. For example:

> Leader: You say you'll feel foolish...you think [she] may try to make you look foolish... you think you will not be able to tell her what to do any more, if you look foolish.

After leaders show they understand these reactions, they may judge that adding a light-hearted comment to the group (e.g. *"You didn't know you'd be signing up for drama school!"*) lessens the group's anxiety. Other times, parents need leaders' help in separating out the difference between imaginative play and daily life. After acknowledging these worries, leaders often are able to point out that younger, 3- and 4-year-old children may need a bit of help with the difference between what is acceptable in play sessions and what is permitted in their home life, but older children know the difference well.

Asking parents not to coach their children

Leaders should remind parents, just as they did for demos, that no one, including the leaders, knows how their individual children will react to practice play sessions. Leaders need to underline that it is not useful for parents to try to anticipate how their children will react, or to coach their children in advance in any way. Reminding parents of the rationale for play sessions—that children lead the way with their own play agendas, which are healing for them when not directed by adults—is timely here. Leaders also can explain that a play session is a unique experience, not only for parents but also for their children. They have not played with their parents in that manner before.

Leaders can emphasize that play sessions are very interesting, because they are designed to offer a different structure for parents' and children's relationships with one another. Therefore, play sessions can evoke very different responses in children from what they might express elsewhere. Leaders can point out that this change in children's behavior may be different from what they did during leaders' demos. In general, leaders should show enthusiasm for the next stage in the program, helping parents to develop a heightened interest in discovering what will happen in their children's and others' practice play sessions.

Logistical details about the next phase in the program

Parents need two practice play sessions with each of their children during Meetings 6–10. The exceptions are auxiliary children, who often need only one practice session per parent, or who wait to begin until home sessions are established (see Chapter 13). Leaders decide on practical arrangements and give parents who are selected to begin their first practice play sessions the following week any additional preparation required. It is important that leaders allow enough time in this busy meeting for preparation of *both* the group and the selected families for the next meeting. Leaders may wish to introduce this phase in the program by saying:

> Instead of the demos we had earlier, we will start with all of you parents having short play sessions with each of your children while the rest of us watch and learn, just as we did today during your mock sessions.
>
> After the practice play sessions, which must start on time, we will have feedback with each parent and discuss what we saw, as well as some more skills training when it's needed.
>
> We plan to schedule two of these practice playtimes for each parent with each of your children who are fully participating in GFT during our meetings. We may have a bit of time for your other children to have a practice play session too; we'll talk about this individually with some of you later.

SELECTING FAMILIES FOR NEXT MEETING'S PRACTICE PLAY SESSIONS

Leaders should aim to choose parents for the first practice play sessions for the following week based on parents' level of skills development, their emotional readiness and their ability to perform relatively easily in front of other parents. Parents should be selected whom leaders anticipate will do moderately well. It is best to avoid the more extreme ends of the continuum of skills development at the outset, avoiding both the "stars of the show" and those who have not developed very much skill. Parents' skills level, rather than children's characteristics, is the better basis for selection of parents. However, it is also best to avoid selection of children who are not able to play easily, if possible.

When leaders prepare for Meeting 5 and identify which parents are ready to do their first practice play sessions in Meeting 6, we suggest leaders have several parents in mind who may fulfill the criteria just listed. During the latter part of Meeting 5, one leader can light-heartedly suggest that certain parents will be first to "bite the bullet," and then suggest a few (or several, depending on the size of the group) of these parents. If one of these parents reacts adversely and refuses, the leader may then go on to suggest some other parents. In our experience, it is very unusual for leaders to have to persevere beyond this brief discussion in order to select parents for the following week. But in rare cases leaders may need to directly appoint parents to start their practice play sessions the following week. It is also important for leaders to remind the group at this point that parents will remember that practice play sessions are an established part of each meeting for the remainder of the program (or until home session video recordings take their place. See Chapter 12.)

WORKING OUT THE PROGRAM SCHEDULE FOR PRACTICE PLAY SESSIONS

In addition to selecting the first families to conduct practice play sessions, leaders try to work out a timetable with as many of the parents in the group as possible for their first practice play sessions. The scheduling of second practice play sessions is usually done after most parents have finished their first sessions. However, in some groups, parents need additional notice, with early scheduling, for both their first and second practice play sessions.

This planning process is familiar to the group because it follows similar lines to the demo schedule in earlier meetings. Similarly to the demo schedule, the practice play sessions during the following five meetings (Meetings 6–10) are primarily for children who are fully participating in the program. Leaders should also keep in mind during this phase, as at other phases, that GFT is a whole family intervention; therefore, inclusion of all children in the family continues to be a goal. Some groups may be able to fit in one practice play session with auxiliary siblings in the family in the usual 2.5–12 years age range. And if time permits, in a later meeting during this phase of the program, a parent or two may have a short, practice play session with their toddler prior to home sessions beginning.

A practice activity or talk session with a teen may also be included during Meetings 9 or 10, if the teen is willing. However, this is a rare event in the authors' experience, due to teens' anxiety and self-consciousness about being observed by strangers. If families and leaders decide at intake that it would be helpful for either toddlers or teens to fully participate in the program, they would then need to be included at the outset, when deciding on group composition and numbers.

Leaders again should remain flexible about scheduling some parents who may have strong performance anxiety or lack skills development. Many times it becomes less problematic, as the group unfolds in Meetings 7–10, to schedule parents who may have more difficulties with their performance, and who therefore may have additional training requirements. And reluctant parents commonly are more willing to volunteer for their practice sessions, once the first week or two of play sessions are undertaken by more willing parents.

SCHEDULING REQUIREMENTS FOR MEETINGS 6–10

It is usual for leaders to schedule two or three practice play sessions per meeting during this phase of the program, depending upon the number of children and parents in the group. Occasionally, if the group is very large, four sessions may be needed in one or two meetings. Leaders should arrange for a time overrun of these meetings with the group beforehand. For the first sessions of each parent with one of their children, shorter sessions of 15 minutes per child are highly recommended. If time permits, practice play sessions can be extended to 20 minutes the second time around. However, leaders have to keep to schedule, and ensure they devote Meeting 11 to preparing the group for home sessions with their children, which start in Meeting 12. As mentioned earlier, for siblings who are not exhibiting emotional problems, one session per child per parent may generally suffice, especially if there are a large number of children in the group.

Single parents with more than two children automatically have more practice play sessions with their children during this phase in GFT, in order to have at least one practice play session with each of their participating children. And two-parent families with one child still have two sessions each with their child. Furthermore, leaders should be careful, if adapting the 20-session model presented here (see Chapter 16), that if any division of a large group is made it still enables each leader to see at least one session with each parent.

SCHEDULING SIBLINGS AT THE SAME GFT MEETING

Similarly to the earlier demos, siblings need to have their practice play sessions scheduled for the same meeting wherever possible. This is not only because it makes it easier for families to participate, but also because sometimes sibling rivalry is fuelled if one or more siblings have to wait for the next meeting for their turn. For example, we recommend having four practice play sessions during one meeting for a single parent with four children in the usual age range.

There may be a few circumstances that prevent this scheduling. First, it may be impossible to fit all the siblings into one meeting, if the sibling group is too large, and therefore leaders must schedule their practice play sessions over two meetings. And if childcare provision is limited, only those siblings who are playing during that meeting should attend. However, for other groups, it may be possible to offer childcare for the entire family, even for families with large numbers of siblings. Provision of childcare is an especially important consideration for single parents who have several young children, but may not have ready access to childcare.

Leaders also need to remember for scheduling purposes that they will be discussing each sibling as a separate case in their feedback after practice play sessions, just as they did after demos. In addition, in two-parent families, each parent should play with each of their children at least once. Therefore parent-child dyads are reversed from the first to the second practice sessions. This reversal is important to establish at the outset, so that each child in the family experiences both parents, and that each dyad increases their positive experiences with one another. For single parents, there obviously are no reversals. However, it is still important that feedback is given for each child, so that a parent experiences each child's needs and presentation uniquely.

SUPPORTING PARENTS AND CHILDREN BEFORE THEIR FIRST PRACTICE SESSIONS

After leaders have lined up parents to conduct their first practice play sessions the following week, leaders help these parents anticipate how their first play session may develop with their own children (e.g. aggressive, talkative, questioning, timid). One of the leaders should ask the parent, *"How do you think [Name of child] will respond?"* and *"Do you want to rehearse anything special?"* The leader then improvises, doing a rehearsal with the parent in front of the group, and going through two or three issues the parent is concerned about during a brief role-play. If a few issues emerge during this rehearsal that are not quickly dealt with, or if there are several major things a parent feels unsure about, the leader should suggest that they attend 15–20 minutes early for the next meeting, and go over these issues in more detail with one of the leaders.

This method of skills teaching is important to adopt for each parent in the group before their first scheduled practice play session with their children. Obviously, if a parent does not have any concerns, it is important for leaders to acknowledge their confidence and forego any rehearsal. After this rehearsal, leaders turn to the large group again. They should mention to the group that they will not intervene or interrupt the play session, unless it is obvious that a parent is in great difficulty with their child or appears emotionally overwhelmed. Leaders should prepare parents to give only a one-minute warning in these very rare cases, instead of the usual five-minute warning.

Next, leaders need to help parents with how to present the idea of beginning practice play sessions to their children before the next meeting. The general explanation—that parents are learning to have special playtimes with their children—is usually sufficient. For more inquisitive children, parents may wish to add that the playtimes are for learning to do things better together. Leaders should remind parents that their children need to be told that these playtimes are a bit shorter to start with, while parents are learning. This can easily be incorporated into the parents' opening statement at the beginning of their first practice play session (e.g. *"These play sessions here are shorter. Our sessions at home will be longer, after we have one or two shorter ones there too."*).

Leaders also remind parents to concentrate on any feelings that may arise for their children during the session itself due to their playtime being shortened (e.g. disappointment). Parents should respond to such comments during the practice play session by empathizing with any of their children's objections (e.g. *"You really want to play longer"* or *"That was too short for you."*). If children compare their parents' session with the demo session they had with a leader, leaders should prepare parents to respond empathically, giving comments such as *"You liked it better with her,"* or if the comparison favors the parent, *"You like it better when we play together."*

Finally, leaders need to remind parents that, just like the demos, the next five meetings (Meetings 6–10) begin strictly on time, so children do not have an unnecessary wait. Parents need to bring their children to childcare and settle their children in, before the meeting starts, just as they did for the demos, rather than bringing them directly to the meeting. Again, one of the leaders will be there to collect the children and bring them to their parents for their play sessions. Leaders end on a positive note, showing their interest in the next phase of the program and encouraging parents in their efforts.

The next chapter turns to these first practice play sessions, in which parents start directly applying their child-centered play skills with their own children.

CHAPTER 10

Beginning Practice Play Sessions

Meetings 6–7

The main aim leaders have during this phase of the GFT program is to ensure that parents display a basic level of proficiency in conducting child-led play sessions before beginning to conduct home play sessions weekly with their children. This chapter considers the meetings in which parents have their first practice play sessions with their children. The next chapter discusses Meetings 8–10, during which parents have their second practice play sessions, prior to home sessions.

Practice play sessions or watching parents' videos of their home sessions continue during the remainder of the meetings, including the meetings after parents begin conducting home play sessions, unless video suffices (see Chapter 12). The timetable suggested here for preparing parents for home sessions should be achievable for almost all the parents in most groups—they will have had sufficient practice to enable them to deliver child-centered play sessions at a basic level in early home sessions. Further refinements of parents' skills and the development of deeper understanding of their children's emotional issues continue during later meetings, after home sessions have begun, as discussed in later chapters.

Considerations for leaders during this phase of the program

The format for meetings with practice play sessions

The format for meetings during this phase of GFT is similar to the format for the earlier meetings (Meetings 2–4) where leaders conducted demos; leaders should schedule all the parents' practice play sessions prior to the break. Leaders also should aim to have all the parents conduct their first play sessions before any parent embarks on their second practice play session during a meeting. However, when the group is a large one, or there was an unavoidable delay for a parent, there may be a mixture of first and second practice play sessions by parents and their children scheduled before the break during a later meeting (e.g. Meeting 8).

After the break that allows for informal debriefing, parents who conducted their practice sessions process each one individually with a leader in front of the group. Then the meeting is given over to other parents' reactions and comments on their observations of these sessions. During the next five meetings therefore, leaders need to allow sufficient feedback time in the group meeting to help each parent process their play session with each of their children, to give direct feedback to the parent involved, and to hear other parents' reactions to the practice play sessions they observed. Further skills training and discussion also are required, since additional training issues emerge from these play sessions and feedback. Finally, leaders need time to offer additional preparation to those parents who are starting their first practice play sessions the following meeting.

Other scheduling considerations

Leaders again need flexibility during this phase of the program to accommodate to unique issues within each group. Scheduling issues may arise for leaders immediately, or may become more obvious as the program unfolds. For example, there may be a parent who has special problems in skills learning, and cannot conduct a child-centered play session with one of their children at a basic, acceptable level with only two practice play sessions. Or there may be a child who is particularly challenging in a first practice play session, or a parent who has missed a meeting. Leaders need to be prepared here, as elsewhere in the program, to tack on an extra practice play session or two prior to a scheduled meeting, or to make extra time for a parent with a particular emotional issue outside of group time, in order to keep to the group's overall schedule, as discussed in earlier chapters. Again, two leaders have more flexibility in scheduling these additional tasks than a sole leader.

Occasionally in GFT, parents voice strong objections to having their play sessions observed by the group, as we mentioned earlier. Leaders should acknowledge these feelings, and suggest that parents should wait and see. They may feel more comfortable after seeing how these things are done in the group. Then leaders re-check their attitudes, after allowing them to wait until several other parents have done their first practice play sessions. Usually parents who fear exposure initially find it less difficult to be observed after they have witnessed the lack of criticism and the supportive atmosphere of the group during other parents' first practice sessions. However, if a parent's feelings remain strong, or if a child has strong objections that cannot be overcome by gentle persuasion by one of the leaders or their parent, leaders should find another solution to this problem. A possible one, if facilities are available, is to set up a camera in a separate room for this parent and child, with the group observing by video link. Or, if this equipment is not available, leaders can suggest that the parent and child come early or stay afterwards to make a video to show to the group next time. Usually this accommodation is only needed for the first practice session, and not for the next one.

Another less than common problem for leaders is when a parent is willing to conduct a practice play session with one child, but initially lacks the confidence to conduct play sessions with one of their other children. In these infrequent cases, leaders may wish to have that parent observe the other parent conduct a play session with that child first, and to then encourage the parent with reservations to conduct their own practice play session, once their confidence has been bolstered by conducting a practice play session with their preferred child.

Leaders already chose parents who have average skills levels and the confidence to perform in front of the group for the first practice play sessions taking place in Meeting 6, and offered extra rehearsal for the few who were not confident beforehand. As the last chapter mentioned, once these practice sessions become routine for the group, performance anxiety tends to decrease for parents, with a few exceptions. Leaders then have more flexibility in choosing parents who are more at the extremes of skills levels for practice play sessions, and parents are usually much more willing to volunteer to participate, after they have seen that parents who conduct play sessions have valued the feedback from leaders, and the group members have shown strong support and interest in the children and parents themselves during practice play sessions.

The logistics of the sessions

As we advised in the last chapter, one of the leaders collects each child who participates in practice play sessions with their parent and returns the child to childcare afterwards. It is helpful to the children if that leader is the one who conducted the demo with the child, allowing the children to feel more at ease before they begin. It also is useful for leaders to repeat the message to each child that this playtime will be a bit shorter, because their parents are learning to do special playtimes before they do them at home. Leaders need to ensure that each play session begins promptly, as emphasized in the last chapter, and that the observing parents watch carefully and quietly.

One of the leaders sitting with the observing parents needs to take notes, as was done for mock play sessions during Meeting 5. It is useful for these brief notes to consist of what the child did, how the parents responded, and what the leader thinks of this interaction. A suggested form for leaders to use in recording these supervision notes is given in Appendix 16. By covering these three areas, leaders have ample information to use during the feedback process with parents after the break, when concrete examples from play sessions are needed. The other leader may take brief notes also, but may instead, when the venue permits, comment very briefly and quietly to the group when parents show child-centered skills clearly in their play sessions. Afterwards parents debrief informally with one another during the midway break; formal feedback with each parent is led by the leader who was taking notes.

Parents' first play sessions

Parents are understandably nervous as they show the group members and leaders what their interactions with their children are like, particularly for the first time. Leaders need to be sensitive to performance anxiety and to some parents' difficulties in acknowledging the limitations of their play session skills during early play sessions. Specific issues that often emerge during this part of the program are explored and illustrated later in this chapter.

Feedback to each parent after their play session

Keeping in mind parents' usual emotional responses to a first session, feedback from leaders should be highly empathic. The majority of the feedback should be positive, without being falsely encouraging. After parents conduct their first practice play sessions, leaders' feedback should primarily help parents with learning CCPT skills. The most effective form of feedback in skills learning, as mentioned already in this book, seems to be starting with positive feedback, moving into corrective feedback, and then ending with more positive feedback (Guerney L., 2003). This sequencing enables parents to focus on what went well the majority of the time, as well as ending the feedback with a hopeful attitude towards their own abilities. In addition, starting with positive feedback seems to help parents to hear the following corrective comments and suggestions from the leader because their emotional defences against failure have not been overly activated or preoccupying, as the next example illustrates.

The above feedback sequencing is important to understand and practice for leaders because it is not the usual order for parents themselves to follow. Parents often start with what was difficult, rather than what went well. It therefore is tempting for leaders to follow parents' lead and start with things that have gone wrong and need correction first, as well as ending with negatives. Leaders also need to pace their positive comments, starting with a couple of things that went well, but saving their strongest positive comments until the end of the feedback. In addition, leaders should remember that, while it is always effective to refer to specific interactions when feeding back positive comments to parents, positive comments also can be global ones and remain effective. However, when leaders are feeding back where they wish parents to make changes, they need to give specific behavioral examples, using their notes as aides memoire, in order for parents to be clear about what they need to focus on.

For example, a leader, in providing corrective feedback midway through feedback to a mother's non-verbal response to her son's drawing, said, *"Remember that Manny kept turning around to look at you while he was drawing? It would be a good idea to sit near Manny when he is doing things he wants you to see."* It would have been less clear and more negative to say: *"Don't sit so far away."*

In general, leaders need to guide parents in processing their first practice play session with them, primarily keeping in mind the learning goals for each parent, but also being mindful of the learning needs of the group as a whole. A summary of the first practice play session for a father of average skills is given next. This is followed by some guidelines on the steps in the formal feedback process with parents, with illustrations from this father's session.

Case illustration of a first session with a parent of average skills attainment

BACKGROUND INFORMATION

Mark is the single parent of Susan, aged 5. He has cared for Susan for two years by himself, after her mother left the family suddenly for a new partner. Mark and Susan have the support of Mark's family, especially his mother and his older brother, but Susan is increasingly showing signs of withdrawal and tearfulness in most social situations, prompting a referral for GFT.

Mark (nervously): *Susan, this is your special playtime and you can do most things you like in here. I'll let you know what you can't do.*

(Susan remains silent and holds her father's hand tightly as she looks around the room.)

Mark (after a pause): *You don't know what to do.*

(Susan shakes her head and looks up at her father. Mark smiles at her and waits patiently with her.)

Mark: You're looking at everything.

Susan: Come over here, Daddy. (She tugs her father's hand and leads him over to the water. Mark stands by while Susan silently pours the water from the bottle to the container and then pours the water into other toy dishes, and from dish to dish many times.)

Mark: You're pouring the water a lot.

(Susan leaves the water and takes her father's hand to lead them over to the doll's house.)

Mark: Are you finished with that water?

(Susan nods and continues her way to the doll's house. She sits on the floor and Mark stands beside her.)

Susan: The furniture is all messed up.

(After silently looking at the furniture for some time, Susan begins carefully arranging the furniture in each room of the doll's house. She places the furniture upstairs first.)

Mark: The beds go upstairs, just like our house.

(Susan continues to sort out the furniture, and moves on to arranging the downstairs rooms.)

Mark: The chairs go downstairs. You like it that way... We have five minutes left for today, Susan.

(Susan silently arranges the kitchen, then tosses aside the toy refrigerator and sink. She continues on to the living room, looking thoughtfully at the furniture for a while, then quickly picks up the couch and places it in the center of the room. She then places other furniture around it.)

Mark: Do you like that couch? You're putting it in the middle of the room. We have one minute left today, Susan.

(Susan speeds up and puts more furniture in the living room until the room is very crowded.)

Mark: You want to finish. You're going quickly.

Susan: There! It's finished. (She looks at the house, sitting back on her heels.)

Mark: You're happy with that. We have to leave now and you're happy you finished.

Steps in providing feedback after parents' first practice sessions

This section gives general guidelines for a leader's formal feedback to parents, with illustrations from Mark's session with Susan.

1. The leader conducting feedback starts by listening to the parent's reactions first, guiding the parent to think about what went well and what the challenges were for them.

2. The leader then begins direct feedback to parents with a positive remark, such as:

   Mark, you managed to stay in there and be with Susan for the whole time. It was very clear to all of us, and most of all to Susan, that you were really focused on her. That is what we want the children to experience. You didn't try to shift her attention to other things in the room.

   Or:

   Mark, you showed understanding of Susan's feelings at important places. You said that she was happy she finished, for example.

3. The leader waits for the parent's reactions to their positive feedback, and insures that they practice empathy with the parent, then moves on to where an improvement can be made. For example:

   Mark, you could improve on what you did in the play session by concentrating on your body's position in the room. When Susan moved from the table in the corner to the doll's house on the floor, instead of standing and watching her, you could sit on the floor near the doll's house, or sit on the small chair near the house. Standing over children can be overpowering frequently. Being at the same level as the child keeps things on an equal plane.

   Or:

   When Susan showed that she didn't like some of the furniture in the doll's house— maybe it will be something else in the room another time—instead of remaining silent, you could show you understand and accept that by saying something like, "You think it's not very good" in an accepting tone of voice.

   NB: The leader did not comment on Mark's two questions to Susan, judging that this error was minor, and could be dealt with in a later session, if needed. Susan had not reacted to the questions by feeling obliged to answer verbally. If she had, the leader could have suggested an alternative response for Mark. For example: *"That couch is important to you; it's going right in the center of the room."*

4. Leaders give highly positive comments at the end of their feedback. For example:

Mark, it was very impressive the way that you managed to show Susan you were interested in the doll's house, and what she was playing with there. You said that was difficult for you because you never have been anywhere near girls' toys yourself, being one of three boys in your family growing up. It was a long time to keep your concentration on Susan, but you did it!

General comments on selective feedback

Leaders need to remember that it is important for them to be selective in the feedback they give parents. Sometimes new leaders attempt to feed back all the details of the play session they have just observed to a parent. However, it is essential that leaders only emphasize the crucial practice points of the session for their feedback. This is done in order to ensure that parents understand and remember these important points for their later sessions. Smaller difficulties, such as a parent following all comments with "right" at the end of sentences, should be ignored; major ones, such as a parent ignoring the child's strong feelings, need to be addressed. Usually, adult learners are inclined to denigrate their efforts when learning new skills. While leaders should remember to be empathic with parents' concerns, yet in general remain positive, leaders should not reassure parents unduly. This rescuing of parents from their emotional responses by becoming overly reassuring encourages a lack of genuineness in parents and in the group as a whole.

Leaders should not imply in any way that they are judging parents as a parent or as a person. *It is vital that parents do not feel criticized.* Partly for this reason, we caution leaders not to link the program or the play skills parents are using in practice play sessions to daily life during this training phase. Leaders should always concentrate on the program itself and the skills that parents are learning. This approach of leaders having the group focus on skills development is much less threatening emotionally to parents than turning immediately to interpreting children's play sequences, and relating their play sequences to daily life.

GFT's approach of initially isolating child-centered play skills from daily life enables parents to learn the skills during their play sessions without having evaluation of their daily parenting cluttering the picture for them. One of the strengths of FT is that leaders frequently describe parents' play sessions as a special way of relating to their children. Because their ordinary interactions with their children are not addressed at this early stage, parents feel less threatened emotionally and can concentrate fully on mastering the skills of the special play sessions. In response to parents who bring up home and school issues, leaders are able to say that these issues are important ones and are addressed later in the program.

The role of other group members in feedback

As stated earlier, leaders aim to ensure that their verbal feedback is a potent way for parents to remember what they did during their practice play session, and then act on this feedback during their next session. It also is vital when beginning practice play sessions that leaders realize that they are modeling for group members how feedback is to be conducted—that is, comments are to be supportive and non-critical. While leaders do not want to inhibit group members from giving feedback, it is very important that parents who have practice play sessions observed by the group do not feel undermined by critical comments. Leaders also select areas for feedback that are crucial and therefore tend to eliminate many unhelpful, extraneous points that other parents might initially comment on. Therefore, we recommend that other group members are invited to comment only after the leader has modeled the tone of the expected feedback after play sessions.

Usually a parent's partner in two-parent families is eager to comment on their partner's session with their child during group feedback. In some cases, it is even more important that leaders first model positive comments towards the observed parent for a partner. This is because sometimes troubled families have developed critical attitudes towards one another's parenting, partly as a result of their difficulties. Leaders need to be practiced in reframing comments and use other person-centered family therapy skills, as well as empathy, during these exchanges. When necessary, leaders need to guide partners towards verbalizing what went well, rather than what was difficult. If an occasional parent is unable to adapt to positive comments towards either their partner or other group members, it is useful for the parent and leaders to meet informally outside the group to discuss this issue more fully, rather than have negativity or rescuing permeate the group's responses to one another.

Sometimes a group member may comment on a skills problem they observed; for example, a parent may enquire about the questions that Mark asked once or twice (i.e. *"Are you finished with the water?"* and *"Do you like the sofa in the doll's house?"*). In this instance, leaders have a fine line to follow. While not condoning the asking of questions, it usually is a mistake to dwell on another parent's criticism of a first practice play session. This could potentially undermine the confidence of the playing parent. Therefore, one of the leaders may wish to point out that, while it is better not to ask questions, there were many other things that Mark did well during his first play session.

An exception to the general rule for leaders of ignoring minor mistakes by parents during their first play session would be if Mark had routinely used questions as an inappropriate means of responding, such as *"You like that couch, don't you? Do you wish you had one like that?"* or *"You want to put the doll on it, don't you?"* A style of response by a parent that is primarily questions does need to be promptly pointed out by leaders, and they need to rehearse immediately with the parent how to change those responses into appropriate ones during their feedback.

The next two illustrations are of first practice play sessions with parents who have widely different abilities. These parents were scheduled for first sessions by leaders after the first practice play sessions had been conducted by parents with more average skills attainment, such as those displayed by Mark. In the first example, the mother has above average skills learning, while in the second the father shows a very poor level of skills development. Excerpts from these sessions, and from feedback afterwards with the leader and the group, are given.

An example of a first session with a parent showing above average skills attainment

BACKGROUND INFORMATION

Ten-year-old Sarah had been bullied at school for a year, before confessing this to her mother, Margaret. Sarah had been complaining of severe headaches and had been through extensive medical testing to no avail, before she finally confided in her mother that several girls had been texting her on her cell phone all the time, and taunting her at school because of her disability. (Sarah had been accidentally injured by fireworks at a display in a park when she was 3 years old. She had lost her sight in her right eye and had been disfigured facially by the accident.)

Sarah's teenaged sister and her father had decided not to participate in the GFT program; they attended the FPO with Sarah and Margaret and were supportive of Sarah receiving help. Another factor that is relevant to the example is that Margaret is a Quaker and has a strong belief in pacifism. However, she decided to allow Sarah to have toy guns in the play sessions, which was a major concession. The example that follows is an excerpt from Sarah's play during the first practice session:

> Sarah (picking up the gun): *You have the other one. We're going to shoot it out in here!*
>
> Mom: *Wanting to play shoot-outs with me.* (Mom gets shot) *You like to shoot me.*
>
> Sarah: *Shut up, you piece of shit!* (Sarah looks up at Mom expectantly.)
>
> Mom: *Trying it out. In here you can say almost anything you want.*
>
> Sarah: *Quiet, you piece of shit!* (Mom remains quiet.)
>
> Sarah: *You shoot me now.* (Mom pretends to shoot.)
>
> Sarah: *You and me are together now. We shoot that robber.* (Mom and Sarah shoot the robber, as directed by Sarah.) *That's a fat bitch we just shot.*
>
> Mom: *You like it in here. You can say shocking things, and do things you aren't usually allowed.*
>
> Sarah (laughing with her mother): *Yeah! Let's go over to the water.*
>
> (Sarah directs her mother to make "water storms" with the water in a container, which showers onto their hands from above. Sarah's exuberant play stays within the container and she and her mother laugh a lot, enjoying the sensation of the water on their hands, and taking turns spraying one another.)
>
> Sarah: *We'll go play with the cars and trucks now.* (Sarah and her mother move over to the vehicles, with her mother tracking how Sarah is arranging the vehicles for the rest of the play session.)

Selective feedback with the mother

Parent 1: That must have been very hard for you Margaret, knowing how you feel about guns!

Leader 1: Yes, we can talk about that first, if Margaret would like to do so. How did the session feel for you Margaret?

Mom: It was difficult at first. I had prepared myself for the guns, and I knew Sarah would try it out, but I hadn't really thought about what I would do if she used rude words.

Leader 1: So that threw you, and you didn't quite know what to do. But, you took it in your stride, which would not have been easy for you.

Mom: I remember you saying that we should try to be as permissive as we can about the words that children use during play. But I didn't want to say that she could say anything she wants, because she might say something I just can't tolerate.

Leader 1: So you chose to say "almost anything." That felt like a good compromise for you.

Mom: I was surprised she just said one more rude thing, and then went on to do something else.

Leader 1: You thought Sarah would challenge you more than that. I thought you did an excellent job of reflecting her feelings. Maybe that's why she did move on. She felt understood when you told her that she liked the room and its permissiveness.

Mom: Yes, I guess she did. I felt I was starting to see what a struggle it is for her to be good, when she has some of those words and feelings inside her.

Leader 2: That really came across. It must have felt good for both of you to play and have fun together in the water.

Mom: Yes, it was so good to see her laugh. It's been quite a while since she was so relaxed. It was almost like she was a little girl again.

Leader 1: You're thinking about when life may have been more carefree for her, and maybe she is tapping into those earlier feelings too.

Mom: Yes, like it was before her accident.

Parent 2: That must have been awful for her and your family. I think you're very brave and strong.

Mom: No, I'm not really.

Leader 1: You don't feel very strong on the inside. You are trying to be a good mom, but it's hard for you to feel strong. Maybe you had a few flutters, like most parents have, for your first play session here with Sarah. You did very well—you were able to do many of the things we have been practicing during your play session, like following Sarah's lead. You did that all the way through the play session and she knows now that you are willing to trust her to choose what to do during the next play session you have here.

Mom: I was amazed by how well it went for Sarah.

Leader 2: It is so interesting for all of us to see how your children act when they have their playtimes. Let's now move on to another play session we saw.

GENERAL COMMENTS ON THIS SESSION

This parent handled her first play session very competently, and the leader did not need to think about what this mother needed to improve for her next session. It was important to acknowledge that the mother had created a permissive environment, had reflected her daughter's feeling very well and, above all, had followed her daughter's lead throughout, despite inner difficulties with guns and language. It was a good chance for the leaders to reinforce these skills for the group, and to touch on the importance of nurturance seeking in play sessions for some children. The leaders empathized with the mother's feelings, but did not turn this feedback into therapy for the mother. (For example, the mother did not mention any guilt feelings she may have had for Sarah's accident, and the leaders did not explore these feelings here.)

An example of a first session with a parent showing below average skills attainment[1]

Jay is a 9-year-old only child whose parents are at their wits' end with him because he refuses to obey them or listen to them. (See Chapter 2 for a further example of this family.) He is increasingly defiant and aggressive with them and other children as he matures. He also steals things from his parents' and friends' houses. Cathy and Ethan, his parents, have taken different approaches to disciplining him. His mother has given up and allows Jay to dictate the rules when she is on her own with him, while Ethan has become the family disciplinarian, backed up by Cathy. Ethan has started setting harsher punishments as he feels increasingly out of his depth with Jay.

The following example is from Jay's first practice play session with his father; the mother had separate feedback on her own session.

Excerpt from Jay's first practice play session with his dad

Leader: Tonight Cathy and Ethan will be playing with Jay next. We will all go into the observation booth as usual, and watch each of the parents have a play session with Jay, and then another parent. Then we will come back together after our break and talk about them. I think I'd like to ask Ethan to start. Will you have the first one?

(Ethan agrees and begins the session with a clear introductory statement to Jay, then sits on a chair with his arms folded. Jay moves restlessly around the room near his dad's chair.)

---

1   This example is adapted from Louise Guerney's commercial videotape on FT, with permission from the publishers.

Jay: What do you want to do?

Dad (clipped and flat voice tone): *You're supposed to play. There are a bunch of toys. Go over and play with those toys.*

(Jay tries on a blank face mask and looks at Dad. Dad stares at him and doesn't respond.)

Jay: That's a dumb toy. Why is it even here?

(Jay tries on a hand wolf puppet.)

Jay: Hey, a wolf! Look at those sharp teeth there... (Jay moves the wolf puppet closer to his dad's face to show him. Dad nods silently.)

Jay: He looks kind of mean, huh?

(Jay pokes some toys on the table with the wolf puppet on his hand and picks up a man figure. He has the wolf puppet fight and bite the man puppet, twisting it hard. Dad looks away and shifts in his chair, but does not comment. Jay removes the wolf puppet.)

Jay: Oh, look! Some dinosaurs!

(Jay sweeps some toy dinosaurs off the table and concentrates on some of the rest.)

Jay: That's a Tyrannosaurus Rex, and we'll use the other one here. This looks like an elephant.

(Dad looks on from his chair while Jay sets up the small figures.)

Jay: This looks like a rhino...they're fighting.

Jay: Hey, look at this one. Kind of neat! Can I take it home? (Jay shows it to his Dad.)

Dad (very firm voice): *No, you can't take it home.*

Jay: Why not?

Dad: Well you know you can't take other people's toys. This stuff and place is used by lots of children.

Jay: But look they have all these!

Dad (warning tone): *Jay!*

Jay (excited and persuasive voice): *But they have all these... They won't miss this one.*

Dad (definite, flat tone of voice): *Jay, you can't take it home. Forget it.*

(As well as aggressively tackling and punching the bop bag in the room, Jay wanted to play horseshoes with his dad, but was overtly angry with him when his Dad corrected the way Jay set the rules to the game.)

Then the time for the play session was over, but Jay's father failed to give time warnings. As is our practice when parents forget to give time limits, a leader knocked on the door and said, "Time is up" so that Jay could hear. As prepared by leaders in advance, Jay's father told him, "You have one more minute." (This one-minute warning is given so children are not hurried out of the room.) With only slight reluctance, Jay left with his father.

Feedback with Jay's dad

Leader: How did you feel about the session, Ethan?

Dad: I felt all right. Sort of hard to get Jay to get started, to know what to do, but when we started to play horseshoes, it went all right, I guess.

Leader: Mmm hmm. You felt OK about the way things went. (Dad nods.) There were no issues that were difficult for you or places where you wondered just how you should handle it, or anything?

Dad: Well, when he wanted to take the dinosaur home, I wasn't sure about that. I tried to tell him not to do it, and it seemed like we were arguing about it, and he wasn't doing what I was telling him to do. So I guess I didn't really like the way that worked out. I didn't know what else to do. He couldn't take the dinosaur home.

Leader: You wanted to enforce the limit, but you didn't exactly know how to do it.

Dad: Yeah, I didn't like the arguing with him.

Leader: It makes you feel very frustrated with him, because you can't get him to do what you want.

Dad: Yeah, he won't listen.

Leader: Even in a place like this, it's still pretty rough.

Dad: I told him… I told him three or four times he couldn't do it.

Leader: So it seems like he doesn't want to be controlled.

Dad: That's right.

Leader: You don't want to have him always under your eye.

Dad: I sure don't!

Leader: Well that's one of the things we are working on in this program, to have children have sufficient control so that they feel responsible to follow the rules even though no one is watching. We would like that to be the way that Jay will behave after play sessions are completed. I think all the parents will benefit from a review of limit setting.

Now let's look a bit more at what went well for you, Ethan, during your play session and then we will turn to Cathy's session in more detail. One of the things that I thought worked very well for you, Ethan, was the opening statement and when you gave him the one-minute warning. You seemed to have real authority when you told Jay that it's time to end the session. Jay listened and came away relatively easily.

Dad: That was easy for me, but Jay's arguing was uncomfortable for me.

Leader: Some of the things he did made you feel very uncomfortable.

Dad: Yeah, he wanted to attack the bop bag all the time, and wanted to play horseshoes the wrong way.

Leader:…lots of things that were difficult for you to accept and follow his lead with.

Dad: I guess I'll try again next time.

Leader: You're thinking about how you can improve your skills. Concentrating on his feelings may work well for Jay. When he said at the beginning: "What do you want to do?", I think he may have been inviting you to do something with him. He seemed uncomfortable there, at the start, and may have wanted you to be with him doing something to make it easier for him. So maybe you can think about how you might reflect those feelings now…

Dad: I guess I could have said, "You don't know what to do," or "You want me to do something with you."

Leader: That is just the right tone of voice, and you are reflecting important feelings he had. Of course he may not react the same way next time, but I think he does want to be with you in the play session. And you showed him that you were trying to be with him too, even though it didn't work out as you had hoped. I can see that you hoped it would be different and are determined to try again to learn all these skills.

Dad: Yeah, it's going to be hard, but I'm a fighter!

Parent 1: You can do it, Ethan. We all have very embarrassing times with our own kids; otherwise we wouldn't be here!

Leader: You're not going to give up, Ethan, and it looks like other parents will be supporting you… Let's turn to Cathy's session now.

Comments on the leader's feedback to the father

The leader started specific feedback to Ethan with a general question about how the session went in his opinion, and invited him to expand on his viewpoint while remaining non-committal. (However, the leader and most parents would have realized that Ethan's session was definitely not on par with the first sessions of other parents in the group.) The father's initial response was that Jay had a problem "getting started", but that overall the play session was acceptable. By using tentative questions at the beginning of the feedback, the leader was able to help the father begin to discuss an issue that seemed difficult for him—his son's need to take a toy away. This led to further discussion of the need to closely monitor Jay's behavior.

It was very evident that Jay's father had serious problems with his limit-setting skill in his play session. Rather than singling out Jay's father for this practice, the leader planned on a whole group exercise on limit setting, particularly because Jay's mother needed this additional training also. Any further emphasis on either parent's lack of skill in this area may potentially have been taken as hurtful criticism of them, particularly when they were both feeling especially vulnerable. It was important that the leader continue detailed feedback with Ethan, after these more inclusive comments about limit-setting training. The leader needed to give more detailed and more positive feedback on his session to Ethan, reserving some corrective feedback for later practice play sessions. (With the number of difficulties Ethan had in his first practice play session, it was likely that more than two practice sessions would be required before home sessions began.)

Because Ethan's relationship with Jay appeared so negative, it was very important that the leader expressed hope for the father-son relationship, given that GFT skills were used effectively. It also was essential that the leader remained the principal person to set the tone of the feedback, and to provide explanations for group members during the feedback. Finally, the leader's comments illustrated how empathic responses always need to take precedence over cognitive or educational responses when strong feelings are raised in parents.

The next chapter continues with Meetings 8 through 10, during which parents hold their second practice play sessions.

CHAPTER 11

Parents' Second Practice Play Sessions

Meetings 8–10

This chapter considers parents' second practice play sessions with their children. Two extended examples are given that illustrate the types of issues that may arise for parents during these meetings. Particular challenges for leaders that may emerge during this part of the program also are discussed. The final part of the chapter addresses the preparations for home sessions by leaders that begin at the end of Meeting 10. This preparation continues for the whole of Meeting 11, the topic of the next chapter.

Second practice play sessions

Format for Meetings 8–10

As explained in the last chapter, the format for Meetings 8–10 is the same as the format for the meetings for first practice sessions, with play sessions before the break and feedback, skills development, and discussion afterwards. Leaders usually have less difficulty scheduling second practice play sessions, compared with the first ones, since parents have relaxed considerably and feel more connected with other parents in the group. They also are more familiar with a variety of play situations and skills applications. Therefore, unlike earlier meetings, leaders usually do not need to prepare parents for their second practice play sessions at the end of the previous meeting. However, a few parents may still need more preparation if, for example, their level of skills development is delayed, or if they have strong reservations about managing their session with a child they perceive as difficult.

There is usually more time after first practice play sessions have been completed for leaders to discuss briefly the collection of play materials for the next phase of the program, home sessions. We suggest that a preliminary discussion is held in Meeting 8, after feedback and discussion of the meeting's practice play sessions. A further discussion is then held towards the end of Meeting 10, as parents ready themselves for their imminent home play sessions.

Shift in group discussions

Typically during their second practice play sessions, parents are still developing their child-centered skills, but they also are beginning to be able to concentrate on their children's play more fully. Play themes arising from their own and other children's play sessions are beginning to emerge and provoke more discussion, but tend to remain less developed until home sessions are under way. This shift in discussion contents is both because parents feel better acquainted with all of the children fully participating in the program, and also because parents have been helped by leaders to develop supportive attitudes towards one another's learning. This supportive attitude is usually highly visible at this point in the GFT program, an attitude that seems to help parents become more open and responsive towards their own children and often their partners. They commonly become more accepting and confident of themselves and their potential as parents within the group as well.

Group members gradually become more practiced and experienced in giving positive and constructive feedback to one another, after seeing this frequently modeled by leaders. Once this style of feedback seems well established in the group, particularly at later stages of GFT when home sessions are under way, leaders need to consciously step back and allow parents to give much more feedback to one another. This is usually most evident at later stages in the program, but can emerge earlier in some groups. Usually, one or two parent leaders also develop in the group over time. It is often difficult to pinpoint who natural leaders in the group are going to be at early stages in the group process, but, by the point of practice play sessions in the program, a group's dynamics and structure usually begin to coalesce. The two examples here illustrate two different second practice sessions, including the emerging roles of parents within their groups during feedback.

Example 1: Jane's second practice play session

BACKGROUND INFORMATION

Jane, a divorced mother of two children, Amy, aged 6 and Billy, aged 4, is anxious to do everything right for her children, and tries very hard to supplement what they learn at school with additional educational toys and experiences at home. This seems partly because Jane feels somewhat guilty that, since the divorce, they live in a neighborhood with poorly performing schools. She wants her children to show good manners, to be popular, high achieving, happy, and contented. Unfortunately, she stated at intake that she was becoming very anxious and depressed because of Amy's difficulties. Amy was pulling her hair out more and more, and lately was starting to pull her eyelashes out too. Another stress for Jane was how much Amy and Billy fought with one another whenever Jane's back was turned. It wasn't just arguing, but real punching and hurting of one another. Jane blamed their weekend contacts with their father; she thought everything was much worse when they returned after their weekends with him. But there was nothing Jane could get their father to do differently, and she had now given up.

Jane's first practice play session was with Billy, who tried to get into all the messy play possible, and stretched Jane's limits on what he could do a couple of times. While Jane managed to set limits and follow his lead, she felt exhausted by the effort to practice new child-centered skills in front of the group. She said she was not looking forward to her second practice play session, this time with Amy. She was worried that Amy would show her up.

EXCERPT FROM JANE'S SECOND PRACTICE PLAY SESSION

Amy came into the play session eagerly and started to play with the doll's house, turning frequently to tell her mother what she was doing. Jane responded by reflecting Amy's feeling of wanting to be there, and her excitement. Amy then turned to the dolls and looked at them.

> *Amy: Can I take their clothes off, Mom?*
>
> *Jane: Yes you can, Amy. I'll tell you if you can't do something.* (Amy starts undressing a doll.)
>
> *Amy: That coat is stuck.*
>
> *Jane: Let me help you, Amy. You might rip it.* (Amy turns the doll over to her mother.)
>
> *Amy: I'm taking these clothes off.* (She picks up the other doll.) *You do that one.*
>
> (Jane readily starts removing the doll's clothes and puts a diaper and pyjamas on her doll.)
>
> *Amy: You can do mine too, Mom. You're already done with that one.* (Jane then changes the second doll.)
>
> *Jane: There. They're ready.*
>
> *Amy: Put them to bed then.* (Amy starts looking through the doll's equipment and picks out a pacifier and a baby bottle.) *I'm giving them their drinks and pacifiers. They have to go straight to sleep and not be noisy. So do we.*
>
> *Jane: We'll be quiet, so they can get to sleep.*
>
> *Amy: You go to sleep too.* (Jane curls up on the floor as instructed and pretends to sleep.)
>
> *Amy: You're sleeping.* (Amy takes one of the pacifiers and sucks on it, lying down with the dolls and remaining quiet for a couple of minutes.)
>
> *Jane (whispering): I'm still sleeping, Amy.* (Amy starts to suck more loudly on her pacifier.)
>
> *Jane: What are you doing, Amy? Please get that pacifier out of your mouth! It is dirty and you'll get sick if you do that!* (Jane gets up and goes to Amy, reaching for

the pacifier.) *You're a big girl, Amy, and you can do lots of things. You don't need to pretend to be a baby!*

(Amy hands over the pacifier and wanders over to the water in the pan. She listlessly pours it back and forth between the bowl and the container for several minutes, looking withdrawn.)

Jane: *You're pouring the water. You like the water.*

Jane: *I can do that with you, too.* (Amy and her mother continue to pour the water together, with Jane talking to Amy in a bright voice.)

FEEDBACK WITH JANE

Leader: *How did that go for you, Jane?*

Jane: *I was really embarrassed that Amy used that pacifier! She knows that she's not a baby any more. Everybody will think that I give her a pacifier to go to bed with.*

Leader: *It was hard for you to have others see what Amy did there.*

Jane: *Yes, I certainly wouldn't allow that at home.*

Parent 1: *We know from our own kids being here that they can do a lot of unpredictable things during their playtimes! My own son really surprised me when he threw that water straight at me.*

Jane: *But she could get sick, she isn't to put things in her mouth.*

Leader: *It was really hard for you to be tolerant of that behavior from Amy. You worry about her; you want to take care of her, so she doesn't get sick.*

Jane: *I have enough to do looking after them by myself! I most certainly don't want Amy or Billy to get sick.*

Leader: *You feel very much on your own; that it's all up to you to make certain Amy and Billy don't get ill. And if they do, your life is much more difficult.*

Jane: *Yes, it is...very difficult.*

Leader: *In the play sessions you were trying not to set too many rules, but that was too much for you. I think we could work on how to make sure you know the bottle and pacifier are clean for Amy to suck on, but it seems to be more than that. You seemed to find it difficult to have her pretend that she is a baby.*

Jane: *Well we already did all of that for real... It was bad enough the first time around, with Amy having colic day and night, her dad never being there to help, and my mom being so ill.*

Leader: *It's painful for you to remember that time in Amy's life because it was so hard for you.*

Jane: *Yes it was. It was terrible.*

Parent 2: Do you think it was a bit difficult for Amy too, maybe?

Jane: Not that hard, she didn't understand most of what was going on…but I guess her tummy hurt, and she may have sensed that I was struggling…

Leader: Thinking about Amy now…maybe thinking that she had it a bit rough too. In Amy's play sessions, one of the things she may want to do is to make things better the second time around by pretending to be a baby again. Remember we have talked a lot about trying to have a few less rules during these special play sessions, so that children can play out things that they have on their minds.

Parent 3: I really feel for you. I can see why it is hard for you to let Amy play at being a baby. I don't know how you can manage it all on your own, when your children fight so much with one another. You'd just like them to grow up, and not be such hard work.

Jane: Well Amy didn't seem angry in her play session. I thought she looked sad later on at the water. I guess I over-reacted when I saw her sucking that pacifier. She couldn't stay with the dolls and baby play when I did that…

Leader: You seem to think that now that you've thought it over; maybe Amy would have done more baby play. And you did recognize her feeling sad too. It was too much for you to say it this time around, that Amy felt sad, but you did see it clearly.

Jane: I hope I can work it out better next time.

Parent 1: We all are making mistakes and hoping for the best the next time around. I think we feel a bit like kids ourselves, trying to do all of this stuff for the first time, and not being brilliant at it. It's hard to see our kids feeling bad.

Leader: You're all determined people, and keep trying, because you really care about helping your children. And helping them with all their feelings, the hard ones and the easier, happy ones. I think Jane and all of you are on the right track. And your comments have been important to hear. Remember, there will be more opportunities to practice after you start your home sessions too.

Now let's go over the things you did really well in the session, Jane. Can you think of some of the things that went well?

DISCUSSION OF THIS FEEDBACK

It seemed evident to everyone watching this session that Jane had a very strong reaction to Amy pretending to be a baby. Because Jane immediately focused on her emotional reactions, it was important that the leader facilitated her to process them by making empathic comments. The leader spent a somewhat longer time than usual on helping Jane think about her own feelings and responding to them empathically, before going on to begin the feedback on the rest of Jane's play session.

After the initial emotional support of Jane by the leader, other group members voiced their own comments and expressed empathy towards Jane and towards Amy. These comments by other parents seemed to enable Jane to turn from prioritizing her own feelings to being able to think about the effects on Amy of her actions and attitudes during this part of their play session. A few key parents began to make highly effective comments. However, the leader still retained the most important role in the group. The leader, for example, drew in the entire group with her comments about the group being highly committed to helping their children. The leader's intent in making this more general, positive, and hopeful comment was to motivate all the parents to continue when their own painful feelings and shortcomings emerged during play sessions. The leader's other general comment was intended to foster group support further by acknowledging parents' helpful comments.

Example 2: George's second practice session with Jimmy

BACKGROUND INFORMATION

Seven-year-old Jimmy has been diagnosed with attention deficit hyperactivity disorder (ADHD) and conduct problems. He has two brothers, 9 and 12 years old. Both his parents, George and Helen, attend the program and have special play sessions with Jimmy and his 9-year-old brother Larry. (Their eldest son Greg is scheduled to have special activity times with each of them later.) George had his first play session with Larry, and Helen had hers with Jimmy. This is George's second practice play session, and his first with Jimmy.

JIMMY'S PLAY SESSION

(Jimmy runs into the room eagerly after listening to his father's introductory message impatiently. George finishes the message after Jimmy starts looking at the things in the room.)

> George: Jimmy, you can do most things in here, and I will be the one to tell you when you can't do something. (George sits down on the small chair in the corner of the room.)
>
> (Jimmy goes from toy to toy, and activity to activity, getting things out and then leaving them on the floor. He spends time rummaging through the dressing-up clothes, and then the toy cars, before moving on to other things. George tracks his actions and says once that Jimmy "wants to see everything.")
>
> (As soon as Jimmy goes over to the bop bag, he immediately attacks it by batting it to the floor, and hitting it repeatedly while straddling it. George gets up from his chair and stands watching Jimmy. George then sits down again on the small chair nearby, remaining silent. Jimmy continues to battle the bop bag, making grunting noises, for a few minutes, looking at his dad from time to time.)
>
> Jimmy (jumping up): I know, I'll fix you a drink. (Jimmy goes to the container of water and pours some into a cup, motioning his dad to come over.)
>
> George: Thanks, Jimmy. I'll pretend to drink that.
>
> Jimmy: No, really drink that.
>
> George: I won't. I'm not thirsty.
>
> Jimmy: I'll drink it then. You don't get any.

(Jimmy returns to the bop bag and pummels it.)

George: You're so strong!

(The bag accidently hits dad on the shoulder as Jimmy pummels it. His dad remains silent.)

Jimmy (launching himself at the bop bag from another small chair in the room): Watch me!

George: You're a tough guy with Goofy [the character on the bop bag]. You want me to see how tough you are. (Jimmy continues to jump on and hit the bop bag for a few minutes and then pauses to have another drink.)

George (still watching): You're proud of yourself. (As Jimmy pours the water carefully into his cup.)

(Jimmy then takes the cup and hits it against the bop bag.)

George: Listen, Jimmy. One of the things you can't do is hit the bag with something that can break it.

Jimmy (stopping his action): You liked it when I hit it with my fist.

George: Yes.

(Jimmy continues to attack the bop bag for several minutes. He then puts on a Spider-Man mask and gives his dad a ghost mask. George puts it on readily.)

George: You're Spider-Man and I'm a scary ghost. Whooo!

Jimmy (turning to his dad): I'm not scared. I want to hug you, Dad.

George: OK. (They then hug one another briefly.)

(Jimmy turns and looks in the mirror at himself in his mask. He waggles his head and babbles in a high-pitched voice to the mirror image.)

George: You like to do funny things… You like being Spider-Man. You like seeing yourself in the mirror.

(Jimmy picks up a toy car near his feet and starts running the car over his reflection in the mirror.)

George: One of the rules is that you can't hit the mirror, OK?

(Jimmy puts the car down, picks up some toy food and pretends to feed himself, while watching in the mirror. He then turns to his dad and pretends to feed him.)

George: That tastes good. That's enough now for me. You need something to eat, Spider-Man. What do you want?

Jimmy (taking off mask): I'm the teacher now. You are at school and in a lot of trouble because you were wandering around the school, and nobody knew where you were.

George: We have five minutes left Jimmy. ...I'm in trouble. I should have told somebody or better yet, I should have stayed in my seat.

Jimmy: You're in trouble. You have to go see Mr. Davis in his office, and he'll tell you off.

Jimmy (shouting at his dad as Mr. Davis): You are not allowed to go on the playground for a year! You were NOT to leave your classroom! And you will have to eat in my office, and not with the other children for a year too!

George: I should have done what I was told. I am being punished a lot.

Jimmy: You get angry and shout back at me.

George: I don't think I should do that. I'll get in worse trouble.

Jimmy: OK, then just pretend that you are angry and don't shout.

George: I feel cross but don't want to get in any more trouble.

Jimmy: I'm off. (Jimmy goes to the bop bag and starts hitting it again, this time with a toy gun.)

George: Remember I said don't hit the bag with anything that will break it. All right? Listen to me. Otherwise we'll have to end the play session.

(Jimmy goes quickly to the whiteboard and draws a target, saying that it's going to be for a game they will play. His dad watches as Jimmy draws the target's circles and then takes the ball that Jimmy hands to him.)

George: You go first.

Jimmy: That was a hit!

George: Let's see how I do. Yep, a hit for me too. Let's see how many we can do. We have one minute left.

(Jimmy and his dad continue to play this game until the end of the session, and Jimmy leaves easily.)

DISCUSSION OF PRACTICE PLAY SESSION WITH GEORGE AND GROUP MEMBERS

Leader 1: You put a lot of effort into that play session with Jimmy. How did it seem to go for you?

George: I was more pleased with what I did this week than what I did with last time. I remembered to set some rules, and I went along with what he was playing.

Leader 1: You think you improved from last time to this time. You were remembering what we talked about working on. You did set limits in the right places—for example, when Jimmy was trying to hit the bop bag with things.

George: I wasn't sure whether I should set a limit on his running that car on the mirror. I decided I would, because it could scratch the mirror. Plus I thought he might just decide to come down hard with it on the mirror.

Leader 1: You decided what rule was needed there, and, now that you are thinking about it afterwards, it sounds like the rule makes sense to you.

George: Yeah, I think we'll keep to that, and I won't allow Jimmy to play with a mirror like that. He can just make goofy faces in it instead.

Parent 1: I think that's a sensible rule too. I'm glad I saw it, so that I can have the same one, if I need it.

Helen [Jimmy's mom]: I'm going to have it too with Jimmy. But what about the way limits were set? Wasn't George supposed to remind Jimmy he said that he could do almost anything, and then say the rule? (Said in a critical tone of voice.)

Leader 1: You noticed that, Helen. It's difficult for parents to remember everything about limit setting when play sessions start, and George did have to set limits a lot, much more than some of you will have to do. We should all take note of how well Jimmy complied when George said them in an authoritative way... no resistance. We're all watching because it helps all of us learn. I think all of the group will benefit from practicing the limit-setting steps later on today. I think it is important that we remember that George was working hard inside his head about what limits to set, and he did manage to set the limits he thought were important.

Parent 2: I think you did a great job, George. I wouldn't have remembered half of what you said, if I'd been put on the spot.

George: Well there were other things I didn't especially know what to do about either. I wasn't sure I could refuse to drink that water Jimmy offered me, and I didn't want to go along with arguing with the head teacher when he said I had to.

Helen: That is the last thing he needs, to see you arguing with a teacher!

Leader 2: Remember when we talked about how imaginative play is just that? Children know the difference between real and pretend by Jimmy's age. I think he wanted to take on the very powerful role of the teacher and see what that was like.

George: But he could get the wrong idea, if I went along. I tried to tell him it was wrong to do.

Leader 2: We have talked about how, in your daily life, it is very important to tell Jimmy what the rules are, and what you expect from him both at home and at school. But that's why this time is a therapeutic playtime. Jimmy seemed to want to figure out what it was like to be the teacher when a child is disobedient in school. I'd encourage you to go along with what he wants here, because Jimmy can start to see different sides of the situation that way. He can see it from the teacher's side, and he can see it from the child's side. Then in his play he can choose, if he likes, to work it out the way that suits him. And maybe it's not just about school. We'll look at it more later, but sometimes there's a deeper issue at work, and for Jimmy *it might be about how adults can manage bad behavior in a way that is just and fair. These play sessions give him the chance to figure things out for himself, rather than him trying (and sometimes not succeeding) to do what adults want him to do. How to get better self-control is a big issue for him probably.*

Parent 3: My daughter has that issue too. She doesn't have Jimmy's problems, but she gets very sullen, if I tell her off. I bet she would love to shout at her teachers!

Leader 1: There are several things all parents have in common that we can work on together here. I just wanted to end by saying how well I thought you reflected some of Jimmy's feelings, George. You picked up and said that he likes seeing himself in the mirror, for example.

George: That seemed a lot easier to do than last time. And I intend to take on the play characters Jimmy gives me, without preaching, next time.

Leader 1: Great! You did respond easily to Jimmy being Spider-Man too. Let's move on to talking about Helen's practice play session with Larry now.

DISCUSSION OF THIS EXAMPLE

The feedback given here by both leaders and other parents illustrates the importance of allowing the parent conducting the play session to be the focus of attention. The example also shows how important it is for the leaders to provide feedback in a supportive manner that does not undermine a parent's confidence and self-esteem. During feedback for the second practice play sessions, leaders continue to model these attitudes to the parent, their partners, and the group as a whole. These leaders seemed to be achieving these aims. During feedback, the group continued to move in the direction of positively supporting its members, enabling more reluctant parents to participate.

Leaders also have to judge what to feed back to each parent, as mentioned earlier. In this case, the leader wanted to help George practice limit-setting skills again and help him follow his child's lead in imaginative play. These issues arose spontaneously in discussion, were elaborated on by leaders, and responded to by other parents in a supportive way. The example also demonstrates one way leaders use concrete examples from the play session in making their comments, and start helping parents think about underlying issues in their children's play. Finally, it shows the importance of ending feedback on a positive and encouraging note.

Special issues for leaders during this phase of GFT

Chapter 3 already outlined some common challenges for leaders in GFT and suggestions for handling them. This section addresses issues that may arise more commonly for leaders during the program's first and second practice play sessions.

Helping parents to be positive group members

As the earlier examples of feedback show, most parents readily model their own responses to other parents on the leaders' responses. Generally, the leaders' tone is picked up very quickly by each parent in the group, and the group atmosphere of joint problem solving and empathy for others' attempts is dominant. However, sometimes an observing parent may become more emotionally involved in a practice play session, and find it difficult to be positive about the skills another parent is learning. For example, George's partner Helen became critical of his limit setting in the feedback. One leader immediately picked up on her tone of voice and, while not dismissing her accurate comment, turned it away from George initially and towards the common difficulty parents have with limit setting. The leader also showed empathy for George's demanding session. Afterwards, another parent reinforced this positive tone with a further comment of support for George, enabling him to continue to freely express his reactions and attitudes about his next planned session. In most instances, quick and light comments by leaders diffuse the effects of overly negative remarks that group members occasionally make.

Very rarely in the authors' experience, leaders need to explicitly teach a very small minority of parents how to be positive group members. Parents' negativity is often fuelled by feelings of inadequacy as parents, which compounds their anxiety when learning new skills. If a parent is tending to undermine group members and is not modeling responses on leaders' cues, a leader may need to take this parent aside and explain further the aims of feedback, while once again remembering to respond empathically to issues the parent raises. It is also useful for leaders to give a few examples of how to make comments in more constructive ways. The following example illustrates this process for a parent, Emily, whose negative remarks had escalated to strongly criticizing another mother, Tracey. Emily commented during the general discussion after an observed play session with Tracey's son that she had *"missed the boat"*; the son's feelings were *"so obvious"* that Emily *"couldn't understand what Tracey had been thinking."* One of the leaders asked Emily to have a brief conversation after the meeting had formally ended:

> Leader: I'm glad you want to participate in the discussion, Emily. But we've found that people really learn a lot better when things are worded in a positive way. It would help, when you give feedback, if you would word it in a constructive way. Could we think about how you might have worded that comment to Tracey tonight about missing her son's feelings?
>
> Emily: Yes, but Tracey always sees something aggressive in what John does, and it bothers me that she never gives John the benefit of the doubt. I just feel like I have to say something because nobody else does.
>
> Leader: You feel bad when John's feelings are mislabeled. You feel like it is important for somebody to take note of it; it seems to fall on you.
>
> Emily: Yes, don't you think somebody ought to say something? I think it's important to correct people, if they are wrong.
>
> Leader: Let's think together about how to word your opinion positively. We really want your opinion, along with everyone else's, and we all benefit when these opinions are given positively. Whether everybody is agreeing or not is not the important thing here. The important thing is that Tracey does not feel criticized, which will help her learn better where she needs to improve.

Emily: Maybe I could say something like "John was feeling sad, I think, not angry."

Leader: That sounds just right. Thanks for talking with me about this, Emily, and we'll look forward to hearing more of your opinions.

Keeping the group on track

Another possible problem can arise in groups where a few parents have major difficulties learning skills and playing with their children during practice play sessions. Earlier chapters mentioned the option of offering an additional, practice play session outside meetings. Leaders also need to remember that, while it is essential to give these struggling parents detailed feedback after their practice play sessions during meetings, it also is important to limit this so that parents who do not have major problems feel important and included in the group. Leaders need to remember that those parents with more serious gaps in their play sessions learn indirectly from feedback to, and watching, parents in the group who have only minor problems. As stated earlier, all group members learn vicariously from one another, including when leaders address minor problems with parents who are developing their play skills more easily.

Bored and discouraged parents

Another reaction worthy of comment, although a rare one in our experience of practice and home play sessions, is when parents say they are "bored" by playing with their child. We again suggest that leaders accept these feelings. They may even wish to acknowledge that sometimes play is more boring for a parent than at other times. Leaders are usually able, based on their experiences of practice play sessions, to pick out the possible reasons for this response. It may be that children's play seems less meaningful if the parent is not involved, if children's play is repetitive, or if children themselves do not seem very involved in their play. Leaders may wish to remind parents that, when nothing much is happening, it is sometimes harder for parents to accept, than when too much is going on! Leaders may also wish to say that play sessions are about what children need from moment to moment, and that this can be different from what parents need.

Overall, leaders need to show empathy with parents who feel playing is a waste of their time, showing they understand that parents may be finding it difficult to have patience and let things evolve. These empathic comments from leaders, which accept parents' feelings of hopelessness and discouragement, often help parents to manage their negative feelings about play more easily. If this attitude persists, however, other troubleshooting (e.g. observing another practice play session, a further discussion) may be required.

Embarrassed parents

Sometimes parents, whose children did not respond well to them during a practice play session, feel very embarrassed by this display of their parenting difficulties in front of the group. If so, it is important that leaders do not rush their feedback with these parents. Clear and detailed empathy is required for the parents' strong feelings, as the earlier example of Jane showed, with leaders addressing at the outset why the play session proved so difficult.

In some cases it is obvious why the play session was difficult. Jane made it very clear during her session that she could not accept her daughter's immature play. During feedback, Jane became able to understand and manage her feelings more easily. At other times, children may have situation-specific reasons that trigger behavior that their parents find difficult to accept. For example, a child may have had a particularly difficult day in school, and was out of sorts before being brought to the meeting. Or it may be that a parent noticed that the ball that the child liked in a previous, practice play session was not available. These latter reasons are more straightforward, and more easily accepted by parents.

As a general rule at this stage in the program, we suggest that it is more helpful for leaders to look for behavioral reasons for children's difficulties in play sessions, and to refrain from focusing on underlying reasons for the session's difficulties in detail. This is done in order to give parents a graceful way to maintain their sense of self-worth when anxiously trying to implement their new play session skills. Yet it also is important that the reasons leaders give are genuine ones (e.g. *"There was a lot of noise outside the room, and it seemed difficult for your child to concentrate."*) and not misleading ones (e.g. *"Maybe he is catching a cold."*). However, in a few cases parents themselves bring up a very strong reason for their child's behavior (e.g. *"The police were called to our home last night."*), which leaders then need to address immediately in the group meeting, as well as perhaps spending additional time after the meeting with this parent.

Preliminary discussion of toys and equipment

After parents have had their first practice play sessions, it is time by Meeting 8 for leaders to discuss the equipment parents should start collecting for their home play sessions. Sufficient preparation of parents in order for them to have time to collect materials and organize their home sessions is needed, but leaders should also be aware that too much emphasis on materials can take away from GFT's main therapeutic and relationship-enhancing aims. Leaders can effectively point out in beginning their toys and materials discussion that the equipment used in the demos and practice play sessions during meetings is similar to what parents will be using at home. Parents are then given a handout on suggestions for home play materials and video recording (where possible) of home sessions for supervision during meetings (see Appendix 17). During this discussion, leaders need to intersperse rationales for the selection and use of toys and materials, along with practical details, both of which are discussed further here. The discussion also deals with wider issues related to toys and materials in the GFT program, in order to prepare leaders for any future issues arising in later meetings, as needed.

Underlying rationale for toys and materials selection in GFT

Compared with the usual playrooms that play therapists may be fortunate enough to work in, and compared with the toys and materials that many children have available at home, particularly in more affluent families, the toys and materials used for FT play sessions are intentionally more basic. Primarily, the toys should be inexpensive, safe, and unbreakable. This less elaborate equipment is intended in order for both children and their parents to concentrate on their relationships with one another, rather than being distracted by elaborate features of any equipment. It also makes storage and reserving the equipment only for home play session use more manageable.

Leaders need to explain these rationales for selection of equipment to parents, emphasizing that the toys and materials are the means towards the end of therapeutic play and relationship building. It is playing with toys that serves as the catalyst to reaching these goals. Leaders should convey to parents that all the equipment listed in the handout is intended to facilitate children to both engage in high levels of expressive play and to interact directly with their parents. Therefore, more complex model-building materials, electronic equipment that fosters solitary play, other things that limit imaginative play, (such as lengthy board games) are not included. The equipment listed for GFT is intended to help children express their feelings clearly. Feelings arising in play, such as aggression, a desire for nurturance, cooperation and mastery, are facilitated by the toys provided. Leaders can add that the toys themselves may give children added permission to express themselves more freely than they may be allowed to do in daily life.

The practicalities of collecting home session equipment

Leaders may have to draw on their own ingenuity to help parents collect toys and materials suitable for home play sessions. One item suggested, the "bop bag," may be more difficult for groups held outside the USA to find than some of the other equipment. Leaders may have to suggest that parents improvise their own homemade bop bags (e.g. stuffed pillow cases with faces drawn on them). Other groups may be able to offer a small quantity of subsidized equipment to group members, particularly for groups composed of a high number of low-income families. Social services and child welfare agencies may be able to contribute a modest sum ($50 perhaps) at referral for clients who are accepted into the program. Parents can pool their ideas for finding inexpensive materials with other group members during their midway breaks, or email or text one another outside group meetings. Parents may be able to find gently used toys at garage sales, yard sales, and jumble sales. Some leaders may be able to take responsibility and provide the basic kit of items for all group members, handing out a "goody bag" to parents when they begin collecting items for their home sessions (e.g. bop bags, sturdy new shoe boxes for making into doll's houses). Discounts may be available for bulk ordering. In general, leaders have the options of either giving out new FT kits or parts of kits, or have each family in the group purchase new, inexpensive items or used items in good condition themselves. Parents should not "make do" with old, used items from home that are worn and uninviting, or still in use at home. Instead, it is important that they and their children have new, fresh, and inviting items that lend themselves to expressive play.

Other advice for parents is that it is more effective for them to collect home play session equipment without their children's participation. This is because children become both curious and excited if they know their parents have new materials. Saving all the new and different items for the first home session helps families' home sessions have a positive start. It also saves parents the difficulty of setting limits with their children when they try to influence their parents' purchases and try to play with the toys beforehand. For these and other reasons, leaders need to stress to parents that the materials used during home play sessions should not be used by children during their usual playtimes at home, and need to be stored securely.

Home video recordings

Making video recordings of home play sessions is highly recommended; however, this may not be feasible for some parents, even though these are invaluable for supervision during meetings, and for the parents' use in self-supervision. Leaders should make certain that low-income parents in particular are either helped to have access to this equipment, or reassured that other forms of recording home sessions are possible and will be discussed later.

Special issues on materials in home play sessions

Some of the following issues are useful to mention during this initial discussion of home play session equipment, while other issues may be more appropriate to mention for some groups during the discussion in the meetings immediately before home sessions begin.

BROKEN TOYS AND REPLACEMENTS

As a general rule, when items become broken in the home filial kit, they should be replaced, if at all possible. If cost is a special problem, the leader or agency may have a small reserve fund to subsidize these purchases. However, it should be noted that the practical side of this issue is often not what is foremost in parents' minds during home sessions. They often are concerned that their children are breaking a toy "on purpose" or because they have not been sufficiently careful. The leader's task is to empathize with parents' feelings, but also to examine with parents the feelings their children are having when this occurs. Parents' punitive attitudes (e.g. *"He'll never learn to respect property, if I let him get away with it"* or *"He's doing that just to wind me up; he'll spite his own face if he has to"* or *"If she breaks anything she is gonna have to pay for it"*) need to be recognized and accepted, and then parents helped to think about their children's feelings. Leaders aim to help parents cope with their children's anger, which is often the main reason for toy breakage, and recognize that in play sessions their children are actively learning how to self-regulate their impulses.

CHILDREN ADDING PLAY MATERIALS OF THEIR OWN

Another general rule for home play sessions is that the materials used by children are the ones provided for them in the filial home kit and that these remain the same during all home play sessions. However in exceptional circumstances, this rule may be bent slightly by a parent, after first discussing the issue with leaders. It seems useful to encourage a parent who observes that their child needs a particular toy or object, or is asked by their child to take something into the play session, to tell their child that they will check with their leaders first. The leaders would then make the decision along with the parents on whether to allow a special toy or object. This decision should be based on the special need of that particular child and its therapeutic benefit. For example, a younger child may have a "transitional object" that is carried everywhere, serving as a comfort object in unfamiliar situations. Such a toy or object may well be allowed to accompany that child to their play sessions.

A less straightforward example, and one which leaders would have to think about more carefully, is one where children insist that one of their usual play objects at home is needed during a session in order to advance their play. Ryan & Needham (2001) give an example of a boy recovering from post-traumatic stress disorder (PTSD) who was ending play therapy sessions with his therapist. He brought one of his stuffed small animals from home each time during his last sessions to play out important themes of resilience and hope. These small animals also seemed to serve as a way to carry the emotionally important issues he had addressed in the playroom into his home life. A similar situation may arise for parents who carry out home FT sessions. However, each child's circumstance differs, and should be examined from a therapeutic perspective by the leaders with parents before supporting these exceptions to the general rule.

Finally, on rare occasions leaders may notice that a child was emotionally invested in a particular toy or object during demos and practice play sessions. If a child has shown devotion to a particular toy in the practice play sessions over the weeks, it might be wise for the leader to suggest that that particular kind of toy be in the play materials for the home kit, and help the parent provide it before home play sessions begin. Providing a toy across settings—home/agency—that has become obviously significant to a child can be critical for their continued emotional expression. That child may feel adrift when beginning home play sessions without that particular toy. An example is a 6-year-old boy, Marcus, with developmental problems who was fascinated with a Tyrannosaurus Rex dinosaur during the demo in an early meeting and in his practice play sessions with his mother and father. All of his fantasy fights during his play had to include the dinosaur either winning or losing. This type of dinosaur was not included in the parents' selection in their home kit. During his first home play sessions with his mother and then his father, Marcus repeatedly tried to find it and then tried to substitute other figures. However, he seemed much less able to carry out his fantasies with other dinosaurs because this particular one was not there. When his parents, after checking with their leaders, added T-Rex, Marcus was able to again use the dinosaurs more easily for fantasy play during his home sessions.

Managing drawings, paintings, and models during home sessions

Leaders should try to encourage parents to adopt a general rule that is workable for them as a family on what to do with products of home play sessions. The rules that play therapists have may not apply wholesale to FT practice. While it is common for some play therapists to keep products made during therapy until the end of the intervention, there also is debate in the play therapy literature about the advantages and disadvantages for children of their therapists keeping all art products from session to session, until therapy ends. Wilson & Ryan (2005) state that this decision will be arrived at by therapists based on their own therapeutic style, and the needs of the children they work with.

For GFT, it seems most useful for leaders to take the position that, while children may not take or use the toys outside the play sessions, drawings, paintings, and models made during play sessions are their own products and are exceptions to this rule. This seems most easy for parents to manage, enabling them to concentrate primarily on reflecting their children's feelings (e.g. wanting to look at it more, liking it, wanting others to like it). This practice also prevents parents from having to introduce another limit to their children's behavior during play sessions, thus reinforcing the permissiveness of play sessions. However on rare occasions, leaders, after discussions with parents, may make an exception to this rule, particularly if children's products are filled with disturbing or very private meanings. In these instances, leaders may suggest to parents that it is more appropriate for these products to remain with the home filial materials from week to week, rather than bringing them into daily family life.

Use of materials acceptable to parents conducting play sessions

As mentioned earlier, the toys and materials suggested for filial kits are designed to give children the strong message that a wide range of emotional expression is acceptable during play sessions. Our discussion of the types of materials to use is based on this underlying principle. However, a few parents may find one or two items objectionable. The most common examples giving rise to problems for a few parents are messy materials (e.g. sand, water, play dough), gender-specific items (e.g. dolls, women's hats, and tea sets), aggression-eliciting toys (e.g. guns, pistols, swords), and items eliciting immature behavior (e.g. a baby's bottle).

In general, it is important for group leaders to stress to parents that the materials during therapeutic play sessions at home need to immediately convey to children that expression of their feelings is acceptable. It is also worth repeating in this discussion that not being able to express feelings appropriately is one of the usual reasons for children's emotional difficulties. When leaders explain that certain children show overly anxious feelings, while others overly inhibit their feelings, and that both of these more extreme reactions can be worked on in play sessions, these explanations seem useful for parents, as long as the issue is primarily an educative one. Giving examples from demos, or having parents themselves point out examples of aggressive feelings, immature feelings, and "feminine" or "masculine" feelings can be effective during this discussion. The child development rationale from Chapter 4, that children depend upon adults to help them express their strong feelings in acceptable ways before they are able to master this task by themselves, also can be effective in this context.

Practical difficulties with materials also can be dealt with directly by group leaders. For example, with water, sand, and play dough, leaders can suggest ways that parents can protect their property (e.g. having a modest amount of liquid in a pitcher for the play session, having a waterproof mat over the carpet, having a baking tray for the play dough). However, it is very important, as we have stressed throughout, that parents' feelings are recognized and accepted by leaders, and that leaders do not use purely objective reasons during this discussion. Parents' strongly held values and experiences underlie their reactions to this topic and should always be respected by leaders. Some parents may have strong beliefs about mess, others about gender-specific activities. It also is important that leaders are not too inflexible in insisting at this point in the program that the complete filial kit must be used. Rather than the materials becoming a barrier to filial training and participation, leaders can state that parents can wait until all their practice play sessions have been completed before they decide that a particular toy(s) should be removed or altered. It is hoped that parents may discover that play items that seemed inappropriate are not as distressing to them as they anticipated.

In general, leaders aim to help the few parents who have emotional issues surrounding the use of particular materials to stretch their boundaries somewhat. It is helpful for leaders to point out to parents that they do not need to generalize these rules in play sessions to their daily lives. These conditions can be met only for their home play sessions, which are held just one half-hour a week with each child. It also is worth leaders noting to parents that the play sessions are special situations and very controlled environments, and children usually find non-destructive ways of using these materials.

Overall, leaders need to recognize and accept that parents often compartmentalize their responses at the beginning of FT training. In our experience, parents commonly lose their more rigidly held beliefs about mess and the expression of feelings during the remainder of their training. For example, a father announced initially, when he observed a demo with another child, that he would not allow his son to play with dolls in his home, and certainly would not allow him to play with dolls in his demo. He believed that dolls taught boys that feminine behavior is good. This father saw no way in which expressing nurturing responses through dolls' play could be therapeutic for his son. Leaders assured him that they took his feelings very seriously, after expressing empathy regarding his position. They also assured him that, when the time came to do home sessions, they would not be insistent that he include dolls, if he still felt the same way. Leaders suggested that further observation on his part of children playing in demos and practice play sessions, including those with his own son (which excluded dolls at his request), would allow him to make a more informed opinion about the positive or negative aspects of dolls during home play sessions.

As the program continued, this father became less distressed with dolls in the sessions and ultimately, when conducting home play sessions with his son, was actually able to use the dolls with him. This proved to be a very therapeutic experience for his son. The father reported that he still did not believe in dolls as boys' toys outside play sessions, but saw the value of them in a therapeutic play situation.

Other issues on conducting home sessions

Most parents naturally begin to think about where and when their home sessions will take place when the topic of collecting materials for this purpose arises. Leaders should give brief information to parents about the importance of an uninterrupted time when holding sessions, and a place in the house that lends itself to play, such as a non-carpeted room, and the importance of reserving these toys for play sessions. Some parents wish to have detailed discussion of these issues at this point. But in our experience it is more fruitful for leaders to say that, for all of these requirements, any problems that have arisen so far for parents have always had workable solutions. Leaders should mention to parents that these requirements will be worked out in detail together towards the end of this phase in the program, before their home sessions start. Leaders also can suggest that parents think about their own possible solutions, in readiness for the later discussion together.

Further preparation for home sessions

After all the parents' second practice play sessions have been completed during meetings 8–10, the last part of Meeting 10 is used to help parents ready themselves for the next meeting, which is devoted entirely to helping parents prepare for home sessions. Building on the briefer discussion leaders had in Meeting 8, when they helped parents with starting to collect home session materials and video equipment, leaders should ask each parent or couple to bring their list of collected materials as set out in the approved list with them the following week, for Meeting 11. (If the agency is providing families with home materials and/or video equipment, then leaders inform parents that these will be available for them to see and take home in Meeting 11.) Leaders also ask parents to come to the next meeting with a suggestion of where they intend to store play materials in order to keep them separate from everyday things, and an idea of the time and place in their home that is workable for home play sessions.

Leaders may need to take an active role helping some parents think about how to keep FT materials separate and reserved only for special home playtimes. Group members often make creative suggestions and engage in problem solving during this discussion. Some suggestions arising from earlier groups have been using the attic or basement space; using the garage or garden shed; putting the equipment in the locked trunk of the car or a locked suitcase under the bed; or taking the equipment to a trusted relative or neighbor.

Leaders should ensure that this discussion results in positive and acceptable ideas for the group as a whole. When parents find it very difficult to imagine where the toys will be left alone by their children, it may be because the parents have underlying difficulties with setting limits with their children, and therefore do not want to enforce such a rule at home. In these cases, leaders need to empathize with the emotional constraints the parent feels (e.g. *"You feel so mean when you have to refuse him."*), then encourage parents to find a solution that does not require direct confrontation with their children over this issue. Instead of focusing on the more problematic issues during Meeting 10, the best use of group time is to assure the group that all these issues will be worked out and finalized during the next meeting.

Place and time for sessions at home

Parents already have been prepared during the earlier discussion in Meeting 8 to think of an uninterrupted space that is easily cleaned for play sessions at home. Usually parents readily come up with suitable solutions, such as using the kitchen or living room on a Saturday morning after breakfast, or using a heated garage or attic room. Sometimes spaces such as hallways can be adapted to this use once a week. However, leaders should caution parents that bedrooms ideally are used for sleeping and restful activities, not play sessions. Leaders can remind parents that sometimes children play out frightening scenes in their play sessions, and it is important not to have this kind of play occur in a space that is later reserved for sleep.

For a few parents, more creative solutions may need to be found, such as having the play sessions at a grandparent's home, or using a family center room. These more complex solutions can be discussed separately after the meeting, then finalized during the next meeting, rather than spending an inordinate amount of group time on this.

Similar to issues raised earlier with materials storage, leaders want to ensure that they have first addressed any emotional difficulties with home space parents have, before practical considerations are explored.

The next chapter discusses Meetings 11 and 12. Meeting 11 is devoted entirely to preparation of the home setting and other features related to beginning home sessions. Meeting 12 is dedicated to processing each parent's first home session.

CHAPTER 12

Transition to Home Play Sessions

Meetings 11–12

The next phase in the GFT program is having parents independently conduct play sessions at home. This chapter considers two important meetings: Meeting 11, which is the meeting before parents begin conducting home sessions, and Meeting 12, the meeting immediately afterwards. We discuss how leaders decide that parents are ready for home sessions, and how to prepare them practically and psychologically during Meeting 11. The next meeting, Meeting 12, is fully devoted to parent reports on their home play sessions—including processing their own reactions and those of their children, as illustrated here. Leaders should note that in both Meetings 11 and 12 *there are no live, practice play sessions.* Weekly, supervised sessions with selected children, either live or via video, resume from Meeting 13 onwards, and continue to be an important component of GFT.

Readiness of parents for home sessions
Criteria for assessing readiness of parents

At this point in the program, leaders typically feel confident that most parents have developed sufficient child-centered play therapy skills to be able to conduct play sessions at home. It is important that skills development is well under way, and that parents will be able to handle issues that may arise within their home sessions without direct and immediate feedback from leaders and other parents. Parents' skills level does not need to be perfect prior to home sessions. Parents should be able to apply basic play therapy skills and avoid major errors; leaders should not wait until parents achieve a professional level of responses. Leaders may wish to remind themselves that there will be many opportunities to sharpen parents' skills as the program continues.

Leaders can feel comfortable about parents starting home sessions, if parents are consistently doing the following:

- Picking up on their children's obvious feelings.

- Following their children's leads most of the time.

- Setting basic limits adequately.

It is also essential that negative responses by parents, such as criticizing their children, attempting to direct them, or setting inappropriate limits, are totally absent. As a general guideline, leaders should ensure as fully as possible that parents begin home sessions at a level of competence that would be expected to lead to a successful session. We have found that, if the first home session does not go well, parents may become discouraged. As we discuss more fully later in the chapter, parents' readiness, coupled with shorter first sessions, generally lead to adequate, or far better in some cases, play session experiences.

The decision to have parents start home sessions is easy to make for leaders most of the time. However in some borderline cases, the decision is less straightforward and dependent on leaders' clinical judgments. Leaders need to decide whether these parents' skills development, while not good, is still sufficient for them to progress at home. As discussed in Chapter 1, supervision is needed by seasoned FT leaders, as well as by less experienced practitioners, from experienced FT supervisors when complex decisions such as these are to be made.

When one parent is not ready for home sessions

There are two different ways to make the transition to home sessions. The most common way is for all the parents in the group to start home sessions at the same time; the other way is a staged transition, to be discussed later. Sometimes, when a whole group transition to home sessions seems most appropriate, one parent is behind the group in the level of skills learned during practice play sessions. We suggest leaders explain that they would like this parent to have one more practice session before starting at home. Generally, these parents accept this suggestion very easily, since they themselves are often feeling less competent. They commonly appreciate the added attention and support.

Leaders should be careful to make their suggestion in a way that is not judgmental. We suggest that leaders identify some phenomenon other than a parent's shortcoming to justify this delay. It is generally fairly easy to provide an emotionally acceptable and valid reason for the delay, citing an event that is obvious both to this parent and others in the group. For example:

> Mary Jane, you missed a couple of the beginning meetings, so it would be good if you had a little more practice that we can observe before you start home sessions.

Or:

> Susan, when you played with Johnny the first time, he was very uncooperative and didn't give you a chance to apply the play session skills as fully as you wanted. So we'd like it if you could have an extra session before you start your home sessions.

When a parent needs extra practice before starting home sessions, it is important for leaders to arrange this with the parent before or after Meeting 11, or, when required, as soon thereafter as possible. This timing ensures that the parent is able to attend and participate in the group at more or less the same pace as the other parents. If an extra session is not possible to schedule before Meeting 12, the parent should still attend, and will profit from listening to the reports of the other parents who were able to start their sessions on time. The parent who is starting later generally becomes highly motivated to get started too, having become inspired by what was reported by the other parents. The extra practice session will have become urgent, and needs to be worked in quickly.

When a staged transition to home sessions may be preferred

The most common way to make the transition to home play sessions is with the group as a whole, which is the main focus here. However, a staged transition may be preferred and planned for from the outset for certain groups, or it may emerge as the most viable option for a particular group during the delivery of the program. For a staged transition, leaders pace the start of home sessions among the parents by beginning the first home sessions with those parents who have mastered play skills well, and who have attended all the scheduled meetings.

This option seems most useful during delivery of the program when:

- there is a real and apparent difference in the number of times leaders have supervised individual parents (e.g. when illness or other urgent issues have prevented several parents from attending weekly)

- there is a wide difference in skill levels among parents

- much more rarely, the children themselves have indicated they have problems with play sessions.

Unlike the circumstances outlined above that emerge *during* delivery of the program, a staged transition to home sessions also can be built into the delivery of the program from the outset. This option may be preferred for groups where open-ended starts are needed, and/or where children with very difficult histories and multiple emotional problems participate. An example of this kind of group is illustrated in Chapter 16, which gives a successful adaptation of the GFT program in Bradford, England, for foster carers and their children.

Preparations for home sessions and their impact on children and family life

Before their first home sessions start, parents should be exposed to all the issues involved in planning home sessions. Flawless structuring is essential for the first session. Once the sessions are in progress, minor obstacles can be handled more easily than in the first session. General discussions about the kinds of issues that may arise, such as those arising from the room to be used, what childcare arrangements are in place, and where other family members will be, are important. Successful home sessions also require discussion of mundane details, such as ensuring that phones are turned off during the session, and that family pets do not intrude. When these discussions are curtailed, some structural element can prevent the session from going smoothly.

It is important for leaders to remember that all of the practical preparations for home sessions during this meeting also give leaders opportunities to help parents think about their children's emotional reactions to introducing a new event into their home lives. Leaders have general discussions with the entire group on the practicalities and possible psychological impact of home sessions before moving on to finalizing home play session arrangements with each family in the group at the end of the meeting. The general attitude for leaders to convey to parents is that these home arrangements are manageable. Leaders should underline that time spent on practicalities and thinking through their children's possible emotional issues that may arise before starting home play sessions enables parents to maintain their weekly commitment to their children.

The structure of home sessions

As already discussed in previous chapters, leaders need to stress again during Meeting 11 how crucial it is for parents to commit themselves to home play sessions being held in the same room, with the agreed materials, and at the same time every week. Leaders should emphasize that parents' commitment to regular sessions is part of what makes home play sessions work as therapy. By holding sessions at the same time weekly, children and parents establish a set routine for the sessions that is part of family life. This regularity means that children can count on their play sessions occurring at a regular time. Parents can also prepare themselves more easily psychologically, just as they have already been doing for the group meetings.

Parents should set up the play space in the same way for each child and each home play session (except for agreed changes for teens and toddlers). Leaders already discussed the kinds of home play spaces that are suitable for sessions and the rationales during Meeting 10. Leaders may need to review some of these during Meeting 11, fielding any general queries that are relevant to the entire group, and leaving more specific queries for individual discussions with families.

The first home session should be limited to the same length as the now familiar practice play sessions—namely, 10–15 minutes. This is in order to ensure that parents are not stretched beyond their capacity in this new setting. After feedback on first home sessions with leaders in Meeting 12, the length of home sessions usually increases to 30 minutes. Once home sessions are established, leaders may suggest that the length increase to 45 minutes for some children. Parents need to be informed that the increase in time will be discussed further during the next meeting, and usually finalized by leaders then.

Scheduling home sessions

The best time of day and day of the week for regular play sessions at home can vary from family to family, but there are general guidelines that need to be given by leaders that help parents decide. Leaders should emphasize, if it is not raised by parents spontaneously, that both children and parents need to be emotionally and physically able to engage readily in play sessions. For example, fathers who work the night shift on Friday night are not usually fresh enough to do Saturday morning home play sessions before going to sleep. For children who have a large amount of homework on week nights, scheduling a play session after all their homework is finished may not be desirable. Other less than optimal times for children, apart from when they are tired or exhausted mentally, are when play session times conflict with other very desirable activities, such as interrupting their regularly watched, favorite TV programs, their weekly pattern of going to a friend's house after school, or having to miss football practice on a Saturday morning. Leaders help individual families think about the optimal time for their home play sessions later in the meeting.

Arranging childcare for sibling sessions

Leaders should help parents think about how play sessions will be managed when there are other children to care for, particularly when children take turns with their siblings for play sessions. In some families, the non-playing parent contributes by caring for the other children during sessions held by the playing parent, or playing parents take turns with one another for childcare. For singleton children with two parents, half-hour sessions with each parent are common. It usually is most expedient if all the play sessions are conducted one after another, in order to avoid setting up the play space more than once a week. Parents also need to put the play space back into its original layout after each session, because it is important that children are not confronted with the remnants of their siblings' play (or their own, for singleton children). Parents should already know that it is the adult's, not the child's, task to sort out the play space; they may need reminding in this new context.

In single-parent families with more than one child, the logistics for home sessions usually entail staggering sessions. If children's ages differ enough, say a kindergartener and a fourth grader, their schedules may allow a parent to schedule each child's sessions when the other child is not in the home, or is in bed. If sessions are held back to back, leaders should suggest having another trusted adult to help single parents with childcare. Ideally this adult would have a close attachment relationship with the children, be supportive of the parent, understand the importance of the children's play sessions, and help them feel settled and relaxed.

Should an older child wait for a play session alone?

As a general rule, we do not recommend that children be left to their own devices while their parent has a play session with a sibling, and we certainly do not recommend that an older sibling is left in charge of a younger one. Feelings of sibling rivalry and abandonment can arise in unattended siblings, apart from any safety issues and the need for the playing parent to remain vigilant to unattended children. Interruptions, which are to be avoided, also are more likely during the play session. However, if there is no suitable adult to help the family, and it is an older, more independent child who is judged by leaders and parents as having the emotional capacity to manage on their own, leaders may choose to make an exception to this rule. Parents should then be helped by leaders to think about setting up their child with a DVD or another enjoyable activity, in order to entertain themselves in a positive way, while waiting for their parent to finish the session with their sibling.

Changes in children's play and responses at home

Another area of preparation is discussing with parents the possibility that some children's reactions may differ from one setting to another, which may result in their home play differing from the play seen during meetings. In addition, the first home session may be different from later ones. The novelty of the experience, for both parents and children, can lead to exceptionally good sessions in some instances and, in a few, to atypical, below average, play sessions. Leaders should emphasize that changes in their children's behavior usually create positive results—for example, some children relax considerably and enjoy their sessions more at home when not being observed. Parents also may feel more relaxed and more able to put their newly developed skills into practice. Leaders can mention that there may be other positive changes—for example, some children may become more talkative and interactive, and others may become more quiet and self-directing than at play sessions during meetings.

A few new challenges for parents also should be referred to. A child may become more aggressive or much messier, for example. A few children may complain that the toys at home are not as good as the ones in the meetings' playroom, and some children start wanting to stay longer. Parents need to be reminded by leaders that they in turn will need to change their behavior and adapt, if their children display these differences, as they already have seen with other parents in practice play sessions during meetings. Encouraging comments by leaders of parents' demonstrated abilities, similar to those made before mock sessions and practice play sessions earlier in the program, never go amiss when preparing parents for home sessions.

Limit setting in home sessions

This discussion of children's reactions often leads to structuring and limit-setting discussions, which is very important for leaders to have with parents. Nothing helps home play sessions go smoothly in our experience as much as parents having clear plans for the structuring of the sessions, and the limits that will be required in them. Parents often raise limit setting as their biggest anxiety about starting home sessions. Leaders need to be empathic about parents' concerns, find out what limits they are worried about, and agree that some of their children may have a reaction when a familiar space is used differently at home. Some children, as parents rightly imagine, do test the new rules directly by their behavior, and a few children test the usual home rules afterwards, just to make certain daily life has not changed in other ways. (This situation is discussed more later.)

During this discussion of limit setting, it is effective for leaders to directly ask parents: *"How do you imagine your child will test you in the room you will be using?"* One parent may reply that her child will go to the washing machine to try to fiddle with the controls, while another parent may think their child will try to leave the room several times during the play session, or another may worry that their child will try to add their own toys to the filial kit. If several parents express concern about their ability to handle these situations, leaders may decide to review and rehearse the limit-setting sequence of play sessions again. But before deciding on this rehearsal, leaders should be certain that parents are fully aware of their power to structure play sessions to avoid having to set limits that may be troublesome to enforce. Some parents may occasionally need to remind their children during the session that *"We play here in this special way for play sessions only."* Practical structuring steps, say, using tape on the floor for play session boundaries, or some other way to demark the safe play area (e.g. a rug) can be given by leaders. Parents themselves often offer other structuring tips, such as trying to cover or make inaccessible or unusable any attractive, yet forbidden items (e.g. the washing machine, the computer).

If no structuring solution whatsoever is possible for items that are prominent and attractive in a family's chosen play space (e.g. washer, video-recording equipment for the session), leaders need to make a clinical judgment about whether a rare exception to the standard opening statement is necessary. This exception is only made in order to prevent an overabundance of limit setting that could interfere with a productive play session. A parent may need to say, for example, in their opening statement, *"[Name of child], this is a very special time. You can say (ALMOST) anything you want in here. You can do almost anything you want, **except play with the computer**. If you cannot do something else, I will tell you."*

Often group members help one another effectively with their anxieties about limit setting at home by recalling similar sequences that occurred during practice play sessions they have held or observed, giving details of how a parent handled these challenges effectively with their child. These spontaneous examples from parents can be added to and reinforced by leaders. As stated in earlier chapters, shared group examples are usually very powerful, and parents are often able to recall, imitate, and replicate these examples of good practice more readily in their home play sessions. In order to put parents' anxieties in perspective, leaders also can remind parents that there will be further chances for skills development, including limit setting, during later group meetings, where necessary.

Play sessions in relation to daily family life

PLAY SESSIONS ARE NOT REWARDS

Leaders need to emphasize that play sessions should never be considered by parents as rewards for good behavior, or withheld as a form of punishment for their children. It is worth talking to parents about how tempting it is to withhold play sessions from children if parents have had a very stressful time with their children during the day, or several times in the week. This wish to withhold play sessions can be especially potent if difficulties occur immediately before a play session is to be held. Leaders should mention to parents that this issue, including how parents can emotionally ready themselves for play sessions during stressful family times, will be discussed soon in the program, once their first home play sessions have been held (see Chapter 13).

PARENTS' DIFFERING ROLES

Another issue leaders help parents think through is their role in play sessions and how that role differs from their usual parenting role at home. Leaders remind parents that play sessions are designed to be child centered but, as the group has already discussed, parents have other roles at home that are equally important, such as making sure family life runs smoothly with regular meals, scheduling, and socializing. Parents also have rules and educational aims at home that need to be carried out. Leaders should recommend that parents' rules and schedules be maintained as usual, and that they confine their play session skills to play sessions, in order to keep changes to a minimum during the first few weeks while home sessions are being established. We recommend that leaders are low key about the possibility of children testing family rules more generally, simply saying that parents should keep to their usual rules at home for now, and bring any worries they have to the next meeting to discuss. Some parents also may need a reminder that children find new experiences easiest when they are not overloaded by change. For example, parents should avoid bringing in a new pet, or having children join a scout troop, until home play sessions are clearly established.

The type and degree of adjustment to home sessions varies from family to family. Some parents have toddlers and teens they intend to include in home sessions later, which will be an additional adjustment for each family member. In other families, partners are not able to attend meetings, and need to be briefed by the attending parents in order to feel as fully included as possible in supporting home sessions. Leaders should discuss the role of non-attending partners with each relevant family at the end of the meeting, in order to finalize the emotional and practical support they are able to provide for the parent conducting home sessions.

AN EXAMPLE OF REVIEWING THE PLACE OF SKILLS GENERALIZATION IN THE PROGRAM

As mentioned earlier, leaders often need to remind parents that, even though they are conducting play sessions themselves at home, the GFT program deliberately delays the introduction of skills for parents' daily use until later. An example of a parent who was tempted to introduce play session responses into her daily living at this point is the following:

> Lisa: Danny responds well to my reflecting his feelings in the play sessions. I am wondering if this would be a good idea to do all of the time. I know that I probably wouldn't be able to put his feelings first often, when other things are important, or if I am upset with him. But, do you think it would be good to do?

> Leader: Absolutely! That is one of the goals of the program, to help parents use empathy, structuring, and limit setting outside of play sessions, and to give children more opportunities to express themselves in daily life. However, we strongly advise that you do NOT try to carry over these skills yet. A little more practice time will ensure success later. We don't want you to experience any failures with skills use because you're not sufficiently practiced. Generalizing skills will be the next step, after you have done some home play sessions.

Parents may need more information about why generalizing is not emphasized until towards the end of the program. Leaders can offer them the following reasons, where appropriate:

- Parents as well as their children need to make adjustments in their lives to accommodate to home play sessions. This comes first and is important for the success of the program. Generalizing skills is an additional area to learn about, better introduced after establishing the home sessions. It's not just children who can get overloaded, as all of us adults can testify!

- The aim in GFT is to help parents become more independent of the group itself, and to develop more regular support from partners, if this is not at a high level already. Home play sessions involve partners more, which should happen before generalizing.

- Parents have sufficiently mastered basic child-centered play skills to start home sessions, but there is more to learn during later meetings about refining their skills. They will develop their skills further, once home sessions are established.

- Children begin benefiting from regular, longer, play sessions at home than are possible during group meetings. Helping children to play about some of their emotional issues more fully is one of the aims of home sessions. Parents will be learning more about their children from home play sessions, and more time in group meetings is devoted to the meanings underlying children's home play in this phase of the program.

- Therefore, generalizing skills to daily life is much easier when parents have increased their skills, involved their families more, and children already have had additional therapeutic play sessions.

Children's' transitions to and from play sessions at home

Leaders should spend a few minutes during this meeting attending to issues about transitions before and after play sessions, in order to help parents maximize the therapeutic benefits of home sessions. Leaders may already have brought this facet of attachment relationships to parents' attention during earlier discussions of demos or practice play sessions. If so, leaders can simply remind parents that attachment theory and research has established the importance of sensitive parental responses when children separate and then reunite with parents, particularly when new experiences occur. For children who have insecure attachment patterns, as many clinically referred children have, they are unable to easily and productively engage and re-engage after separation from their parents. Parents' sensitive responses are more crucial in these circumstances. Leaders themselves can draw on their experiences of their own play therapy sessions, if required, when as play therapists they facilitated children's positive disengagement, and then re-engagement, with family members before and after play therapy sessions. However, examples from the group's shared experiences are invariably more powerful and more easily remembered by parents.

For this discussion of transitions, leaders may need to focus parents' attention on the practicalities of the transitions, and have parents think about what their children will be doing immediately before and after their home play sessions. Parents may need help to ensure they structure the time well (e.g. not interrupting their children's play midway through a computer game to start a session; having enough time for a bedtime story after the session). Parents also can be taken through what their children may be feeling immediately after the play session. Sometimes children miss the close attention they had from their parents during their play sessions. For these children, it usually is desirable that their parents continue to provide closer attention immediately after the session, at least until children have settled into another activity. Leaders can help parents, especially single parents, think about how to establish routines with their children that allow closer involvement and emotional availability from them before and after play sessions (e.g. shutting the door to the play session room and tidying up later).

The order of playing for families with siblings

Unless the family has worked out a preferred routine themselves, we usually suggest parents reverse the order of playing with their children from week to week, when they have sessions back to back. For example, Dad plays one week with Suzie first, and Mom is with Johnny second; Dad plays the next week with Johnny first, and Mom is with Suzie second. This order minimizes the potential sibling rivalry issue of *"Who gets to be first?"*, which often arises when working with siblings. We also suggest that parents reverse the child they work with each week, as the example just given illustrates, in order to avoid the potential for exclusive pairings in the family.

Preparing children for home sessions

Once parents have been prepared for home play sessions sufficiently, leaders need to help parents structure this new experience for their children before the sessions begin.

An example of a parent preparing their child for home play sessions, such as the one that follows, is useful for leaders to give to the group; a few families may require more individual help with this during the last part of the meeting.

> *Leader: Here's an example of what parents can say to prepare their children for home play sessions. Remember that younger children, and some older children too, may need to have this information a bit at a time, and not all at once. Your children also may want to say something to you about home play sessions, or ask questions, so try not to rush what you say. And try to pick a quiet and relaxed time to talk with them, so they can listen more easily.*

> *Parent: Starting on Tuesday afternoon, after you have had your after-school snack, we will be starting to do our special playtimes at home. I've been learning to do these during the meetings when you came with me. We will play for a short time the first time, so I can practice here at home. It will be for 15 minutes and we'll stop before your brother comes home from school.*

> *I have been collecting toys for us. Those are the ones we will use. They are played with only during our playtimes together. We will play in the basement, where I have put a big rug.*

> *So that I can learn more, I will be making a video each time, and writing down a few things. I'll show this to my group. Mary and Bill, our leaders, and the group of parents will help me learn more that way. We can talk about special playtimes at home again before we start, if you want.*

Recording home play sessions for supervision and discussion

The last general issue leaders need to discuss with the group, and finalize with each family later in the meeting, is how parents plan to record home sessions. This in turn has implications for the way in which leaders supervise home play sessions during subsequent meetings, discussed later in this chapter. In order to supervise home play sessions adequately, leaders need to monitor and understand each child's therapeutic progress during home sessions, and to help parents maintain and increase their skills levels in an active way. These two rationales are helpful for leaders to offer to parents at the beginning of their discussion on recording home sessions. The recommended ways of recording home play sessions outlined next address these two aims.

Both video recordings and written reports by parents of their home sessions with each of their children every week are highly recommended. The information on videos is a much more accurate and fuller account of each home play session than written records alone. Videos also facilitate better discussions during meetings when parents present their home play sessions to the group, and allow parents to share the play sessions with their partners at home in an immediate and fuller way. Leaders should encourage parents to use video-recording equipment for home sessions, and confirm that they know how to use it. Video equipment needs to be set up by parents in a static position before each home play session, and taken down afterwards. One of the rules is that children do not play with this equipment during sessions.

Written records, which are not onerous to complete, allow parents to think about the contents of each of their sessions. They also provide an important aid for parents in sharing information with their partners, and with leaders and group members during meetings. Parents need to be reminded that their play sessions are therapy for their children; therefore their written notes and videos are confidential, and need to be stored securely at home. They are to be shared only with their partners (and not with their children, without discussion with leaders beforehand), and with leaders and other members of the group during meetings.

Processing of home sessions by parents

Parents are asked to process their weekly sessions prior to attending each group meeting. They are asked to watch their recordings and make written notes on the home play sessions recording form (see Appendix 18) for each of their play sessions.

WRITING UP HOME SESSION NOTES

Leaders need to hand out and review the written recording form with the group, explaining that the form is intended to help parents pick out the main things that happened, and to capture the tone of the session for the group and leaders. Parents need to give themselves clues to the contents of sessions on the form, in order to remember examples from each session when they talk to the group. It is important for leaders to stress that each parent who has a session needs to fill in a form, in order to ensure that parents are conducting their home sessions on schedule. If leaders' work commitments permit, they may offer to collect all the parents' forms after each meeting and comment on them, and then return them to parents during the next group meeting. If this more intensive supervision is offered, leaders should be certain that their written comments are constructive, and are neither critical of parents' skills nor their children's behavior. While it can be an additional burden for leaders to write comments on parents' reports, it does seem to increase the number of regular submission of home session reports. Leaders' comments seem to serve as reinforcements, as parents look forward to seeing what leaders have written.

PREPARING PARENTS TO SHARE VIDEO EXCERPTS

Leaders should prepare parents for the next meeting, Meeting 12, stating that they will be eager to check with each parent about how things went for them and their child. It is a special meeting, with each family having a turn to talk about and show their video of a small part of their first sessions. For the meetings after that, families take turns being the family in focus to show and talk about their play sessions.

Parents are asked to choose five minutes, or short segments totaling five minutes, from their recordings of each of their children's first sessions to show the group. (Leaders need to make certain that they have instructed parents to mark their videos for the places they want the group and the leaders to watch with them during the next meeting.) Leaders should explain that everyone in the group will want to see how the first home sessions went. Therefore, it is important for parents to pick segments that show children interacting with their parents, where parents verbalize and respond directly to their children. Segments that are not as useful are ones where their children are very quiet, perhaps drawing a picture, and not interacting closely with their parents. These quieter times might be important to look at later, when each family takes turns being the focus in meetings.

If it proves impossible for any of the parents to access video-recording equipment, or if any parent or child feels strongly undermined or threatened emotionally (e.g. a child who may have been abused using video), then written reports alone, using the home play sessions recording form, have to suffice. Leaders need to help these parents not to feel criticized or unduly different from others conducting home play sessions. Because written reports alone are inevitably shorter and less "meaty" than those accompanying videos, leaders should emphasize that stand-alone written notes need to be completed by the evening after each session, in order for parents to maximize their ability to remember their session accurately.

It is important that practice play sessions at the meetings be continued for parents without video recordings, in order for leaders to supervise parents' play skills development closely. In groups where all the parents use home videos, discussed in more detail later in this chapter, leaders should remind parents that occasionally the parents in focus may be asked to have a live play session at the meeting for supervision.

Special issues arising for parents in home sessions

Next, some ways leaders prepare parents for some important, yet less common, challenges that may arise during home sessions, either at the outset or later on, are discussed.

Preparing parents for children who refuse home sessions

It is important that leaders manage to allocate a short time during Meeting 11 to discuss how parents manage any children who are reluctant to participate in home play sessions. Parents should be reassured at the outset of this discussion that, in general, children are excited to have home play sessions with their parents, but that leaders want to cover all eventualities. Leaders may be cognizant of possible "worst case" scenarios, but these are not useful to use. It is important instead that they help parents manage their anxieties about trying something new, and facilitate a positive group attitude towards each parent's success, rather than reinforcing or increasing parents' anxieties.

Very rarely, children have cold feet about playing with their parents at home. While there is no research available to date that can be cited about the reasons children sometimes refuse to participate in home play sessions, leaders all have clinical experiences of play therapy or FT on which to draw inferences. Sometimes, for example, refusal may be due to the oppositional attitudes children have adopted in order to preserve their autonomy in the face of excessive parental emotional demands. Other times, children who refuse initially seem to be the "hard to warm up" children described in temperament research; they find change and new beginnings more difficult to master than other children. Or practical arrangements may not be quite right for the play session at home. Leaders need to underline during this discussion that children *do* want to have loving relationships with the most important people in their lives, their parents, and therefore these hiccups, if they arise, can be managed and lead to good outcomes.

Leaders need to prepare parents on both a practical and a psychological level. Leaders and parents usually have an idea of whether particular children may find the transition to home play sessions more difficult. A few children may already have shown their reluctance to come to demo sessions or to their practice play sessions. However, these children can sometimes surprise both professionals and their parents by their unexpected enthusiasm for home sessions. Likewise, occasionally a child who has enjoyed play sessions on site can unpredictably bristle at home sessions. Therefore, leaders should make parents aware that there is no guarantee that all children will make the transition to home sessions immediately and smoothly, but it is common that they do.

Leaders also should point out during this discussion that sometimes children settle down well with home play sessions at the beginning, but then start to opt out. Some of the same things talked about regarding starting home sessions, summarized here, also apply to these later cases, with leaders assuring parents that this issue will be addressed again at a later meeting, if it arises.

Specific steps for parents if children resist home sessions

Leaders should give parents the following advice, if their children show reluctance to participate in their first home play session:

- First, make certain that parents can handle their own disappointment and frustration, without their feelings having an impact on their relationship with their children. Parents should make a note of how they feel, if this happens, so that they will be able to share these feelings with the group next time. Leaders can point out that everyone in the group wants to share in the parent's feelings, and learn from that experience, if it does arise.

- Second, if parents have picked up clues from their children that they are not so enthusiastic about taking part in home play sessions, parents are advised to set up the first home play session for only a short amount of time, 10 minutes, rather than 15 minutes. Leaders need to discuss this individually with parents and finalize the allocated time in the last part of the meeting. Slow to warm up children in new circumstances may need to have a short session for exploration and testing the water, before they feel able to settle into home play sessions.

- Parents of these slow to warm up children have adjusted their expectations to a short ten-minute, first play session. It is important that parents enforce the time limit agreed with leaders and not extend it. If, for example, a child goes very reluctantly into the first session, and starts asking the parent when she can leave, it is important that the parent should have a realistic response. A rule leaders suggest to parents is: "*We have to stay at least five minutes and we can stay no longer than ten minutes this first time. Then our time will be up.*" Parents should set a timer or a watch/clock alarm to go off at the end of the five minutes. This timing must be done in order for children to realize that parents really mean what they say, and are not trying to manipulate their children into playing longer. When the time signal goes off, the parent indicates that the child may leave, and the parent indicates that future sessions are longer. If the child should decide to stay past the five minutes, the child is free to do so, and the timer set only once again for five more minutes (that is, ten minutes in total).

- If the shorter ten-minute session is recommended for the first home session, leaders should remind parents that this is a temporary limit and that parents are free to make the session longer, up to the recommended time of 30–45 minutes, after the first shorter session is successful, and after it is discussed during Meeting 12. Leaders should remind parents that solutions to other problems with duration of sessions arising later on will be worked out in meetings by leaders and parents on an as-needed basis.

- If a child unexpectedly objects to starting their first home session, and it was not discussed with leaders in advance, parents should feel free to tell their children that it is necessary for them to stay for five minutes this time. The child can choose to play up to the 15-minute limit allotted for the first home sessions, since the parent had prepared their child for a 15-minute session already.

- Leaders should reinforce with parents that it is very important for their positive relationships with their children that children are not seduced into, overly persuaded, or tricked into attending or staying in play sessions. Strong parent-child relationships, one of the goals of GFT, will be undermined if these ploys are used.

Preferring one parent over the other

Another eventuality, that leaders should prepare parents for in a low-key way, is when children refuse to have play sessions with one of their parents, and readily have sessions with the other. It is critical for the success of FT at home for leaders to take time to mention this possibility during preparation for home sessions. However, it is not desirable to have a lengthy discussion at this point in the program. It seems most enabling for leaders to remind any parents whose children do not wish to have a first home session to tell their children that they are required to stay for at least five minutes with each of their parents. Aside from following this principle of a minimum of five minutes, and having this parent keep notes on their feelings, to be discussed next time, we think it is wisest not to dwell on one parent being favored over the other at this point, since it may be a one-time occurrence. There are many possibilities for children's resistance and preference for one parent; for example, a child may be slow to adjust to home sessions, or cannot cope with two sessions back to back. If this problem arises again, leaders should above all be empathic and then help the parents review all possibilities, including the ones just mentioned.

Responding to serious and urgent emotional issues, including allegations of maltreatment

Leaders are aware that every group has the potential for children to re-enact traumatic events and to make allegations of mistreatment during their home play sessions. Preparation for the latter already has been addressed at the beginning of the program (see Chapter 2 on mandated reporting requirements). In groups composed of families with children who have a history of maltreatment (e.g. children who are fostered or adopted after their infancy), there is a stronger possibility that allegations may arise, particularly when traumatic play is engaged in during sessions. In our experience, it is more likely that re-enactment of traumatic experiences by children will occur after play sessions are established at home, when children relax more fully and are less scrutinized by leaders and other parents. Since home sessions are not directly supervised by leaders, parents need preparation by their leaders for ways to respond to highly traumatic re-enactment and to allegations of maltreatment.

In many groups this preparation can be brief and factual. At the same time, leaders need to reflect any uncomfortable feelings arising in parents, and answer any questions that may surface. Leaders should aim to contain parents' anxiety around these topics, which already may be raised because of the impending transfer to home sessions. Leaders need to remind parents first of all that their home sessions are therapy for their children. As such, it is possible that children, once they feel more understood and confident, may confide in and play out with their parents many issues that are troubling them, either currently or from the past. Parents need to know that leaders are available for supervision for any very serious emotional issues, including allegations, as they arise in home sessions, and that parents should contact leaders as soon as possible. Leaders need to underline that parents should not wait until the next meeting for feedback and supervision in these circumstances, and provide parents with contact information for emergency supervision.

In addition to giving their own emergency contact details, leaders should remind parents that for any allegations that seem to be current and potentially very harmful to their children's well-being, parents need to tell their children that they will be contacting the leader and the child welfare agency *after their play session is finished.* Leaders should remind parents that, during the remainder of such a play session, they need to internally manage their own feelings, even though this may be very difficult, until they have discussed the situation with the leaders and/or the agency. In other cases where allegations seem to be related to past events that do not put their children at risk currently, parents should again contact leaders. If allegations are ambiguous, parents should inform leaders no later than the next group meeting.

Above all, during sessions with fresh revelations of mistreatment, parents should behave as follows:

- Continue to be very empathic. It is important for parents to concentrate on reflecting their children's feelings, including their anxieties, sensitively and fully, and to give them emotional support during the session and afterwards.

- Refrain from asking detailed questions to get their child's report of issues "straight." This is not the job to be done in a play session by a parent. A protective service worker will be put in touch with their child in most instances. This specially trained child case worker is the best person for fact finding.

For GFT with families where children already have a history of mistreatment prior to their current placement, or where children are known to have experienced highly traumatic events, leaders should consider preparing parents more fully for traumatic play enactments before home sessions begin. Responding to traumatic enactments is discussed more fully in the next chapter.

Finalizing home session arrangements

Leaders need to allocate enough time before the end of the meeting to focus on each family's practical arrangements for home sessions. Group members often have valuable contributions to make when practical dilemmas arise for individual families that have not been covered in earlier discussions, in addition to leaders' contributions. Leaders need to have a short review of each family's list of required materials, planned separate storage arrangements for materials and recordings, home space for sessions, time of day and day of the week for sessions, childcare arrangements for siblings, type of recording of sessions, and toddlers or teens to be included after home sessions are established. Leaders can use the checklist for home play session arrangements in Appendix 19 for each family. Leaders also should ensure that their own playback equipment accommodates parents' videos.

Sometimes a few families may find it more difficult than others to decide on these practical arrangements, even with supportive comments and suggestions from leaders and other parents. After a few minutes' discussion, leaders may decide that these issues are most usefully discussed on an individual basis after the meeting finishes, rather than spending a disproportionate amount of group time on them, as mentioned already. Finally, leaders pass out any last materials for home sessions, perhaps loan video cameras to families to record their sessions, and remind parents to bring their marked recordings and written notes to the next meeting, along with their Manuals. Leaders also need to give their final encouraging words to families about starting home sessions as the meeting ends.

Meeting 12: processing first home play sessions with the group

The meeting after the first home play session is organized differently from previous and subsequent meetings, and is a very busy meeting for leaders. During this meeting, almost the entire time is taken up with discussion of the first home sessions, and with troubleshooting any problems that have arisen. There is only a short time at the end of the meeting for arranging which families will present play sessions in depth at the next meeting. We suggest that leaders make a schedule during Meeting 12, as families present their first sessions, of families in focus for the next few meetings. The way to select families in focus is discussed later in the chapter. Modifications can be made in the schedule, if it should prove to be unworkable, in later weeks.

This meeting's strong emphasis on home play sessions is because the overriding aim of leaders is to firmly establish this important phase in the program. It is also because there is a great deal to discuss following the transition to home. The meeting is primarily concerned with developing parents' play skills within this new home context. The emotional contents of children's play are not emphasized yet. Themes in children's play are an emerging topic during subsequent meetings, once home play sessions have been established. (The topic of play themes is taken up in the next chapter.)

Parents are very eager to share their experiences of their first home sessions with other group members and leaders. Parents also invariably are very interested in one another's home sessions. They want to know others' feelings about their sessions, and how they handled challenging situations and "teething" problems. Leaders should make maximum use of this enthusiasm and curiosity. It is highly likely that parents who are excited by what happened in their home play sessions are able to share valuable contents of their home sessions with the group. Leaders too are naturally curious about how these first home sessions went. By their genuine interest in home sessions and by their comments on the sessions' contents and parents' feelings, leaders reinforce and contribute to this positive group atmosphere.

It is vital for group cohesion and the establishing of home play sessions that leaders find time to discuss first home sessions with everyone in the group, including watching all the five-minute video segments, or short segments totaling five minutes, that parents bring. Leaders ask parents in turn to report to the group from the home session report form they filled out and their video recording. Leaders should ensure before the group begins, as stated earlier, that the electronic equipment in use at the meeting is compatible with parents' recordings, that they are able to operate their equipment easily, and that it is in full view of all the group members. Problems with the quality of some video recordings (e.g. positioning of the camera, quality of the equipment or videos themselves) also may emerge, all of which need to be addressed by leaders with parents briefly in order to prepare them for their next home sessions. It is useful for one leader to be responsible for the equipment, while the other leader has overall responsibility for feedback. Before the five minutes of video are watched, one leader helps parents discuss the session, as they use their written feedback form for reference, and the leader asks the family what went well (e.g. Did the child engage? Did the parents see where they displayed their own skill in following the child's lead?). Then the other leader plays the selected segment(s). The first leader should ensure that their beginning and ending feedback is positive, as before, and the leader may highlight one area for further work, as needed. Above all, leaders should remember to primarily convey their encouragement and support for parents' efforts throughout their supervision of first home sessions. Leaders then swap roles as they discuss the first home sessions with the rest of the parents in turn.

Deciding on lengthening home session times

Leaders need to help each parent with each child pair to decide on the length of time for subsequent home sessions during this meeting. For parents who have successfully made the transition to home sessions during their first session, leaders should suggest that these parents hold longer, 30–45 minute sessions for each child in the family, starting with their next home session. Leaders should underline that it is important for parents to keep with this decision on length of sessions for all their home sessions.

A brief discussion of the feasibility of 30- versus 45-minute sessions for each parent and child pair often suffices, but in some cases more thought is required before this decision can be made. Forty-five minute sessions are frequently desirable for children aged 7 and older. However, if a child does not seem to want to play the 45 minutes, then a 30-minute period would be scheduled. Similarly, if children under age 7 seem to need 45 minutes to complete their session work, then 45 minutes can be scheduled for those children. Another factor to consider is the stamina parents have, and the commitment they can make to the sessions, especially in families with several children. The important principle is that the session be definitely scheduled for one length of time or the other, subject to children leaving early if they so choose, and not changed from week to week. Given this predictability, children can learn to manage their playtime activities more easily for themselves.

Trouble shooting for home sessions

Leaders must keep each group member's needs to the forefront during this meeting. Every parent needs both an opportunity to feed back on their first session, and opportunities to explore possible reasons for their children's reactions to first play sessions, both their positive and challenging reactions. This sharing of challenges and successes has a motivational and collaborative effect on group participants. Parents who had difficulty starting their home session are eager to share these with the leaders and group members. And leaders need to help iron out any practical difficulties in collaboration with parents on challenges that have arisen. We suggest leaders brainstorm with parents about the source of the session's difficulties—whether it was with the place, toys, duration, time of day, or the parent's style, to name a few. Then leaders need to plan for success by having the parents keep the next week's session to 15 minutes (or less, if needed). Shorter sessions with defined times typically reduce parents' struggles conducting the sessions at home, as discussed already.

Parents who do not conduct home sessions on schedule

In some groups, parents may not have managed to conduct their first home play session on schedule during the week. This usually emerges during the group meeting itself, when these parents do not have any play session material to share with the group. It is important that the leaders manage their own disappointment internally and listen with empathy to the reason(s) for this delay. It also is essential that leaders take the position that this program is therapy, as already emphasized. Parents attend because their children need home play sessions. Leaders then should establish with the parent whether missing a home play session is likely to happen again (e.g. *"I had to work overtime again this week, even though I asked to leave on time."*). If so, leaders need to help these parents modify their practical plan for conducting home sessions, in order to guarantee that parents start during the following week. (An informal survey among parents attending GFT at Pennsylvania State University revealed that the most common time for home sessions was Sunday morning, even for churchgoers. In some groups, leaders may wish to suggest that parents may find it more manageable to conduct their play sessions on Sundays.)

Usually the group's enthusiasm for their home sessions, and their children's disappointment when they were promised a home play session they did not receive, spurs on parents who are slower in organizing their play sessions at home. However, if a parent does not conduct a home play session by the second week of home sessions, leaders need to draw this parent aside and establish the cause(s) for this two-week delay. For example, maybe a parent finds it impossible to ask an elderly family member to remain in her room while the parent conducts a play session with a child in the main living space. In these unusual cases, leaders may be able, for example, to offer an open playroom at the meeting site for the parent to use, instead of conducting the session at home. However, leaders also need to reinforce the point that this program is therapy for children, and, if the parents do not conduct home play sessions, their children will not be able to make enough progress. If parents remain unable to conduct home sessions, leaders should contact the referrer, and hopefully an alternative treatment can be offered. If self-referred, leaders might suggest a short parenting program instead that does not involve weekly play sessions.

Helping parents when children refuse their first home play sessions

As stated earlier, children rarely refuse to participate in their first home play session in the authors' experience. However, even though leaders prepared parents for this possibility during Meeting 11, the rare unsuccessful parent is still likely to be devastated by what they perceive as overt rejection of themselves by their children. These parents naturally compare themselves with successful parents in the group, which can make the sting more painful for them. This sense of rejection can be even more acutely felt by a parent if their child attended one parent's home play session, and refused to attend the second parent's. Leaders need to empathize with these parents, and try to help them identify the causes underlying the children's refusal, as well as ways to handle it for the next scheduled home session, as discussed earlier.

AN EXAMPLE OF REFUSAL

Eight-year-old Gemma is an only child who was adopted by middle-aged parents when she was 3 years old. Her adoptive mother Heather gave up her career in order to care for Gemma. Her father Carl is a police officer who often works shifts and overtime. Both parents have shown strong commitment to attending GFT and learning to offer play sessions to Gemma. She has shown very insecure behavior during her practice play sessions with her father, and to a lesser extent with her mother, before home play sessions began. Gemma completed her first home play session with her mother, but refused to enter the room for her session with her father.

Leader (to Carl, the father): It must have been very difficult for you to have Gemma refuse to come into your first home play session, even though you had thought this might be a possibility.

Heather (interrupting): It was something I was so much hoping wouldn't happen. I wanted Gemma to get a lot out of her Dad being there for her again.

Leader: You wanted it to work well too. You really felt for him.

Heather: There wasn't much I could do. I didn't want Gemma to feel naughty about not going in.

Carl: We did try to manage things and then talk about it together afterwards. We thought she'd prefer to have her mother, but we thought if we let her mom go first, she'd manage to come in with me too.

Leader: You thought that strategy might have worked. You're both looking very upset when you're talking about this.

Carl: I...feel like giving up. I really want to have more time with Gemma, and I thought this would work.

Leader: You want very much to get closer to Gemma, and to have special time with her. But you don't know if you can go on doing this.

Carl: I don't like to give up... I'm not a quitter... but...

Leader: You'll find it really painful, if Gemma tells you again next time that she won't come in, but you don't want to give up on it either.

Carl: No, I guess I don't. I guess you can't guarantee that she won't hurt my feelings again, then? (Laughs.)

Leader: I wish I could! It matters a lot to you that it works next week. I have a suggestion that might work, but as you say, with no guarantees, I am afraid. If this suggestion doesn't work, we will think of something else that may be easier for you and Gemma to do together for the next few weeks. Maybe it can be a special activity together, or coming here for more practice playtimes, before trying again at home.

Carl: I did think that if I had an even shorter time with her, maybe she wouldn't resist the idea so much. I know she's not used to me trying so hard to spend time at home with her on her own.

Leader: You've already thought of a possible solution. Let's refine that idea of yours a bit before you try again next week, and work on how to reflect Gemma's feelings and accept them right at the beginning of the session... You seem to think you can handle your feelings of disappointment next week, and still keep trying, because Gemma is so important to you.

Carl: I let things slip, after the time I spent with her when she was little, so I guess I have to put in some work now to help Gemma see she's still important to me.

Another parent: I'd find that so difficult. I really admire the way you're willing to put yourself on the line again.

Leader: It's really coming across that Gemma is very important to you, and worth some hurt feelings on your part.

Carl: Yes, she is. I guess I might have hurt her feelings too, and I know she didn't have an easy time before she came to us.

This example illustrates how important it is for leaders to empathize with parents and give them hope for the future under these exceptional circumstances, and how leaders can collaborate with the parents to achieve a positive outcome. It also shows how effective other parents can be in supporting and validating fellow parents.

Partner's doubts about the program

Another issue that very occasionally arises after a first home session, of doubts about the program, is illustrated next.

BACKGROUND INFORMATION

Dorothy has been a faithful attendee at all meetings, and held her first play session at home with her son Stewart, aged 9. Her husband, who is not participating, finds all of the home arrangements rather a nuisance, and complains that he doesn't see how all of the things that Dorothy is doing are really helping Stewart. Stewart has been having behavioral problems in school and the neighborhood, and is difficult to manage at home.

Dorothy herself recognizes that starting home sessions is causing quite a few changes in the family routine. This has been hard on the family, since the other children need to be cared for, and a special spot had to be created for her and Stewart to play. While Dorothy feels she has gained from what she has learned so far, she herself wonders if all the accommodations they've had to make are going to have a payoff. Stewart did not show great interest in the home session, and was only minimally interested in the practice play sessions that she conducted during meetings.

Dorothy (reporting on her first home session): The session went all right, I guess. No difficulties, but nothing much happened. I'm really wondering if all of the trouble we've gone through to get these sessions started at home is going to have any return.

Leader: It seems like it may be more trouble than it is worth to have these home sessions.

Dorothy: Well, I liked playing here, but it's a lot of trouble to keep everything structured as you suggest in our house. My husband is already complaining about having to come home early to watch the other kids for Stewart's session. He thinks that we're not going to get much accomplished with all this playing.

Leader: With your husband so uncertain, and even complaining of the inconvenience, you can't help but question this approach.

Dorothy: No, I really can't, because we have been coming for about ten weeks and I really haven't seen much change in Stewart.

Leader: You've really only done one short home session so far, but you have done everything that you were instructed to do before that, and you don't see anything much happening. You'd like to see some sign of progress.

Dorothy: Yes, I need to have something to keep me going over these hard places.

Carrie (another parent): I can understand how you feel, Dorothy. I feel somewhat the same way as you, but I'm optimistic that when we get home sessions going we'll see some real progress with our two children.

Dorothy: I think that this may work very well for some of you, but I am not optimistic the program will work for Stewart.

Leader: I think Carrie is right. It takes several weeks of play sessions before you can see measurable changes in children. They have had years of practicing behaviors that parents want them to change. Some children show very rapid changes, others seem to need to hold onto their behaviors for now.

Research on this program shows very positive results, and we have every reason to believe that Stewart will respond well to home sessions, assuming you can carry everything out as expected. By the time the program has finished, you probably will see, and your husband as well, some pleasing changes in the way Stewart manages his behavior. You've got things all set up for your home sessions, even if your husband is not thrilled about it, and we'd like to suggest that you do at least four home sessions before you make a firm decision. It is always possible to make some additions to play sessions with Stewart, like working with his school, if that seems needed. We'll discuss our options more, after you've done your next home session, and we all see your video.

Dorothy: I think I really need to give it more time, as you are suggesting, before we decide that it's not going to work. It would help me if Stewart would be a little more enthusiastic about his next home session. I think he might be, because he didn't get to play with the things he wanted to in the short session we had. The next session will be longer, as we've agreed, and he'll have a better chance to use the toys.

Leader: I think that is a good decision, Dorothy. We're all hoping that you'll feel more encouraged after the next home play session. Do you think it might help for either you or one of us leaders to talk with your husband about his doubts?

Dorothy: I can explain to him what you just said. I think he just gets discouraged about Stewart, and feels helpless about changing him, just like I do.

Leader: We'll be interested in what he thinks. You'll begin to notice that, when Stewart gets engaged in his longer play sessions at home, he'll be leading the changes in himself, and you'll be able to understand what he's thinking and feeling better. Home play sessions really are at the heart of the therapy that children are offered in this program.

This example illustrates one kind of doubts parents experience from time to time during the program, when changes they hope to see in their children have not yet occurred. Since home sessions have not been fully instituted at this point, the leader pointed out that the heart of the program had really only begun for Stewart. The leader also ensured that consideration was given to the husband's feelings and doubts, since his cooperation is critical to Dorothy's successful home sessions.

Parents wanting to include younger and older children

During Meeting 12, some families are eager to begin including their toddlers and teens immediately in home sessions. Their feelings need empathic responses too, such as: *"It's important for you to be fair to all your children."* However, parents should be encouraged to wait a couple of weeks for these additional sessions, until their home play sessions and skills are better developed. Again, this advice is intended to prevent parents from being overloaded, as they begin this new home session phase in the program more independently.

Preparing parents for subsequent meetings

Leaders explain to parents that all subsequent meetings, except for the last one, Meeting 20, will be looking at home play sessions. For the next seven meetings, the first part of the meeting concentrates on a few families' play sessions at a time, and then the group catches up briefly with everyone else's ongoing home play sessions, as well as looking in more detail at external issues that arise. After a while, meetings also help parents generalize their skills to daily life.

Scheduling issues when selecting families in focus for subsequent meetings are discussed in the final part of this chapter, after first looking at options for leaders in supervising play sessions during these meetings.

Format variations for meetings

There are different ways in which parents' home sessions can be supervised by leaders during the next several meetings. The three main options for leaders to consider adopting for the group as a whole are:

Option 1: supervision via practice play sessions during meetings and home feedback sheets alone.

Option 2: supervision via practice play sessions during meetings plus videos and home feedback sheets of home sessions.

Option 3: supervision via videos and home feedback sheets alone.

The features of each option are listed next.

OPTION 1: PRACTICE PLAY SESSIONS AND HOME FEEDBACK SHEETS

This option was the one used traditionally in GFT, before video recordings were readily accessible to families. It still may be the preferred means for leaders to provide supervision for groups that have to forego video recordings due to budget limitations of the families themselves or the organization, or for other good reasons. For these groups, parents should be prepared to make detailed written reports of their sessions immediately after they conduct each session at home.

For the meeting immediately after their first home sessions, all families present from their written notes and receive feedback. Then there is a general discussion of issues with leaders and the group, and further skills training, as needed. Meetings 13–19 start with practice play sessions of 15 minutes each for the children from families selected as the families in focus for the meeting, followed first by supervision of these sessions, and then discussion of these families' home sessions. Afterwards, time is allocated for reviewing all the other participants' home sessions, based on each parent's written sheets, and, finally, time is allocated to addressing other issues of relevance for the group, including skills training. Leaders reconfirm families in focus for the next week's meeting, altering the planned schedule where necessary.

OPTION 2: PRACTICE PLAY SESSIONS, VIDEOS AND HOME FEEDBACK SHEETS

Parents bring both their home session videos with marked segments and feedback sheets to each meeting for discussion and supervision. This alternative combines regularly scheduled, practice play sessions for designated families in focus augmented by viewing segments totaling 15–20 minutes of their home videos and feedback sheets. Afterwards, as many other families as possible in the group show their short, pre-selected segments of home sessions and hold discussions based on their feedback sheets. Additional skills training also can be scheduled. This option provides the most comprehensive coverage of each parent's and child's progress, and may be preferred for certain groups needing more intensive supervision. However Option 3, discussed next, has to a great extent replaced this format.

OPTION 3: VIDEOS AND HOME FEEDBACK SHEETS

All parents make video recordings of home sessions and fill in home feedback sheets after each session. They bring both their home session videos and feedback sheets to each meeting for discussion and supervision. Leaders ask the designated families in focus to show 15–20 minutes in total of unedited recordings of their home sessions. The remaining families select small segments of their home videos that went well, or were problematic, for their briefer supervision in the last part of the meeting. Skills training also can be scheduled.

Selected families' videos serve in the same capacity as live, supervised sessions during meetings. In addition to videos tracking parents' progress in home sessions, there are several other advantages. First, this format allows the group to spend all the available time on home sessions using videos, with the advantage of having more lengthy discussions of home sessions each meeting.

Another advantage is saving time during the meeting itself, without sacrificing depth. In most instances, it is just as useful for supervision purposes for the group to watch play sessions recorded at home, as it is for the group to see them live. Only one feedback and supervision time is needed for the home play session, instead of separate feedback times for a live, direct supervision plus a briefer supervision of the home session. This option is especially useful for leaders to consider when there are a large number of children in the group. Third, videos have an advantage over live play sessions and written reports because they can be stopped and started where needed. Finally, using home session videos during the next seven meetings, rather than engaging in live play sessions, also is helpful for parents who have practical difficulties bringing their children to meetings.

However in certain cases, as mentioned earlier, leaders may decide that live, direct supervision of a parent and child is important. Examples of when live sessions are inserted are when one or more parents are unable to do home video recording, and/or when leaders or parents think that watching a session live might assist in troubleshooting. Therefore, leaders need to remind parents that sometimes it is helpful to see live play sessions and receive feedback directly, but the general plan is to have supervision based on their home videos. (NB: For these occasional live play sessions, leaders need to remember to organize child attendance and childcare needs beforehand for the following meeting, as they did earlier in the program.)

Selecting the next meeting's families in focus

In general, it is important for leaders to allow enough time in subsequent meetings to address each selected family's current issues, ensuring that all the participating children and both parents in families are included. The parents selected for playing their lengthier videos and/or having live play sessions consume the bulk of the meeting times, with parents who are playing short segments of home sessions, or reporting verbally, filling the remainder of the time. The general rule is that struggling families need to take priority.

We suggest leaders plan together after Meeting 11 their views on which families in focus to select for Meeting 13, and receive clinical supervision to talk through scheduling dilemmas after Meeting 11, where required. Leaders also should draw up a tentative list of families to focus on for Meetings 13–15. Two to four families need to be scheduled per meeting, depending on the size of the group. The scheduling of families has to be somewhat flexible initially, usually aiming for deciding on families two or, at the most, three weeks in advance, and consulting with parents about their expected availability, if practice play sessions with children are needed. The group can be told that future scheduling beyond these two or three weeks will be related to play session issues for children or parents. In meetings with live, practice play sessions, outside issues concerning family life and families' availability also need to be considered.

In some groups, when all the parents' first home play sessions went well, judged by their video excerpts and/or written records and comments during the meeting, the tentative schedule planned by leaders after Meeting 11 need not be altered for the next week's families in focus. Other times, it is apparent to leaders during Meeting 12 that a parent's skill level deteriorated during the transition to home, which resulted in difficulties in their home play session. It is essential for leaders to select these parents for in-depth supervision during the next meeting, Meeting 13, in order to quickly address these deficits and adjust their tentative schedule where necessary.

Flexibility for future meetings' families in focus

As stated previously, some flexibility in selecting families to focus on in later meetings is needed. At times, issues raised by parents in the meetings suggest that some families might need more immediate feedback on their home play sessions. Or sometimes parents request supervision before their turn on the schedule; such requests should be honored. Other times, parents are concerned about problems at home or at school, even when their play sessions have gone well. Leaders usually agree that more in-depth supervision might be useful to these struggling families. The difficulties these families encounter commonly are instructive for all the parents in the group. The next meeting's concentration on these families also increases group cohesion and participants' empathy for other parents' issues. However, leaders also need to assure the group that the order in which families are selected will be given to them in good time, to enable them to make practical arrangements, particularly where live sessions with children are needed.

Finally, leaders should remind parents to bring their up-to-date written reports and/or videos to all the rest of the meetings, to augment discussion of home sessions, just as they did during Meeting 12.

The next chapter explores issues arising for leaders as home sessions become an established routine for parents and their children, and in-depth supervision of children's play becomes established.

CHAPTER 13

Early Home Play Sessions
Meetings 13–15

As underlined in the last chapter, helping parents conduct home play sessions effectively is a major task for GFT leaders. Home play sessions continue weekly until the penultimate meeting, Meeting 19, of the GFT program. This chapter outlines the issues that arise in meetings during early home sessions for families, before they concentrate more fully on generalizing their skills to daily life, which is the topic of the next chapter. Ways to help parents consolidate their therapeutic skills, discuss play themes that often arise in home sessions, and handle other issues that may warrant further input by leaders are considered in this chapter, including how shorter play sessions with young children and special activity times with teenagers are introduced.

Early home sessions
Leaders' aims for Meetings 13–15

One of the main aims of leaders for the next few meetings following the transition to home sessions is to ensure that parents' play sessions are continuing in a productive and practical way at home. For parents who seem to lack consistency, or who are not as proficient in child-centered play skills, leaders aim to increase these participants' effectiveness in using their skills. Usually this process is completed for all participants within two to three meetings (e.g. by Meeting 14). Once a family's home play sessions are well under way, and for some parents this happens immediately, leaders concentrate on helping parents understand their children's play themes, develop their child-centered play skills further, and start thinking about daily life parenting issues together. An additional task for leaders, which starts in Meeting 14 for the majority of families, is to help parents with very young children and teenagers to offer them special, one-to-one, times at home.

For early home sessions, as mentioned in the last chapter, leaders should adopt the strategy of giving priority during meetings to parents who seem to be struggling. As explained in the last chapter, in Meeting 12 leaders draw up a schedule for supervising the families in focus that is somewhat flexible, and able to be adapted to the needs of particular families.

The general format for home play session meetings

During the next seven meetings (Meetings 13–19) devoted to home play sessions in a 20-week GFT program, leaders schedule in-depth supervision of families in focus play sessions in the first part of the meeting. Regardless of whether video or live supervision is chosen as an option, leaders again aim to have the first hour of the meeting for supervision of play sessions for 10–15 minutes each per child per parent, depending on the size of the group. This is always paired with the type of feedback leaders have used for practice play sessions. For live play sessions, feedback is given after all the live sessions are finished. Feedback with videotaped sessions is done during and/or after the video is played. For early home play sessions, feedback and/or presentation of video recordings by selected families may occupy meeting time both before and after the midway break.

Once home sessions are well established, leaders confine feedback to before the break, and use the time after the break to look in more detail at other therapeutic issues, including helping parents develop more advanced skills and more understanding of the underlying emotional issues, or themes, expressed in their children's play sessions.

After parents begin to understand the needs and issues their children are expressing in play sessions, leaders use this foundation to discuss daily parenting issues of interest to most parents. Issues such as children's difficulties at bedtime and during school time commonly arise spontaneously during feedback, as the following example of Peggy and her son Tommy indicates, and can be easily expanded. Leaders should again use experiences that arise spontaneously in groups to address themes and daily life parenting issues; these can be ideal learning opportunities for the group.

Finally, leaders should allocate the last half hour of the meeting to supervising the remaining parents' ongoing home play sessions. Whenever live play sessions are held in meetings, leaders should remember to ask the families in focus to report on their home sessions first, before turning to the remaining families' home sessions. All the parents should have brought their up-to-date video segments and/or written reports to share with the group.

Shorter discussion of remaining families' home sessions

For the last part of the meeting, we suggest leaders ask the remaining families if anyone in the group has particular issues about their home sessions that seem important to discuss. Leaders then suggest that those parents with more pressing issues start the general discussion. Small segments of their home videos and/or written recording forms that went well, in addition to any problematic issue, should be addressed during these briefer supervisions.

Leaders also should be aware that, particularly while home play sessions are being established, a few parents may take up a disproportionate amount of a meeting when they are having difficulties with their home sessions. Leaders should keep this disparity in mind when providing supervision, in order to guarantee they provide some attention to all group members' home sessions, even though this time may be curtailed. This inclusivity is in order both to continue to promote group interest and cohesion, and to keep up to date on all participants' progress. Similar to other parts of the program, leaders need to be good timekeepers in order to allow each family to take part in this general discussion, rather than having one or two parents monopolize the time. For smaller groups, time management of sessions in order to include all participants is not as urgent an issue, compared with larger groups.

In the early meetings after home sessions begin, leaders may need to actively encourage a few of the more reticent parents to use their written reports and show short video excerpts. It is also facilitating to the group, where the emphasis is on helping parents who are struggling, to ask families who are succeeding in home sessions to report and/or show parts of their home play session videos to the group during the last part of the meeting. These parents are able to model successful sessions for the group, giving hope to other parents and ending the meeting on a positive note.

Ongoing home session supervision

Leaders' supervision of home sessions using videos and/or written reports starts as usual with key questions about how the play session went. Following the format familiar to participants from their earlier practice play sessions during meetings, questions on what went well and what was challenging are discussed. Leaders take parents through their written report of sessions first, and then use video, where available, for more in-depth supervision.

For early meetings after home sessions have begun, leaders may need to more actively guide parents in selecting contents from home sessions to be brought for discussion. Leaders need to prioritize issues that are clinically relevant to particular children and their parents, but also keep in mind the overall clinical and learning needs of the group as a whole. For example, leaders may suggest a parent selects a limit problem that is applicable to any group member, rather than a situation that would be unique to a particular child. Leaders also may need to give parents further help in selecting segments or talking about times during home sessions that were challenging, if a parent is not forthcoming, or the reverse—if a parent is overly critical of their skills. For example, some parents may fail to show the difficulties they had with transitions between activities, or starting and ending sessions, and a leader may ask one of these parents for further details or suggest watching their video at a key point.

If a video segment or reported session seems to be getting tedious for the group (e.g. when children are silently engaged in a routine activity), leaders may choose to skip a chosen segment, or ask a parent to move on in their account. But leaders should always check with a parent before moving on. If a parent does not agree to this, they will undoubtedly have a good reason for choosing to report the entire episode, and time should be made for this.

Sometimes parents' reports from their written records alone, where video is not available, are too detailed and go beyond the length of time allocated for them in the group.

But, more commonly, parents do not give enough detail about the play sessions. Leaders need to help both sets of parents with their reporting style—for example, highlighting a briefer part of the report that worked well for the former, and helping reticent parents to expand on their examples.

Addressing parents' competence in early home sessions

During early home sessions, leaders aim to increase struggling parents' practice of child-centered play skills, and help them empathize more fully with the issues their children express. Other parents may have well-developed skills, but need more urgent supervision because of outside issues. The examples below illustrate leaders' responses to such issues.

An example of skills development

Fred's mother shows a video sequence in which her 7-year-old son plays out a monster attacking the doll's house. The mother watches him without comment. The leader pauses the recording and comments:

> Leader: An empathic response can be used here to show you understand him.
>
> Mom: I can always think of something to say afterwards. It's difficult when I'm right there in the play, and trying to follow what Fred is doing. It's always so busy with his play, now that he's at home doing his sessions!
>
> Leader: You're very pleased that he has taken to his play sessions at home so well. But you weren't expecting that fast pace. You know what you want to say now, but it's much more difficult to do while all that action is going on during the session. (Other parents in the group affirm that this happens to them too.) It's also more difficult to think of these responses when the feelings are shown through the toys, and not directly in Fred's face and body. We'll think more about how to do this when we are all together later in the meeting.
>
> Mom: I wish I would have said: "That was scary."
>
> Leader: Excellent! That is very helpful; you can think about what you wanted to say, and try to apply it next time, if a similar situation arises.

With other parents, leaders may instead quickly suggest an empathic response themselves, or choose to stop the video and have the parent or group think for a minute about what a good response for this play sequence might be.

A competent parent with outside behavior management issues

In contrast to this example, the following one shows a parent who quickly became competent in applying her play skills to home sessions. Therefore, leaders were able to concentrate on the underlying issues her child was addressing, and other concerns she raised within the home play sessions and outside of sessions, rather than helping her to refine her play skills.

BACKGROUND INFORMATION

Eight-year-old Tommy's mother, Peggy, complained during Meeting 13 that she had been receiving calls recently from school saying that Tommy was picking on another boy. Along with this, Peggy reported that Tommy was aggressive in his first two home sessions. She showed the group a short segment of this behavior during the meeting. Leaders decided to select Peggy for in-depth supervision at the next meeting. They asked her to select a 15-minute, uninterrupted, video sequence of the following week's home play session that had examples of Tommy being aggressive, rather than showing a brief excerpt from an episode. At the beginning of Peggy's supervision during Meeting 14, leaders asked her to look at her record of her last home session first, giving highlights on what had happened. Then she showed her 15-minute segment to the group.

Leader 2: What we watched was a very smooth session. How did you feel about it, after watching it here with us? What went well? What was challenging for you?

Peggy: I think it was a good session. I didn't have any problems, really. I would have preferred that his play was not so hard and aggressive. It seems like he has a lot of aggression coming out. He has always been a kind of problem at school, but I never got phone calls before. I'm wondering if all the aggression in the play session could make him worse in school. I'm not sure what to say to Tommy about school either. He would probably say that the teacher was exaggerating or something like that, and then cry, if I suggest that he stop bothering the other boy. Sometimes I wonder if this other boy is just a complainer, or if this teacher just has a "big eye" on Tommy and watches for him to do something.

Leader 1: So, you really don't know what to believe, and it's distressing when you don't know what's really going on. You want to be fair to everybody concerned.

Peggy: Yes, I do. So, did you pick up anything from the play session? It was sort of hard to be there when he was playing so aggressively.

Leader 2: Tommy was aggressive in the play session. That is for sure. You said it was hard to be there, setting those limits quickly when you needed to. But he was not out of bounds. You set the limits perfectly, and he abided by them. You made accepting statements, which seemed to be just right, with him. It is not easy to be close to a lot of bop bag punching, rolling, and jumping. It was hard for you, but you allowed it because you wanted to permit him that kind of outlet in the play session.

Peggy: Yes, he's been through a lot, what with his dad walking out on us last year, and not even sending Tommy a birthday card, or calling him, or anything last month.

Leader 1: You think he has plenty to be angry about, and you understand why he is. Children have a lot of reasons for playing aggressively. You linked it to his dad. Was there anything that made you think that was what was behind his play?

Peggy: The way he squared up to that bop bag, and kept punching it. It reminded me of his dad, the way he gets so fired up and angry. I hope Tommy doesn't take after his dad.

Leader 1: *You're worried, when you see Tommy's play, about him turning out like his dad. You're doing play sessions to try to help him manage his aggressive feelings better, among other reasons. You'll remember we talked about common stages in play therapy in our earlier meetings. Aggression often happens by the midpoint in these play sessions. I expect that he will become calmer in a session or two.*

As far as the play session we watched, I saw Tommy trying to work out his angry feelings. That was the main issue in his play. I think that after he has dealt with most of that in his home sessions, he will not be expressing anger as much outside the sessions. However, it may help with the school problem if you knew whether the other child perhaps quietly annoys Tommy in some subtle way. We know that Tommy is not good at handling his feelings yet. Does he ever complain about the other boy bothering him?

Peggy: *No, but Tommy says that he doesn't like him.*

Leader 2: *We generally don't see the anger in play sessions creating anger in daily life. So, I don't think that we should believe that his aggressive play is responsible for him annoying the other boy. Play session anger seems to be contained in the play space. In fact, some children use the play session as the time to work out their anger, and restrain themselves outside the play session.*

Leader 1: *I would suggest that you talk to the teacher, to see if she can shed any light on how these events at school occur. You may want to tell Tommy that you are talking to his school to see how he can be helped to get along better with the boy you mention.*

Peggy: *I will. They actually reported last year that he was having some trouble at playtime with that boy.*

Leader 2: *Let's see if things settle down in the next couple of weeks, after you talk with his school, and after Tommy has a few more play sessions that we will talk about. If not, we will try to set up a call ourselves to the teacher, with your permission. If we all have information from her, along with what you have learned when you see her, we may be able to sort out the reasons for his problems together. With play sessions, the problems at school could well diminish, with changes in Tommy. In fact, we would expect that.*

But, if there are bigger difficulties with the teacher, or the other children, changes in Tommy may not be able to correct the situation. More environmental changes may have to be made to support the changes Tommy makes himself. In our next meetings, we'll be looking at how changes in family life, and school too, can support changes you see in your children's play sessions.

COMMENTS ON THIS EXAMPLE

It was important for leaders to watch Peggy's home session more thoroughly to establish whether she was handling Tommy's aggressive play during a home session competently and setting limits appropriately. In this instance, the video showed that Peggy was able to keep Tommy's aggressive play within effective limits. The entire group benefited from hearing again about the leaders' experience of the calming effect on children's aggression when they have the opportunity to be aggressive in play sessions, and are accepted, rather than punished or criticized, by their parents. Leaders used this supervision to underline that aggression is a typical and helpful phase in play sessions that will commonly diminish after a peak period, if it is handled correctly by parents.

In the authors' experience, there also have been many instances where children who were very aggressive in play sessions became less aggressive in school, including behaving better in the playground, and standing in line without pushing other children. Therefore, we believe that the link between aggression and play is generally the opposite of what parents fear might be the case; it seemed helpful to Peggy and the rest of the group to be reminded of that. It was also important that leaders began to explore the possible underlying reasons for Tommy's aggression, which in this case the mother herself was able to share readily with the group.

Nor did leaders rush in to try to rescue the mother or Tommy at school; instead they tried to empower the mother to manage this issue herself, with the added back-up of asking leaders to help, if the problem persisted. Leaders took this opportunity to refer to aggression as a theme in Tommy's play. They will continue to provide input on play themes over the next few meetings, as addressed later in this chapter.

Including toddlers, teenagers and other auxiliary children in home sessions

Once families have established their play sessions at home successfully with the main children in the program, leaders help parents offer time to their other children (referred to as "auxiliary children" earlier). Siblings in early and middle childhood, who do not have emotional issues that warrant close supervision of play sessions during meetings, may begin to have their own, weekly home play sessions, after this is discussed with leaders. These sessions are not video recorded but parents fill in written notes briefly, following the home play session format for each play session, and bringing these notes to all meetings. Toddlers and teenagers need more adaptations, to be discussed later.

The main reasons for offering regular, special times to siblings were discussed with parents earlier, but may need repetition here. They are as follows:

- To enhance these children's development by providing ideal conditions for progress during one-to-one times with a parent. For example, both toddlers and teenagers have opportunities to extend their autonomy and mastery of chosen activities in developmentally appropriate ways.

- To promote these children's attachments to their parents, including helping parents understand their emotional expressions and needs, and helping these children feel that their parents are closely attuned to their emotional lives.

- To provide a "whole family" intervention, thus avoiding potential worries of favoritism and rivalry in siblings, as well as guilt in parents for not offering special attention to all their children.

Preparing families for home sessions with toddlers and teenagers

Leaders prepare parents by reminding them that, due to the differing developmental needs of their children, their time with them needs to be adapted accordingly, but the skills they practice remain the same. It again is important for parents to offer weekly sessions consistently at scheduled times. This regularity serves several purposes: first, it helps toddlers and teenagers develop an awareness of the pattern of these sessions; second, it reflects these children's importance in the family—the time devoted to them is as regular as it is for their siblings, who have play sessions; and third, it ensures that parents are viewed as reliable and trustworthy by their children.

For both toddlers and teenagers, materials and activities need to be age appropriate, which requires some adaptation, to be discussed later. Unlike home play sessions, the special times are not usually video recorded; parents again rely on written reports alone for feedback in group meetings. A suggested written form for "special times" is included in Appendix 20. These weekly written reports with each toddler and teenager should be brought to meetings by parents, along with their home play session recordings and written forms.

Home sessions with toddlers

Leaders commonly recommend shorter, 15-minute special times for toddlers on a designated day each week, rather than the full half hour. A blanket or mat with age-appropriate toys and materials is always needed as a visual reminder to young children of the boundaries of their play space. Parents need to select fewer and younger toys for toddlers than they use for home play sessions, but again should try to keep these toys separate and use them only during special times.

Leaders can remind parents to use gestures, facial expressions, tone of voice, and other non-verbal communication in fuller, and very clear, ways for this age group (Ryan & Bratton, 2008). When children are primarily non-verbal, following their non-verbal directions can result in very creative and satisfying special times. Examples of adaptations for toddlers are important to give parents. One suggested example is when a toddler hands his father a toy phone. For toddlers, this commonly indicates that the father should start talking on the phone to his child, while the child responds as fully as they wish. The father should then continue until his child seems satisfied that the conversation is over.

For this age group, rules and limits need to be reinforced by parents' actions, tone of voice, and frequent repetition, rather than using the 3-step limit setting parents learned for home play sessions. Reflection of toddlers' feelings around limit setting remains important. Leaders should briefly review with parents how they intend to verbalize their toddlers' basic feelings, and the age-appropriate limits that will be needed. Leaders need to point out that parents should not expect their young children to adhere to rules as quickly as more mature children, and that young children need a more "hands on" approach to keeping them within the play space in the room. For example, parents may need to repeat the limit of staying on the mat during the play session several times, along with helping their toddlers physically return to the mat, particularly during early sessions. However, when toddlers go off the mat, it also may be a strong indication to a parent to empathize with their children's feeling of *"You've had enough"* and end the session early, especially if toddlers persist, after several attempts to steer them back, in leaving the play space.

Home sessions with older children and teenagers

As an introduction to this topic, leaders can point out to the group that one of the options for families at the end of GFT, and, very rarely, an option when a child in the leaders' opinion seems to have completed their therapeutic work earlier than Meeting 19, is to change from play sessions to "special times." Hearing about how these special times are introduced to teenagers can prepare the group for this later option.

Including toddlers at this point in the program is often greeted with enthusiasm by parents. However, some parents seem more daunted by including their teenagers. Parents' initial reaction may be that their teenagers will not want to spend special time with them every week, not even the 30–45 minutes recommended by leaders. They may say that their teenagers have independent social lives, and want to be with their friends, rather than at home. Similar to other parts of the program, in these instances, it is important for leaders to show empathy for parents' reservations and reflect, if relevant, that parents may be worried that their teenagers will reject their offer of special times. It is also important for leaders to assure parents that special times are adapted to teenagers' interests.

Typically older children (11–12-year-olds and teenagers) feel that they are beyond playing with toys—that they would feel silly—and might identify the term "play sessions" with the toys used by their younger siblings (Ryan & Wilson, 2005). Therefore, we recommend parents use the term "special times" when offering a time for interacting with teenagers that is equivalent to the play sessions of their younger siblings. Leaders can give examples to the group of successful times parents have spent with their teens from other groups. Many interactive activities work, depending on teenagers' interests. Art and craft activities, hair and makeup sessions, cards or board games, interactive computer games, baking together, and shooting baskets or golf-putting practice are a few of many possible activities. Leaders should advise parents to have in mind activities that lend themselves to special times together and are sustainable, rather than activities that are special treats, or that are too ambitious to be practical over the longer term. Activities should be ones that are possible to engage in for half to three-quarters of an hour a week for the remainder of the program.

Another consideration in selecting suitable activities with teenagers is to avoid activities where there would be a heavy teaching role for parents. An example of an activity that young teenagers might enjoy with parents would be working in their parent's workshop together. This would be a good opportunity for parents to teach their children about using tools. However, there would be many rules and cautions for a parent in teaching woodwork, which cast the parent in an authoritative role. Therefore, this kind of activity would not be recommended for special times. And while teenage interests will dominate the choice of activities, suggestions agreed to should be manageable emotionally and physically for parents too. If parents are being stretched beyond their toleration point to engage in special times, the sessions will not go well. To guard against this, parents should think through what the activity entails for them, before agreeing to what their teenagers suggest.

INTRODUCING THE IDEA OF SPECIAL TIMES

We recommend that parents introduce the notion of special, weekly times with teenagers by saying:

> *I'd like to spend some time with you also, as I do with [Name of child]. I suspect that you would want to do something very different from playing the way s/he and I do. I'd like to know what you think would be an enjoyable way to spend some time together. I was planning on about a half hour [or 45 minutes] here at home, on our own."*

Should the teenager say, "*I don't know, I don't think there is anything,*" parents should reflect these feelings, while keeping their own feelings in check. Negotiating acceptable activities, or accepting non-participation, can be an important part of parents' recognizing their teenagers' autonomy, as well as an opportunity to reflect their mixed feelings. Parents need to think about how to apply their child-centered play skills throughout the negotiation process with their teenagers. Leaders may wish to role-play this process, with a leader in the role of the parent, and either a parent or the other leader playing a teenager. Leaders using role-play are able to demonstrate directly to parents that it is important to reflect teenager's feelings throughout this negotiating conversation, and to stay within parents' personal boundaries about acceptable activities at the same time, as our example below shows.

AN EXAMPLE OF A NEGOTIATION ROLE-PLAY WITH A "TEENAGER"

> *"Parent"* (leader in parent's role): *Now that I've learned to do home play sessions with your younger sister, I'd like to spend some special time with you too.*
>
> *"Teenager"* (leader in teenager's role): *Naw...that stuff is for her. I don't want to play.*
>
> *"Parent"*: *You are too old for all that. You wouldn't like it. We can think about something we could do together on our own that is for teenagers.*
>
> *"Teenager"*: *Well, I have to be out on weekends. I'm not going to be stuck at home.*
>
> *"Parent"*: *You're not sure this is a good idea... You haven't thought about it before, and it's important that you have a lot of time with your friends... Let me tell you some more about this idea, before you make up your mind. I would like us to spend about a half hour a week having time on our own at home. We can have the time when it's quiet and your sister has gone to bed, maybe on Thursdays at 9 p.m. I have been thinking about what we could do together. I came up with doing hair and makeup together, bringing all our hair things and makeup down and trying it out together, or doing art work together.*
>
> *"Teenager"*: *I know! I'll go to that social networking site on the internet and we can email one another instead.*
>
> *"Parent"*: *That's something that really appeals to you, but I'd like to spend time right with you, and not just on another computer... I can see you're disappointed.*
>
> *"Teenager"*: *Can we do something on the computers though?*

"Parent": You're really interested in having fun with me on the computer. I wonder if we can think of doing something together, maybe accessing websites together that give us glamorous hairstyles to try out, or a computer game...

"Teenager": Maybe we can do that some weeks, and other weeks we can find things to draw together. That would be good.

"Parent": You're coming up with some ideas of your own.

GROUP DISCUSSION OF THE ROLE-PLAY

Leaders should guide the discussion afterwards on this kind of role-play, if parents do not spontaneously comment themselves, on the way the "parent" reflected the "teenager's" feelings, and the ways the "parent" was both structuring and limiting their special times together during the negotiation process. Role-playing the negotiation process with a teenager, and the subsequent discussion, serves several purposes for the group. It actively helps parents who will be engaging in special times with their teenagers to think through how to begin, it prepares parents of younger children for the future, and helps the group become interested in and empathic towards parents who are starting sessions with their older children. Another highly relevant purpose, as mentioned above, is to prime the entire group for how to discuss with their children the option of changing from home play sessions to "special times" at the end of the GFT program.

ISSUES ARISING IN SPECIAL TIMES WITH TEENAGERS

Once special times are agreed, during these weekly special times parents are asked to practice their child-centered skills by allowing their teenagers to set the pace, reflecting their feelings and setting limits as required, following the 3-step procedure learned in play sessions. Leaders may decide to mention that sometimes parents find that they involve themselves more fully in complex activities with their teenagers than they would in play session activities with younger children. This may make it more challenging for parents to practice their child-centered skills, until they adapt to this difference. It also is crucial that teenagers are given the chance to engage in an enjoyable activity without parents having hidden agendas, or attempting to educate, monitor, or question them. Leaders may also wish to point out that parents often find that their therapeutic skills are used on a verbal level, which more closely resembles counseling, rather than play therapy, with their teenagers. In fact, in the second author's experience, sometimes teenagers request special "talk time" with their parents weekly, rather than wishing to engage in any activities, once they realize their parents will follow their lead in conversation.

Another issue that arises during special times with teenagers that parents need supervision with is when teenagers do not fully commit to their special times initially, or decide later that they want sessions only intermittently rather than weekly. Often teenagers' lack of commitment can be felt as a personal rejection of a generous offer by their parents. Leaders need to help parents recognize that teenagers' transition from childhood to greater independence from their parents is often done in a piecemeal and incomplete manner, with teenagers vacillating between too much independence sometimes, and more dependent feelings at other times. Parents also are vulnerable emotionally, usually having to move from more immediate involvement in their children's lives to a position of standing on the sidelines, watching, waiting, and trying to trust their teenagers to make worthwhile choices. Leaders should encourage parents to continue offering the time each week, even though it is not always taken up by their teenagers, and to bring this issue to the group meetings for discussion. Parents' personal feelings of usefulness/uselessness, authority/helplessness, and competence/ incompetence, among other issues, are likely to be challenged by these sessions with their teenagers. Leaders can help parents to view their teenagers' reactions to special times within this developmental context, which is outlined further in the next section. It may also become clearer to parents during these discussions that special times, similar to home play sessions, have a developmental aim, as well as an attachment aim.

In summary, leaders provide valuable supervision of teenagers' sessions to parents, with the whole group learning from and supporting these parents. However, if more serious clinical issues arise in any parents' special times with their teenagers, similar to toddlers, leaders should take these issues to their own FT supervisors, and consider making another type of referral, when required.

Play themes

The underlying emotional issues in children's play, called "play themes" by play therapists, are an emerging focus in group discussions after home play sessions have been established. Once skills are practiced by parents at a competent level, and their confidence increases, then more time during meetings can be spent on thinking about the underlying meanings of their children's play sequences. Both the leaders and participants are in increasingly privileged positions, because more intimate family details are shared in the group when parents explore possible meanings of play during these meetings. Sometimes leaders need to remind parents at this stage in the program about confidentiality, asking them again to respect the privacy of families' details, and not to relay them to others outside the group, even though these topics may potentially be very interesting to discuss with others.

Leaders already have forewarned parents when preparing them for home play sessions that the contents of children's sessions at home may differ from their practice play sessions during meetings. Once parents have adapted to their home sessions, they begin to more thoroughly search for meanings to their children's play, especially if they are puzzled by what is being played out in more than one play context. When parents themselves talk about the possible meanings of play in group meetings, it often sparks off other parents thinking about their children's play in a new light. For example, one parent was struck by her child creating an airplane accident with toy planes during a home play session, leading her to wonder if this play was related to his overhearing her talking to her own parents about their near accident at the airport during their recent vacation. This led another parent to think about how his child's decision to hop on one foot around the play space might be related to an earlier accident that resulted in a temporary lack of mobility.

It is always interesting for leaders that parents have a rich fund of personal information about their children and families to draw on, compared with professionals. Parents often are very quick to see connections in their children's play to real-life events. In the authors' experience, parents usually are adept at understanding the meaning of what their children are doing in play sequences, especially when other parents contribute their insights. However, it is when parents remain at a loss that leaders need to step in and facilitate parents in developing possible meanings for these play sequences. Some suggestions for leaders are outlined next.

Beginning to focus on play themes

In the early stages of parents becoming interested in their children's underlying, emotional messages, or play themes, it has been most successful in the authors' experience for leaders not to actively search with parents for possible emotional meanings of their children's play when these meanings are not obvious to the parents. It can be unproductive for leaders to ask a parent *"What do you think your child means here?"* We realize this is particularly tempting for leaders to do with some parents who may appear to under-analyze their sessions. A parent may, for example, frequently state: "*We had a lot of fun,*" and stop there. When this occurs, leaders need to deliberately refrain from adding additional meaning to these parents' interpretation of their play session. Instead, leaders should continue to empathize with these parents' feelings, affirming that they felt close to their children, and happy about the way things had gone in their play session. Because the group as a whole is increasingly focusing on play themes, commonly these parents soon become interested in the underlying meanings in their children's play, without any direct intervention on the leaders' part.

Once again it is important that leaders use readily accessible terminology for the emotional issues arising in children's home play sessions. If instead, leaders use psychological terms for children's behavior, this labeling of behavior can quickly lead to parents curtailing their developing ability to explore their children's behavior and meanings fully. Using play therapy terms, such as the term "play themes", also can be counterproductive. These terms may inhibit parents who struggle to understand underlying meanings of play, and may encourage other parents lying at the opposite extreme to react to their children's play in sessions in an overly cognitive or clinical/diagnostic manner. For example, one type of play, in which children play at a much lower level than expected for their chronological age, is often labeled "regressive" in the psychotherapy literature. Because this term is usually interpreted pejoratively, we suggest that leaders, rather than labeling this play as "regressive," instead call it "seeking nurturance/nurturance play" or "wanting to be taken care of."

It also is important that leaders continue to empathize with parents' feelings, as appropriate. For example, a father may be worried about his son's latent sexual identity difficulties when the son engages in younger, feminine play sequences. In this case, leaders should help the father process his own feelings first. It may seem from the information available that his son is reliving past experiences that did not feel quite right to him. The son may be playing out how it feels to be masculine and feminine, in order to sort this issue out again, now that he is older. Leaders may be able to say simply:

James is showing you that he needs you to accept him. You can follow his lead here with what he wants. When he asks you to put on a scarf, he seems to want you to play an old woman, and he's playing a young and helpless girl. Often children whose leads are followed this way go on to other things soon. Let's see how this issue of helplessness develops for him.

Aggression too may be difficult for parents to accept easily in home play sessions, just as it may be in practice sessions during meetings. Again, leaders need to help parents express their own feelings and expectations, along with helping them understand the emotional messages their children seem to be conveying. A parent may say during discussion: *"Ed is angry because I don't give in to him."* The leader may first of all empathize by saying that this seemed to create uncomfortable feelings for the parent, which in turn may open up the parent's thoughts on what the interaction is like for Ed himself.

AN EXTENDED EXAMPLE OF A DISCUSSION INVOLVING PLAY THEMES

Martha's parents were one of the families in focus during Meeting 15. Six-year-old Martha had a congenital condition that led to serious difficulties digesting food. This resulted in three major operations for her, with another one due soon. Both her mother and her father had weekly home play sessions with her.

Dad: We know Martha's hospital visit the day before her home play sessions this week was feeding into the way she played out a hospital scene with me. We've talked about it, watched the video together, and we still can't figure out what it was all about.

Leader 1: I'm glad you brought the video sequence for all of us to watch together. Let's look at this sequence and what follows it, as you suggested.

(The hospital play on the video was fragmented. Several different roles were taken by Martha, or abruptly assigned by Martha to her father—nurse, doctor, ambulance driver, cleaner. They all seemed to be hurrying to take care of a baby doll in a bed. This scene shifted very abruptly to the baby being at home, playing with toys and singing loudly. Then Martha went to the sand, where she pretended that she was making a magic potion for the baby. This sand play lasted several minutes.)

Leader 2: That was a very intense session.

Parent 1: It was really hard to follow.

Leader 1: What did you make of it, now that we've watched it together?

Dad (worried tone and expression): It is even clearer to me now that Martha's play was about her feeling anxious, the way she kept moving from being a nurse, to me being an ambulance driver, to her being a cleaner at the hospital. But I'm still not sure what else she was trying to play out there.

Leader 1: It's made you and Lorraine [Mom] feel more anxious and confused, watching it again. You want so much to help Martha by making the right responses.

And I expect it's an anxious time for you and Lorraine too, so it's hard to remain calm and give Martha all the support she needs.

Dad: It's been going on for so long... I just wish it were over and done with.

Parent 2: It must be hard to feel you can't do anything. You just have to wait for what will happen. I wonder if Martha was rushing through everything in her play, trying to get it all over with too.

Dad: It did feel very rushed.

Mom: She did the same thing in my play session with her this week, as you'll see. With me, she was the doctor in the operating theatre for a short while, then she was visiting someone else in the hospital.

Parent 3: Maybe she's trying to play out bits of what she worries about, but doesn't want to spend too long on it, in case it scares her.

Dad: I wonder if she worries that she'll scare us too! It is hard to take on these different roles in her play, but it does make me feel I'm doing something, not just waiting.

Parent 4: You did a good job. I thought it was interesting, too, the way Martha played out the baby singing at home. And I thought it was very positive that she was making the magic potion herself for the baby.

Mom: I didn't really notice that play. The singing was so quick, and I didn't link the magic potion with the hospital play.

Leader 1: Sometimes it's easy to miss some of the positive things in children's play, when you are worried yourself. What do you think Martha was feeling when she played out the singing and the magic potion?

Dad: It seems like she was trying to do something for herself. Thinking about being at home, and thinking about a magic solution. But they didn't seem to be real solutions that would work.

Mom: Martha did seem to show that she felt helpless, choosing a baby to look after.

Parent 2: But she seemed to be the one looking after the baby. Maybe she's being positive, imagining she is going to feel all right again.

Dad (brightening): Yes, she did seem to be working on ways she can feel positive. Maybe she's trying to find ways to trust herself, the hospital and us that things are going to be all right...

Mom: That could be true! You know, yesterday she asked me to tell her what she was going to be able to eat for the first time, after she came home from the hospital.

Leader 1: You are starting to think about how much trust she has in you, and how hopeful she is herself.

Dad: That makes sense to me. I really want to have my next play session with her now!

Leader 1: You think it is a good thing that Martha's home play sessions are happening. I think you are both doing such a good job, sharing your worries with one another and trying not to burden Martha. You did a good job following Martha's lead in the session we saw, even though that was difficult to do. So I'm sure you will be able to do that next time too. Martha may or may not keep playing out a hospital scene next time, but we'll be glad to keep a close eye on things next week with you.

Dad: It's really helped me a lot, to think about Martha's play session together. It doesn't feel so jumbled now. I just have to keep doing what I was doing this week, if Martha decides to play hospitals again.

COMMENTS ON THIS EXAMPLE

By watching the video together, the group was able to experience Martha's play session very directly. The leader initially helped the parents process their difficult feelings and provided the parents and the group with a more general understanding of Martha's play themes (e.g. commenting on her trust in herself, the hospital, and her parents). The leader did not need to directly address some of the underlying feelings of the parents, because it seemed evident that the couple was able to support one another, and use the support of other parents in the group effectively. Nor did the leader need to dwell on the underlying meanings of Martha's play during feedback, since other parents' comments seemed effective and insightful. It is common at this stage in the program for other parents to regularly provide support for one another. The example also demonstrates how parents are indeed experts in knowing their own children, and can usually link their daily experiences with them to understanding play themes at this point in the program.

Children with earlier, difficult life histories

For children with more complex or unknown early life histories, particularly children who have been fostered or adopted and separated from their birth families, leaders may find that there is more need than usual for these parents to think of possible meanings behind their children's play sequences. For example, with 10-year-old Jane, who had been adopted aged 2, her adoptive parents found it helpful to think more deeply with leaders and the group about Jane's play sequences. It was striking that 10-year-old Jane spent several play sessions playing hide and seek with her father, then returning to him to be held in his arms and rocked. She also developed a game in which her father was told to hold the tunnel she dived into, while Jane told him to remain silent. Jane was silent and unavailable to him for some time, hiding in the tunnel. Her father was somewhat distressed and felt excluded in these play sequences. Both parents wondered if the play could be related to their family pet's recent death, which had shaken Jane. When the leader wondered if Jane's early experiences had influenced her play too, her parents became thoughtful and agreed that it was possible that these play sequences may be related to Jane's earlier experiences before adoption, as well as to more recent events.

As this example of Jane illustrates, in general, leaders want to help parents, where needed, to think symbolically, rather than taking all their children's play contents too literally. Even when there is a clear and direct link to children's known life experiences, leaders may want to help parents consider emotional issues more broadly and in more depth. Sometimes it is easier for parents to consider the underlying symbolism of children's imaginative play—for example, a child playing that a baby doll is distressed and lonely—than it is when parents are directly involved in a behavioral enactment, such as the example of Jane herself hiding in a tunnel and directing her father's responses. In either case, it is important for leaders to encourage parents themselves to think of meanings, and then supplement this exploration, when this seems needed.

The next section is intended to give leaders a general developmental framework for thinking about play themes, to aid them in their discussions with parents.

Play themes: their uses during GFT

Leaders will already have discussed many of the ideas on which children's play themes are based with parents during demos and practice play sessions. At this point in the program, leaders aim to reinforce and extend parents' capacity for thinking more broadly and deeply about their children's emotional needs and expressions during home play sessions. By helping parents understand their children's underlying emotional needs and expressions as captured in play themes, leaders aim to help parents develop a more complete understanding of both their children's imaginative play in home sessions and their children's needs, motivation, and behavior in daily life. Leaders are already familiar with the concept of play themes from their own play therapy practice. Identifying play themes and using these themes to discuss children's needs and emotional progress can be a complex process at times for therapists. Ryan & Edge (2012) examined this process and set out a developmental framework for understanding themes. This article's concepts are adapted here for use in GFT; this is intended to provide leaders with a transparent and broad framework that is not overly complex to use with parents on play themes.

Identifying themes

Play themes can be identified in several ways. Children may repeat a play sequence several times in one session, or spend a lot of time on one thing, or repeat the same play from one session to the next. Often they show that they are very involved in their play, and that it is important to them. Their behavior at home and school also may seem to reflect the same issues, not only their play.

Some themes are expressed in fantasy form such as good guys (policemen, spacecraft captains, etc.) versus bad guys (e.g. pirates, robbers, evil spacemen). Young children, as well as those in their middle years, often play out this prevalent theme of good and bad, suggesting that trying to deal with the development of their conscience is very common and a long lasting developmental task for children. Other themes, for example, helplessness and lack of hope, may be expressed in more concrete play, such as a child making sure that all the trucks and cars crash into one another and are left in a heap each session. In other words, themes can be expressed in many forms; probably there is no end to the creative and varied ways children can devise to play them out. Later in this section, a general framework for ordering and understanding play themes developmentally is described.

There are several aspects of play themes that leaders can weave into their discussions and supervision of home play sessions. These include the following:

- Children are not expected to have a conscious understanding or an ability to discuss the underlying meaning of their play sessions. Children spontaneously play and do not typically figure out what their play signifies. However, occasionally older children may spontaneously relate what they play to what they are thinking about. Parents may need reminding that they should not ask their children questions about underlying issues or themes that emerge in home play sessions.

- A play theme is used as a window of understanding for parents to see underneath their children's behavior and play during their weekly sessions. While parents sometimes identify themes during home sessions, themes are often better understood when watching videos again and discussing play session contents at GFT meetings.

- Play therapists think about play themes in different ways; there is no right way to do this. Parents too can use what is useful to them from play sessions and their lives with their children when they think about their children's emotional issues.

- Parents have the advantage of being "experts" on their own children's lives and often understand the context for themes better than therapists.

- Sometimes play themes may be very obvious, but other times they may be difficult to see or difficult to accept. Parents may have to have a "wait and see" approach at these times, as now illustrated.

A "WAIT AND SEE" EXAMPLE

Eleven-year-old Kim's stepfather, Hank, had discussed their early home play sessions during each meeting with the group. For three weeks, Kim had started her session by setting up the hero and monster figures in the same way, stationing them inside and outside the doll's house. She then conducted a battle between the good guys and the bad guys for the whole of her sessions. Hank had been able to accept Kim's need to repeat her play for two weeks, but by the third week, he began to have serious doubts:

Hank: I don't think it's doing Kim any good, just letting her keep playing out those battles.

Parent 1: You feel you may be harming her by just following her lead.

Hank: Yes. It seems to be reinforcing her bad language at home too. I know we already talked about how important it seems to be for Kim to play out good guys and bad guys doing battle, and that lots of kids do this kind of play, but I still think this is about seeing her mom being beaten up time after time by her dad when she was little... But nothing seems to be shifting and I think I should start telling her how it should go.

Leader 1: You feel very discouraged and wonder whether another approach, where you tell her what to do in her play, may be better. You think you understand why Kim has this powerful emotional issue of a battle between good and bad guys, but you want her to get this play over with.

Hank: Yes, I guess I don't want to see what damage it caused her, seeing her dad beating up her mom. It makes me so angry with him, but there's nothing I can do about that now.

Leader 1: You feel sort of helpless about changing the past. And now you feel helpless about changing Kim's play about the past.

Hank: Yes, I guess it's my own issue maybe. I really want to help Kim. And she does seem to trust me to watch her play, even though I have to keep reminding her to watch her language at home now.

Parent 2: I can see you're thinking a lot about all of that. Kim keeps playing out bad guys sneaking up on good guys, but she's trusting you to see it all while she plays.

Leader 1: Trust seems to be a big issue for Kim; you've said you think she learned to mistrust her dad when she was little, and that makes it harder for her to trust you. You are trying to be very trustworthy for her, but it's hard. Now you have to trust in the method of play we are helping you to use, and to trust in Kim to work things out. I think she needs you to keep to the same rules in her play sessions and keep to them at home, as you are doing, but it's hard for you to wait and trust in it all.

Parent 3: It would be hard for any of us.

Leader 1: Yes. We all want to support you as much as you need in your sessions with Kim. We'll look in detail at what happens in Kim's next session and watch your video together during our next meeting.

In our experience, once children play out battle scenes in that intense way for enough time, they start working out solutions for themselves. We'll see how Kim is responding next time. It's also important to remember that it's very common for children to conduct battles between good and evil forces in their play sessions, and that this kind of play has different reasons for each child. There are a lot of times during children's conscience development when they struggle with the conflict between good and evil, and it can come out in their play.

DISCUSSION OF THIS EXAMPLE

Hank seemed to be helped to continue his "wait and see" approach by the leader's and other parents' comments during this discussion. He was able to openly acknowledge his helpless feelings and suggested historical reasons for Kim's protracted battle scenes. This discussion was deepened by referring to trust versus mistrust, one of the developmental themes examined more fully next, as an important underlying emotional issue for Kim, and one that also resonated in Hank's responses to her. In addition, the leader was able to draw on experiences of children's resolution of their own themes in play therapy to help Hank maintain his "wait and see" attitude. It was also important to the group's understanding of emotional issues that the leader referred to how common "battles" between good and bad are in children's play sessions across a broad age span as part of their conscience development, and not only due to witnessing domestic violence.

Common themes classified by age

One way leaders can help parents think about play themes and ways to understand their children's behavior is to use descriptors of behavior connected to children's normal development (Erikson, 1977; Ryan & Edge, 2012). The descriptors presented here are based on the assumption that children work on deeper emotional issues that depend on their age and stage in development. For example, the first and most important developmental issue for children is developing trust in their carers. Children may return to some of their earlier, important emotional issues later, such as trust, if new or difficult events occur. Or children may jump ahead out of sequence to an emotional issue more common later in their development, if their life experiences are not the usual ones.

Sometimes play session issues seem to be related to early developmental issues that are being reworked; say, a 6-year-old child who plays out the emotional issue of trust in his mother that usually arises for 1-year-olds. Children seem to continue to work on important, early developmental issues when they have not been resolved satisfactorily. For example, if children develop strongly negative feelings, rather than more predominantly positive ones, towards their parents, they may continue to address the developmental issue of trust throughout their later development, to the detriment of other emotional tasks, until that issue has been reworked more positively (Wilson & Ryan, 2005). At other times, themes expressed in play sessions seem more common during later emotional development—for example, an 8-year-old child who plays out a theme of confusion about her gender, which is usually an issue for teenagers. The next sections give an overview of some developmental issues that arise as themes in home play sessions and special times.

EARLY DEVELOPMENT: TRUST/MISTRUST, AUTONOMY/ SHAME AND DOUBT, INITIATIVE/GUILT

One of the most crucial needs children have from birth onwards is to trust their parents and to see themselves as lovable, trustworthy, and important to their parents. Emotions that children often express and show in their behavior when they trust important people, and think they are important to others, are happiness, hopefulness, and a sense of curiosity about the world. Play themes parents can expect to see when their children have resolved these issues in their emotional development, which often occurs when they are ready to end their play sessions, include looking after others well, feeling satisfied, being well looked after, having enough themselves, and being saved and comforted when bad things happen.

The play theme of mistrust may have been prominent earlier in play sessions, with children showing that they felt unimportant to their parents. They may have shown play involving fear, rage, and a sense of hopelessness and sadness, and may have shown their need to reject others, or shown their anxiety about close relationships because they are mistrustful. Themes of death, chaos, and destruction, of never having enough, and of feeling very lonely and empty may have been prominent. For example, 6-year-old Diane, who had been hospitalized several times during the past year, worked on this early developmental theme during her home play sessions. In her early home play sessions, Diane played out many different scenes in which animals were lonely and afraid, including a powerful play sequence of a pony eating a poison mushroom. In her later sessions however, she made a comfortable bed for her pretend pony, who was given delicious carrots to eat, as well as showing other signs that she again felt trust in her parents and trust in herself.

As children reach toddlerhood, they start becoming more independent, and make a start at seeing themselves as more independent from their parents. They begin to learn to get what they need for themselves. In their play themes and behavior, children who have resolved issues of autonomy show a sense of independence that is appropriate for their age, and a sense of being important as a person in their own right. Their play themes and behavior may show a sense of power, mastery over difficult things, and satisfaction.

Five-year-old Len chose to play a ring toss game with his father during several of his home sessions. At the beginning, he became easily frustrated and needed to win quickly, moving to stand on top of the post when tossing his rings, while directing his father to move further and further back. In later home sessions, he began to set his own rules for the game, saying that he was younger and needed five turns, while his father needed only one. As he illustrated in his other play during home sessions—including racing cars to win unfairly against his father, and throwing bean bags to his father that could not be caught—children who are struggling with issues about independence may show in their play and behavior a strong sense of weakness, anger, and frustration. Later, when Len developed a better self-concept as a winner, he no longer found it necessary to adjust the rules so that he could win. He became better able to tolerate a loss in games.

As children become more independent and more able to have choices about things they can do, they also start to develop a sense of right and wrong. They can imagine themselves as all kinds of characters, including characters based on real-life figures such as their parents and teachers, as well as fantasy figures, such as princesses and gladiators. Children show creativity and initiative. Their play sessions can show themes about keeping rules, helping others, and being good, and an interest in playing out different adult roles. A 6-year-old girl, Sandra, who in previous home play sessions had taken on the role of an evil witch and assigned her mother the role of a wicked fairy, decided this time that her mother as the wicked fairy would be loved and helped, with Sandra herself taking the role of a loving mother. This play theme was age-appropriate for Sandra, who seemed to be starting to resolve this developmental issue positively in her play sessions.

Some children can show strong feelings of guilt, for not being good enough, and blaming themselves and others. They may escape into excessive and intense imaginative play, or show an inability to play freely because they do not want to let their bad feelings slip out. Play themes may be about harming themselves, others and property, conflicts about good and evil, defying rules, and evil in others, or they may be about sneaking to get what they need, and being very concerned for their own safety. For example, 9-year-old Patrick, who recently had moved to a long-term placement with a foster family, deliberately threw a cup of water at his foster father and then laughed with both excitement and fear, appearing to be waiting for a negative reaction. Patrick, unlike Sandra in the last example, had not positively resolved his earlier developmental issue of independence satisfactorily, nor had he resolved the issue of trust in his new carers. These earlier developmental issues, which seemed to be very negative for him, needed to be reworked in more positive ways in his home play sessions with his new foster carers.

MIDDLE CHILDHOOD: INDUSTRY/INFERIORITY

Children's main task in middle childhood is to learn to work in school. They need to get along with other children and their teachers, to work and play with other children, and develop their own skills. They display feelings of persistence, feeling clever, and feeling able to accomplish things for themselves as well as with other people. Play themes include an interest in learning skills and accomplishing tasks, and sharing interests with others. Seven-year-old Mary, for example, instructed her mother to be her audience as she danced in a concert with "other girls," and to applaud loudly at the end of her performance. This play sequence was very age-appropriate and positive for Mary with her mother. Children who show more negative play themes may express feeling stupid, worthless, and unable to accomplish tasks or enjoy friendships and cooperation, or they may have a strong emotional need to please others or to continually prove their skills and knowledge. For example, 9-year-old Martin spent his entire play sessions for several weeks drawing a model racing car in great detail. Each time he was very frustrated with the result, and destroyed his drawing before he left. Therefore, while expressing an age-appropriate play theme, he also showed that it was a predominantly negative rather than positive one.

ADOLESCENCE: IDENTITY/ROLE CONFUSION

Parents who have older children and adolescents to whom they are offering special times, and parents whose children display overly adult-like behavior and concerns, benefit from thinking about play/emotional themes for this age group. Parents often recognize that their teenagers are trying to fit into their peer group and into wider society as well, with an interest in what their adult lives may be like, and an increased sense of independence, as well as an ability to review their earlier lives in more detail than when they were younger. Teenagers may express pleasure in remembering their younger lives and hopes for the future, as well as pleasure in belonging to their family, peer groups, and society in general. They also may be trying to work out what values and ways of relating to other people are important to them, and what their sexual identifications are, all of which are positive and age-appropriate themes.

Teenagers who are struggling with this stage in their lives often show either a rejection of or a longing for their childhoods, feelings of alienation and despair for their future, and continual questioning of their own, others, and society's values, with a sense of excitement over delinquent behavior and cynical mistrust of others. They may show overly mature or overly young themes and behavior. For example, 15-year-old Bob was emotionless and withdrawn during the activity he had chosen to do with his father, which was playing a computer game about football together. However, one week he became animated and began describing to his father an escape a friend of his had had from the police. With a smile on his face, Bob then started to give details of his friend's episodes of fire setting, drug taking and stealing to his father, which was emotionally challenging for his father to respond to. Again Bob's theme is age-appropriate, but he expressed very negative themes that were not emotionally adaptive. Leaders chose to closely monitor Bob's and his father's special times again the following week, in light of Bob's reactions.

Using these descriptors of behavior in processing themes

Leaders can use these descriptors with parents to discuss their children's play themes and underlying developmental issues, helping parents adjust their understanding and responses in keeping with their children's underlying emotional needs, rather than reacting too concretely to their children's behavior. These descriptors also are useful when reviewing children's progress during play sessions with parents. When children show predominantly positive, age-appropriate themes, it is one indication that home play sessions have been therapeutic for them and may show their readiness to finish. Other evidence from earlier play therapy research (e.g. Guerney B. & Stover, 1971) showed that children's behavior altered from aggressive to less mature themes involving receiving protection and nurturance, and then to more reality-oriented and mastery themes during the course of their play therapy sessions. This progression in themes also is useful for leaders to keep in mind with parents during home play sessions and when reviewing children's progress.

An example of a child's themes changing with improved adjustment

Brent, aged 7, who displayed aggressive behavior in school and in his neighborhood when home play sessions began, entered a pattern after a couple of warm-up sessions of putting his mother, in the role of a robber, in jail for several sessions. He handled her roughly and gave her harsh punishments, pretending to be her jailer. After a few weeks, a new theme entered this play, with Brent adopting the role of a kinder and more nurturing jailer, bringing tasty, comforting foods to his mother. Shortly afterwards, Brent asked to have his mother put *him* in jail, and bring him all these wonderful foods.

Brent's parents said they found their leaders' and other parents' comments very helpful during this period. Leaders guided his parents towards deeper understanding of the meaning of Brent's role-plays from their knowledge of play themes, as presented earlier. Brent's initial theme of mistrust, characterized by his aggression and control, was discussed and his parents' difficult feelings recognized and empathized with by other parents. As Brent's role-play developed, leaders were able to guide his parents into understanding how the role-play was evolving into Brent starting to trust his mother to nurture him. Brent's parents rejoiced during a later meeting and reported to the group that, as this more trusting theme emerged in his play sessions, Brent had become less aggressive in school, to the point where he was no longer under threat of suspension. Leaders anticipated that Brent was soon likely to begin to express himself more industriously and independently in his play sessions, with age-appropriate mastery and reality play themes becoming more predominant.

Common challenges arising in home play sessions

Special issues often arise during home sessions that are demanding emotionally and physically for parents. This section of the chapter examines some of the potentially difficult issues that arise for parents after play sessions are well established at home. Leaders may need to reinforce, when problems arise, that it is the parents who are the therapeutic change agents, and therefore it is very important that they keep up their home play sessions, despite setbacks. Leaders should try to help parents stretch themselves towards what their children need from them as much as possible, similar to other parts of the program. In addition, leaders want to enable parents to solve problems themselves that arise in home play sessions as much as possible.

Helping discouraged parents

It also is important, when leaders supervise parents' home sessions, that they are sensitive to parents becoming over-stretched physically and emotionally. Leaders need to recognize when parents begin to feel resentful of the play sessions and special times, and when they feel overwhelmed by their children's needs. Sometimes when parents are stretching their tolerance and understanding to their limit, they may become defensive in order to protect themselves, and may revert to an earlier attitude that their children are solely responsible for any difficulties. Empathy should be offered readily by leaders when parents feel overwhelmed, and other group members can be encouraged to offer support. Some practical suggestions may be required too in exceptional cases, such as shortening sessions to 20 minutes, or alternating sessions between two children. A few such solutions arrived at by leaders and parents under these circumstances may appear somewhat hampering or unfair to the children. However in the authors' opinion, it is better to compromise on non-major points, rather than having some parents either become so discouraged that they do not want to continue their play sessions, or overly dictatorial and authoritarian in their attitude towards their children in their play sessions. Parents should not be expected to sacrifice themselves too much to the process of GFT.

Our suggestions for emotionally taxing issues

Some emotionally taxing issues for parents and their children, along with suggestions and solutions, are discussed in the following sections. Most of these potentially difficult issues already are familiar ones for leaders in their own play therapy practice, and they already have developed ways in which they have resolved them. However, parents are not professional therapists. Leaders usually find that their own FT supervision is invaluable in these circumstances. It can help them separate out their own reactions and personal solutions from those they need to offer to parents.

CHILDREN "TRASHING" THE ROOM

Sometimes parents object to the amount of time it takes them to clean up after their home play sessions. We suggest leaders empathize with parents' feelings, and try to help parents think about the meaning of this play to their children, and the feelings that are being expressed. When required, leaders may need to facilitate a problem-solving approach. Solutions may range from shutting the door of the room and picking up the toys later, to limiting the child to two containers of toys for dumping out per session, or, if necessary, eliminating the problem toys (e.g. small bricks). The latter may be a solution if the child does not seem to play with these problem toys during sessions. However, if the child has shown that these toys are important, then we suggest that another solution should be found. As stated earlier, leaders should try to compromise with something that is of lesser importance to the play sessions' success.

Leaders also may want to help parents practice CCPT skills, such as reflecting feelings and limit setting, as appropriate. They may offer the comment that sometimes it is a phase children go through before they have more control, or that they are testing their parents' tolerance in this way before accepting that the rules are indeed different. Leaders may wish to underline that, in general, if children are purposely destructive of toys in home sessions, then a limit needs to be set.

CHILDREN REFUSING TO CONTINUE THEIR PLAY SESSIONS

Occasionally, children may decide after, say, five play sessions not to come to their home play sessions any more. Leaders already mentioned this possibility when they prepared parents for home sessions (see Chapter 12), stating that they would return to this issue if it arose later. In these cases, we suggest that parents have an observed play session at the next meeting, for leaders to troubleshoot the problem. If an unplanned practice play session needs to occur during the next meeting, this may require other parents rearranging their schedule for the next meeting in order to accommodate this family's more urgent need. If rescheduling is not feasible, then we suggest that the parent and child come in early, or another time, before the next meeting. It is important under these circumstances that a leader supervises the practice play session directly, rather than via video, in order to judge whether it is the child's or the parent's issue (or both) that seems to be driving the child's refusal.

If issues arise during a play session that are unexplainable to leaders, then they need to try to find out what is happening at home, school, or the neighborhood, and ask questions of the parent in order to understand the dynamics of the situation. For example, in a foster family, 8-year-old Angie suddenly refused her last two play sessions. After the leader asked, *"Is there anything that happened recently at home that may have upset Angie?"*, her foster parent revealed that Angie's foster sister was moved from their home recently to a placement in kinship care. During Angie's play session after the move, she didn't talk about it, but she started not wanting to play in her next sessions. It was clear to her foster parent that she was suffering a loss, and everyone in the group agreed that her major loss could have some bearing on her not wishing to play. After considerable empathy with the foster parent from both leaders and group members, suggestions were made as to how the parent might engage Angie again. The leader decided to take the parent's role in a role-play to work directly on this difficulty, as shown in the following example.

> *"Parent" [leader as parent]: Angie, you seem to be feeling kind of down because Grace was moved away. I think it would be very helpful if you could have a play session with me, even if you're not really feeling like doing it. I would really like to have our playtime together.*
>
> *"Angie" [foster parent as child]: (Silent, just looks at her Mom.)*
>
> *"Parent": It is hard for you to talk about it. I'm going to suggest that we come into our play area for five minutes. I will set the timer to go off after five minutes. When it goes off, you are free to leave. If you decide you're not ready to leave, you may stay longer.*

("Angie", dragging a bit, goes into the play area and idly handles the toys... After five minutes, when the timer goes off, she makes a move to leave.)

"Parent": *You've had enough for today. You want to end now. We can do it this way again next week, if you want to, and you can decide to leave or stay longer.*

In the example of Angie, it was clear what the problem was. If leaders are unable to distinguish what factors are responsible for a difficulty, we suggest that the parent go back to shorter sessions, and renegotiate these with their child. Leaders should stress that it is better for parents not to give up easily on home play sessions; they should aim to contain parents' strong feelings of helplessness and discouragement. Parents need to be given hope that their child will start play sessions again, and leaders often have to reaffirm that children have a strong wish to have positive experiences with their parents. In the first author's experience, there have been parents who have kept coming to group meetings when their child stopped playing, and then had the happy outcome of their child beginning play sessions again after a short time. In general, almost all of these kinds of problems can be salvaged, with patience by parents and support from leaders.

PARENTS FAILING TO CONDUCT HOME PLAY SESSIONS

When preparing for home sessions, leaders emphasized that home play sessions are not rewards for children's good behavior, and that the topic of parents conducting play sessions when stressed by their children or by other events would be returned to during a later meeting. Returning to a discussion of this topic when it seems timely, leaders first need to empathize with parents—sometimes it is tempting for parents to withhold play sessions when they have had a very stressful time with their children during the day, or when stressful times have occurred several times in the week. It can be especially challenging for parents to offer play sessions when difficulties with their children (or partner or other stressful life events) occur immediately before a play session is scheduled. Second, leaders should make it clear that home sessions need to be held weekly, even during stressful times. Parents may need to be reminded that, because their sessions are for therapy, it is when things are difficult that play sessions are often most effective for their children. Third, leaders usually need to help parents with more specific strategies for readying themselves emotionally for home play sessions when stressed. Many times, other parents in the group are excellent sources of ideas for effective ways they have discovered for themselves to maintain emotional and physical readiness for home play sessions.

ILLUSTRATIVE EXAMPLE

Nine-year-old Ben's father told the group that he did not hold a home play session last week because Ben had taken the paint tin and deliberately dumped it on the family car.

Leader: *You're very angry right now, just thinking about it with us.*

Dad: *Yes, I am! It will take a while to get over. I may have to get the car resprayed. Ben certainly didn't deserve a play session to do what he wanted after that damn behavior.*

Parent 1: I would have been furious! I would have felt like grounding him for at least a month!

Parent 2: Me too. The expense of it all! I would have made him pay for the respray.

Leader: I think any parent would have been very upset by this behavior of Ben's. Maybe Ben was very angry himself when he did it. But it is important to remember that play sessions are offered on a regular basis, regardless of how children act outside the home play session.

Dad: Well, you just come over and do it then, if there is a next time!

Leader: You're angry with me for suggesting this. You think it just wasn't possible for you to do a session yourself.

Dad: No, no way.

Leader: You know your limits. I do think though that it's important for all of us to remember that play sessions have the power to heal, and you are doing them to help Ben manage his feelings and behavior better. Children's impulsive, destructive behavior can be decreased when their angry feelings are under control. This control can happen through therapeutic play.

Dad: There's a lot of healing and making amends that Ben DOES have to do, right now!

Leader: You think Ben has big problems, and that worries you a lot. I know it isn't obvious—or maybe even believable—to you, but usually children who have done something like Ben has often use the play session to work through the damaging situation.

Dad: I guess I have to take a lot on trust here, but I just couldn't do it right away.

Leader: You feel you have to trust me about the way Ben may use the play session. You also know that you would have been too angry to go straight into the play session with Ben and do a good job. In those circumstances, it sounds like you need to calm down first. It is possible to postpone the session for an hour or two, or even a day, if time demands.

Dad: I would have liked to just go into the garage and do some things by myself for a while.

Leader: You have a way to calm yourself down, if anything else gets really out of hand. If anything like this happens again, and we all really hope it doesn't, be sure to tell Ben that you will play with him when you are calmer. It may be important right now to think about how to feel calmer before your next play session with him, because it might bring it all back for you… I think all parents sometimes feel pushed beyond their endurance, so this is useful for all of us to talk about. How do other parents put aside their strong feelings in order to do their play sessions? (The leader opens up the discussion to other parents, returning to Ben's dad later.)

This example shows how important it was for leaders to respond empathically to this father's underlying emotional issues, supporting him, acknowledging his anger with leaders, and helping him engage in problem solving the difficult situation when he was ready, along with reinforcing the importance of holding the play session as promised. The leader then used the situation to brainstorm with the father and other parents, at the same time as helping other participants examine their own emotional responses to stressful pre-session experiences with their children.

CONTRASTING LACK OF PROGRESS OF ONE FAMILY WITH PROGRESS IN ANOTHER

At times, parents who are struggling to accept their children's behavior and emotional needs may begin to compare their children's lack of progress with other families' apparent successes. For example, a frustrated parent may ask (or imply): *"Why is my child still so aggressive, while the other kids are making progress in their play sessions?"* When these comparisons arise, it is crucial that leaders first of all reflect parents' feelings empathically. It also is important for leaders to maintain, as they have throughout GFT, that children work through issues at their own pace, while at the same time acknowledging that this pace can feel too slow sometimes for parents. There are often changes parents want their children to make quickly in GFT that they hope will result in the family's lives becoming much easier.

If parents continue to be dissatisfied with changes that they perceive as only minor in their children, leaders can point out that children's changes may be meaningful and useful, without immediately being apparent to anyone. Leaders can ask for examples from the group of different kinds of changes parents have noticed in their children, including ones that seem minor right now. If other parents are not able to give this kind of example, leaders should offer examples themselves from ongoing home sessions for the group to consider. For example, leaders may mention that one child may be working on independence issues, while another child may be working through issues about friendships and how to play cooperatively.

RESPONDING TO TRAUMATIC PLAY ENACTMENTS

The previous chapter discussed the preparation leaders give parents for possible allegations of mistreatment that may arise during their children's home play sessions. Parents were asked to contact leaders for a full discussion immediately, where possible, and not wait until the next meeting. This section discusses play enactments by children in home sessions of apparently traumatic experiences, which may or may not include abusive experiences, and which arise in leaders' supervision of home sessions during meetings. When traumatic play contents arise during meetings, leaders should be aware that this topic is one of the most emotional topics for parents to manage in play sessions. Throughout their supervision of these sequences, leaders need to be highly empathic to parents feeling out of control and anxious. Parents' understandable reactions will be over and above the considerable emotional demands traumatic enactments can engender in professionals because of parents' highly intimate and protective role with their children. Parents' reactions also are stronger because they often more readily connect this play with real events in their children's lives than professionals can.

Yet, for both parents and professionals, traumatic play enactments can be fragmented and obscure, especially when initially explored by children in play sessions. For enactments portraying maltreatment, leaders need to judge whether such enactments are of sufficient clarity and seriousness that the leaders and parents need to make a report to their child protection agency. And in the very rare circumstance that parents themselves seem to be implicated by their children in their play, leaders also have to consider reporting these to their child protection agency.

In order to help parents process very difficult re-enactments of trauma, leaders need to see the videos of these play sessions in full, if they are available, or help parents report as fully as possible on the play sequences, if written reports alone are used in the group. Sometimes leaders need to consider with parents whether the traumatic issues enacted are of sufficient seriousness for parents to need additional, personal supervision outside of group meetings, as well as continuing with home sessions and group supervision. Leaders need to judge whether these parents can be sufficiently objective, and feel sufficiently supported, to handle such highly emotional material in home play sessions. If not, such parents may be offered use of facilities provided by leaders, who will need to directly supervise play sessions outside of meetings and give additional input. Under these extreme circumstances, home play sessions would be stopped temporarily until the parents were able to manage them at home again.

EXTERNAL SUPERVISION FOR LEADERS

We recommend that leaders always receive FT supervision themselves when such issues arise, which should include discussions of implications for parents continuing in the group, implications for the children involved and potential disruption to their therapy, and opportunities for leaders to address their own emotional reactions.

APPLYING CCPT SKILLS TO TRAUMATIC ENACTMENTS

There are a few general concepts that leaders should emphasize when parents discuss home play sessions that have traumatic contents. First, leaders should stress how important it is that children trust their parents sufficiently that they are able to play out very difficult events with them. Second, leaders need to help parents to apply their child-centered skills to traumatic play as reviewed next, skill by skill.

Skill 1: Parents accepting and reflecting their children's feelings with empathy. Using this skill is a very important part of the parents' role during traumatic play. It is also very emotionally demanding for parents. It is particularly difficult for most parents when:

- their children's traumatic play is directed towards themselves in an extreme way (e.g. within an aggressive or sexualized role-play)

- they have not fully processed the event themselves (e.g. a mother who has recently separated from her partner after chronic domestic violence; a father whose driving resulted in his child's serious injury)

- the play challenges deeply held values or beliefs (e.g. hurting a defenceless person or animal, sexualized play).

Leaders need to help these parents during supervision to name, understand, and then empathize with their children's feelings. Showing parents places in their video where they applied this skill is effective, with parents then guided towards finding another example of where they might have used this skill further. While parents need leaders' help dealing with their own strong feelings, leaders also often need to provide parents with a better understanding on a cognitive level of how children work through traumatic events in their play sessions (see Wilson & Ryan, 2005).

Skill 2: Parents following their children's lead. Children who engage in traumatic enactments often have fragmented, highly sensory, and highly emotional contents in their play. This type of play can be difficult for parents to follow for several reasons:

- It is difficult for parents to make sense of the play and follow their children's lead because the play moves quickly and unpredictably from one event or type of play to another.

- The play can be marked by high anxiety and play disruption, leading to abrupt endings and rapid shifts to another activity, leaving parents feeling out of control and anxious themselves.

- The children may show very immature or atypical behavior, such as curling up on their parent's lap for an extended period of time after the play, which can in turn engender increased anxiety in parents.

Leaders should support parents in their efforts to follow their children's lead, making full use of video material, where available. Leaders usually need to make specific suggestions to parents of how to use this skill more fully in the future when traumatic play emerges. They also need to help parents understand that their children are making their first attempts (or further attempts) to process these very difficult events for themselves, as the example of Kim illustrated earlier in this chapter. Any examples that have already arisen within the group of children playing out traumatic scenes can be useful to refer to here. Leaders should emphasize to parents that children feel understood and accepted when their parents are able to follow their traumatic play sequences. This is because one of the most important roles for adults during children's re-enactments of previous trauma in their play seems to be conveying to children, both verbally and non-verbally, that their play is important to carry out (Ryan & Needham, 2001).

Skill 3: Parents structuring play sessions for their children. Parents need to adhere to the familiar structure of play sessions during sessions with traumatic re-enactments, to ensure their children feel secure.

Skill 4: Parents setting necessary limits to their children's behavior. Leaders should remind parents that children who are enacting traumatic play contents usually are more fully immersed in their play than usual because the events enacted often have not been processed on a more mature, cognitive level. Parents find that they sometimes are the ones to have the "thinking" and "managing" roles in this kind of play, and not their children. It is very important that children feel emotionally contained and safe during their re-enactments of trauma, since the traumatic play itself is an enactment of events in which children felt out of control and very unsafe. Therefore, limits to their children's behavior are very important for parents to maintain. Some limit-setting situations that may need further discussion are addressed next.

PARENTS TEMPTED TO EXTEND THE PLAY SESSION TO ENABLE THEIR CHILDREN TO CONTINUE THEIR TRAUMATIC PLAY ENACTMENTS

Parents may be tempted to forego finishing a session on time, if their children continue to enact important play scenes beyond the last minute of their session, despite the parents' usual time warnings. If this occurs, leaders need to reflect parents' feelings of wanting to be helpful, and also reinforce the point made earlier in the program (e.g. Chapter 4) that children feel safest when they know that the usual rules to their sessions apply. Often leaders also need to discuss with parents how they can handle any spillover to home life that resulted from a session's traumatic play.

In more extreme cases, leaders' suggestions on responding to traumatic play can be carried out effectively by parents, and yet their children continue to engage in traumatic play beyond the end of the session. It is important for leaders in these rare cases to discuss and work out the best strategy for each case with their FT supervisor. Where it is clear that children themselves cannot regulate their own heightened responses, leaders may need to help parents introduce a new rule. The rule may be, for example, that these children do not engage in role-play during the last five minutes of their play session. Depending on the situation, children may be told that they can *"do most other things"* or that *"We will have a quiet time for five minutes before we end. You can choose to either draw with me, or do some other quiet thing. Next time you can do most things you want in here."*

PARENTS ASKED TO TAKE ON A POTENTIALLY ABUSIVE ROLE

Traumatic re-enactments can be highly arousing and emotional for children, and younger children in particular may struggle to maintain the distinction between their imaginative play and reality. Leaders sometimes need to help parents maintain this distinction, rather than expecting their children to do so when they are highly aroused. Leaders also should discuss with parents that they need to place a limit on any requested role or action in which they feel very uncomfortable, whether the discomfort is due to their own emotional reactions to a previous event, or to their perception that they are being placed in a re-enactment of an event as, for example, an abuser.

Parents should reflect their children's feelings as usual, and then set a clear personal limit on a role they are asked to take. Sometimes parents also may need to suggest an acceptable alternative, if children seem unable to manage this for themselves. For example, the second author and her colleague (Ryan & Courtney, 2009) discuss their work in individual FT with fostered and adopted children and their families. They give an example of 5-year-old James who was having home play sessions with his adoptive mother. James had been severely neglected and abused, which may have involved the use of restraints. In one of his early home sessions with his mother, he asked her to cover his mouth with a Band-Aid™ from the doctor's kit:

Intuitively his mother responded: *"I wouldn't like to do that to a little boy, I will put it on your chin instead and we can pretend."* James was satisfied with this alteration and it did not interfere with his continuing his play sequence... This example shows how important it was for both James and his mother to have her clearly recognize with him that she was not going to enact potentially abusive experiences as his mother, even in role-play. This stemmed from her need to be certain that James was helped to clearly differentiate his own earlier experiences from his play enactments (Ryan & Courtney, 2009, p.126).

This example also demonstrates the balance parents need to maintain between taking part in traumatic play re-enactments that are needed by their children to work through their experiences, such as taking the role of a very neglectful or abusive mother, and also ensuring that their behavior is not interpreted as abusive by their highly emotionally involved child. Any role in which parents are asked by their children to engage in direct behavior that may be interpreted as abusive by them and/or others (e.g. *"You lie on top of me while we are in bed.")* should have a limit set. Most children are capable of finding their own solutions to these limits in their play enactments; however, in a few cases parents may need to be more specific about where children can redirect their efforts, while still maintaining the role-play, as shown with James earlier. In addition, parents need empathic and helpful supervision from leaders, and support from other participants, while engaging in these difficult home play sessions.

The next chapter examines how leaders help parents generalize their skills to daily life, the last stage in the GFT program before ending.

CHAPTER 14

Generalizing Play Session Skills and Preparation for Ending

Meetings 16–19

In the last phase of the program, leaders concentrate on helping parents apply their play session skills, along with other parenting skills, to daily life, which is one of the main goals of GFT. Leaders formally help parents generalize their play skills to daily life during Meetings 16–19, while continuing to work with them to understand underlying emotional issues expressed in their children's play sessions.

Similar to other parts of the GFT program, this phase of GFT has a strongly therapeutic aim. Leaders continue to concentrate on children's play themes and parents' reactions during supervision of selected families' live and/or video-recorded play sessions at the beginning of the meeting, while the last part of the meeting is allocated to reviewing the other families' home play sessions.

Before the last part of each meeting, after the midway break, leaders help parents generalize their play skills, and introduce other parenting skills to them. Leaders should aim to have some flexibility in the time allocated for this part of the meeting, to address more general issues that might arise and would be of interest to the entire group, such as discipline at home. It is in this part of the meeting that leaders also introduce the topic of ending the program, by Meeting 18 at the latest, as discussed later in this chapter.

Generalizing play skills to daily life[1]

Towards the end of the group process, leaders have an eye to transferring and generalizing parents' play skills to daily life, along with ending the program itself. In general, for a

---

1   The sections on generalizing are adapted for FT from Guerney, L. (2013).

group that is competent in conducting play sessions and has seen most of their problems reduced, leaders are able to start helping parents generalize their skills by Meeting 16. Signs of readiness are parents being able to discuss and understand their home sessions in more depth, including their children's play themes, and to accept their children's feelings in play sessions.

Most parents already have discussed concerns about their children's behavior outside the playroom, as earlier chapters illustrate, and are primed to work further on their concerns in the last phase of GFT. In addition, leaders will by now be very familiar with parents and their emotional reactions to new learning. Leaders are accustomed already to empathically responding to parents' feelings, an important part of this phase of the program also. And parents themselves usually feel able to honestly explore difficulties in parenting with leaders and group members. This openness is important for leaders to maintain in the group, as parents share more details of their daily problems during the generalization phase in the program.

As mentioned earlier, leaders already prepared parents for this part of the program by commenting on and giving examples of where CCPT play skills are transferable to home life during previous discussions, before play sessions were well established at home. However, leaders took the stance earlier that play skills need to be well established, along with parents having a greater understanding of their children's underlying emotional issues, before generalizing play skills to daily life. Now leaders affirm parents' progress and take on an instructive role in teaching parenting skills, demonstrating to parents that they as leaders have substantial knowledge of the kinds of situations parents encounter in their lives where such skills might be useful. Above all, leaders need to establish that parents themselves have the ability to think through and apply play and other parenting skills, with group help to begin with, in their daily lives.

When parents show early ability in generalizing their play skills

For parents who do not have more serious problems with their children, particularly parents who attend for primary and secondary prevention goals, sometimes formal instruction in this phase of the program need not be extensive. Some parents seem to grasp play skills readily and in turn transfer these skills to home sessions quickly, as mentioned in previous chapters. A few of these parents may have mentioned during earlier meetings that they used structuring or reflecting their children's feelings empathically in their daily lives to good effect. It can be surprising for new leaders to realize the extent to which parents often begin to generalize the FT skills and attitudes without direct training by leaders. This seems to occur more easily within GFT, compared with individual FT, in the authors' experience, because group members' comments often facilitate other parents' generalization skills. The two examples that follow are good illustrations of this phenomenon.

EXAMPLE 1

Seven-year-old Sophie's mother and father had complained often that she started arguing with them regularly when it was time for her to go to bed. In the group discussion after an early practice play session with Sophie and her father, her parents stated that they had decided together that, instead of reacting argumentatively themselves to Sophie, they would watch out for what Sophie was doing immediately before her bedtime, and maybe they could figure out what was setting her off. Sophie had been very grumpy yesterday evening, her dad said, yet again refusing to get ready for bed. They wondered if she was worried about the darkness on the staircase, and did not want to go upstairs on her own. They suggested to her that she take her flashlight up with her and use it until she turned on her ceiling light. They would then come up, turn off the ceiling light, and read to her, using her flashlight, before putting on her night-light.

The leader, after reflecting the parents' strong desire to help Sophie, stated that this was a good example of applying the structuring skill parents were learning, along with thinking about the reasons underlying Sophie's behavior. The leader added that applying this skill, along with other parenting skills, would be something that the group would look at in detail later in the program. The group would benefit from being reminded of this example later on.

EXAMPLE 2

During the meeting immediately after parents conducted their first home sessions, Julie reviewed her home session, which went well, and then mentioned that the other day she had "*let slip out*" something she had said during play sessions. She explained that, when her son Robert was putting away several of his board games in the cupboard, she could tell he was getting fed up, even though he hadn't said anything. She related to the group that she had spontaneously said: "*You're getting annoyed with those games,*" just as she would have done during a play session, "*and it worked!*" She said that Robert had then turned to her and said: "*I'm not going to blow up. Don't worry Mom,*" and he continued to calmly sort the games out.

The leader reflected Julie's pleasure and commented to the group that some parents might find that they have taken the play skills to heart and are spontaneously using them effectively from time to time with their children. The leader said that they could use this example of reflecting children's feelings when they were looking more fully at how all the play skills can transfer to daily life in a couple of weeks.

When parents apply their play skills too early

As the earlier examples imply, leaders have to strike a balance between encouraging and affirming parents' efforts and positive outcomes when they generalize a play skill at an earlier phase in GFT, and discouraging parents from taking too much initiative before they are able to successfully implement their new skills more widely. There will be other parents in many groups, unlike the parents discussed here, who try to apply play skills to their daily lives prematurely and do not succeed. This lack of success usually leads to the parents feeling discouraged about their own effectiveness and the effectiveness of GFT. Leaders should provide empathy and may hypothesize that these parents were unsuccessful because they had not grasped the skills sufficiently, or may not have understood the underlying reasons for their children's responses adequately.

In unsuccessful cases of premature application of CCPT skills, it is frequently limit setting that parents attempt to practice first, in order to try to gain more control over their lives. However, limit setting is usually a more difficult skill to implement, because parents need to keep their own stronger feelings in check, to clearly understand their children's motives, and to learn limit-setting skills thoroughly. Furthermore, as set out next, for successful generalization of limit setting, we recommend parents first are encouraged to use other parenting skills before resorting to limit setting, a similar attitude to what is practiced in play sessions themselves.

Steps in training parents to generalize their skills
Introducing the generalization phase of GFT to parents

Leaders often successfully introduce generalization of skills to parents by saluting them for mastering their home play sessions and now being ready as a group to think about how these skills can be applied in daily life. It is essential for leaders to relate this part of the program to the problems with their children that parents mentioned at referral and during the earlier parts of the program. Leaders may need to bring up issues themselves at times, when parents do not address them spontaneously. However, usually parents are very eager to raise parenting problems at home, and typically feel confident that they can make progress on them now.

Leaders should plan to briefly review justifications for each of the play session skills covered in the earlier, training phase of the program at relevant points in their generalization discussions. They again should underline for parents that, until they feel sure of using their skills more widely at home, it would be best to use their skills in simpler situations; otherwise, parents tend to tackle the problems that seem more difficult to them immediately. This strategy of working on tractable problems is necessary for leaders to mention here, in order to ensure that parents are successful in their first attempts at generalization.

Leaders should aim to elicit parents' ideas as much as possible during these discussions, as well as helping everyone draw on shared group examples from discussions and play sessions. At this point in the program, parents are much more able to lead discussions and give examples themselves, as well as to problem solve for their own circumstances. All of these characteristics of later meetings are ones that leaders should foster and facilitate because they enhance parents' increasing independence and confidence in using play skills in their daily lives.

It is often most effective for parents when leaders utilize specific problem situations described by them to demonstrate how a given skill can work to solve a problem arising in daily life. Along with a short explanation, leaders can often improvise a role-play for a more vivid illustration of generalization. If, for example, a parent complains of not knowing how to handle an exchange with their child, a leader can take the parent role and assign the child part to the parent (unlike earlier phases of the program, when parents took on only parental roles). In acting out the situation as the "child," parents can often learn to empathize with their children and see more experientially how using the skill effectively can lead to changes in children's attitudes and parent-child interactions. Reversing these roles, with a leader or another parent taking on the child's role, can be helpful too, in order for parents to experience the effects of their own use of these skills on another person. Which role to assign parents should be based on leaders' judgments of parents' emotional needs and competence.

Leaders also need to review child development principles, in order to weave these concepts into discussions on generalization of skills. Some of the most important concepts to emphasize to parents are the same ones that were used earlier when introducing CCPT skills in the first part of the program (see Chapters 6–8). The overarching concepts to reinforce in skills generalization include the following:

- Children's developmental readiness needs to be taken into account when parents have expectations about what their children are capable of, and how their children should behave.

- Children have things in common with other children, as well as unique characteristics that influence who they are and what they do.

- Children's environments make a difference to who they are and what they do. More optimal environments lead to children who are more able to achieve and more able to feel content.

- Important new events and traumas can disrupt children's development.

The generalization of skills outlined next gives the order that seems most useful for leaders to use when introducing generalization of each skill. However, leaders also should adapt to the examples and motivations of their own groups as much as possible within this ordering. Therefore, they need to be very familiar with how parents in general are able to generalize all their play skills, and which skills are most relevant in common scenarios from daily life, in order to adapt to the unique needs of each group of parents.

Generalizing the skill of empathy

Showing empathy for their children's feelings is one of the main play skills parents learn in GFT, and a skill that parents are very familiar with at this point in the program. Leaders start with the skill of empathy in generalizing usually because of its high importance, and help parents make ample references to play session examples, as they generalize this skill.

Leaders may need to remind parents that, just as in play sessions, if their children show very extreme behavior in daily life, particularly behavior that puts their children at risk of harm, parents need to deal with that behavior as the priority, perhaps before their children's feelings are addressed. Therefore, extreme temper tantrums, running away, extreme withdrawal, serious aggression, and self-harm need more immediate action by parents to keep their children safe, before children's feelings can be understood and reflected on.

REVIEWING JUSTIFICATIONS FOR EMPATHY AND ACCEPTANCE OF CHILDREN'S FEELINGS

Parents' attitudes towards their children's feelings are very important in daily interactions. Key points about parents' attitudes that leaders should make at relevant places in the group's discussion on generalizing empathy include the following:

- Parents have seen in their play sessions that responding to their children's feelings usually is perceived by their children as non-threatening and non-rejecting.

- When parents recognize their children's feelings, it helps their children understand how they feel and builds their self-confidence.

- Children are encouraged to use direct verbalization, not inappropriate behavior. (One parent remarked: "*Now that Robert **says** he's angry, he seems to have less need to throw a tantrum.*")

- Feelings are not labeled right or wrong, so all children's feelings are allowed.

- Parents, by showing they understand, build up their children's trust and confidence in them as parents.

- Parents showing understanding increase their children's willingness to respect their parents' feelings and ideas. (This chapter later discusses when "I" statements by parents are effective in daily life communications with their children.)

- Understanding of feelings does not always determine the outcome for either adults or children. (There are other considerations too, discussed later.)

- Parents must genuinely accept what their children are feeling, however different from their own feelings.

- Parents must be confident that children can grow to handle their own feelings and find their own solutions to problems.

General attitudes that leaders help parents to internalize while practicing empathy and acceptance of their children's feelings in daily life are to:

- accept rather than criticize

- accept rather than reassure

- accept rather than suggest a solution

- accept rather than moralize

- accept rather than threaten with a punishment

- accept rather than put a child down for feeling a certain way.

STEPS IN PARENTS SHOWING EMPATHY

Leaders need to review with parents the steps in showing empathy that they already apply in their play sessions, and that they now are to begin to apply in daily life.

1. Listen carefully to what your child is expressing and look for feelings. Verbal messages from children may not be the same as their feelings underneath. And sometimes children do not say directly how they are feeling.

2. Identify your child's feelings.

3. Say something that shows you accept and understand your child's feelings. (This is *especially important* when parents have strong and opposing feelings about the matter.)

4. An accepting voice tone and the right words are important in showing understanding.

EXAMPLES OF GENERALIZING EMPATHY TO DAILY LIFE

Leaders may wish to introduce an example of their own, as well as eliciting examples from the parents themselves, after introducing generalization of empathy. For groups who do not generate examples themselves readily, the following brief examples may help parents think of examples from their own home life and guide leaders in teaching this skill. For a group that needs even more input, leaders may want to give a choice of two responses, one showing empathy and one not, then discussing these alternative responses before calling for examples from the group.

Example 1:

> Tom (defiantly): *Forget about taking me to school tomorrow. I'm not going! That stupid old teacher! She's always picking on me!*
>
> Two possible responses by Dad are: *"She's picking on you again. That's terrible."* (a non-empathic response) *or "Your teacher really makes you angry!"* (an empathic response).

Leaders with groups needing prompting can ask which response showed understanding of Tom's feelings and then help the group discuss how this parent sets his own feelings aside. Leaders ask parents to think about the range of feelings that may have been aroused in the father (e.g. anxiety or panic, loss of control, helplessness, anger, a wish to argue or control the situation, or agreement with his son). It is useful for leaders to point out that it would have been confrontational for the father to have immediately replied: *"You're going to school, and it's my job to get you there!"* And leaders should emphasize that showing understanding of Tom's feelings doesn't mean that the father agrees with Tom's solution, to not go to school.

Example 2:

> May (shouting): *I hate you!*
>
> Two possible responses by Mom are: *"I don't know why you are so angry. I told you that I wasn't going to let you have another ride on the Big Wheel."* (a non-empathic response) *or "You're very angry with me. You're disappointed that you didn't get what you wanted."* (an empathic response).

Again, leaders should encourage parents to think about the feelings the mother may have to put aside in order to accept May's feelings.

Example 3:

> Helen: I don't think I'll go to that party of Claire's tonight.
>
> Parent: You'll have fun! (a reassuring response) or "You're not sure you want to go to her party." (an empathic response).

Leaders should help parents understand that the first response not only failed to accept Helen's feelings, but told her how she should be feeling. Many times this response is based on how the parent would feel or what is socially desirable, rather than accepting their children's expressed feelings.

An additional step: "I" statements

Unlike play sessions, in daily life it is important for parents to both identify their own feelings and judiciously express them to their children. However, parents need to empathize with their children's feelings first and foremost in most situations, as they have learned to do in play sessions. Leaders also should caution parents when necessary that "I" statements when expressed by parents do not automatically mean that children become considerate of their parents' feelings, even though they may learn to express their own feelings more clearly. Learning compassion for others is a developmental process that all adults can attest takes a lifetime to perfect!

Developmentally, children first begin to feel empathy for others within primary attachment relationships (Schore, 2000), and "I" statements from parents allow children opportunities to develop their capacities further. Feelings expressed by parents genuinely and non-confrontationally create opportunities for children to take into account their parents' views as they act independently and act interdependently as well. When parents add simple reasons to explain to their children why they feel as they do, in situations where the reason is unclear to children, this helps their children to develop emotional understanding of others and of themselves.

As discussed earlier in Chapter 9, parents using "I" statements (also referred to as expressing congruent feelings by Ryan & Courtney [2009]), is commonly facilitated in GFT during the last phase because parents first need to understand their children's needs and feelings, and to follow their children's lead, before helping their children recognize their parents' feelings. This emphasis on placing children's feelings first also coincides with the main role of parents more generally, which is to provide a nurturing and safe environment within which their children can develop. As Erikson states in his theory of emotional/social development, parents' needs for caregiving and generativity are satisfied when they are able to provide well for their children's needs (Wilson & Ryan, 2005). Children's attachment needs generally should take precedence over parental needs because of children's vulnerabilities and care-seeking needs. Parents do not have symmetrical attachment relationships with their children; rather they are complementary, with different goals and behaviors (O'Sullivan & Ryan, 2009; Ryan, 2004). Therefore, parents reflecting their children's feelings need to remain dominant within parent-child relationships in daily life, similar to play sessions.

In keeping with GFT principles, leaders help parents to first of all convey their positive feelings towards their children using "I" statements. This can be followed by leaders discussing with parents when other, less positive, feelings may be appropriate for parents to share with their children. Leaders may wish to caution parents not to start a statement to their child with the words: *"I feel…"* because there is a tendency for parents to think they have stated a feeling when they begin sentences in this way, when they have not. Similar to play sessions in which parents reflect their children's feelings clearly, leaders should help parents to state their own feelings directly (e.g. *"I love it when you smile that way."*)

When helping parents use their own feelings in important communications with their children, leaders facilitate parents to do the following:

- State their feelings clearly, as they state their children's feelings clearly in play sessions.

- Give children the reason behind their feelings, and state the reason in a simple way. Try to be specific.

- When giving a negative feeling, make an explicit and clear statement about a difficulty with their children, but do not accuse, condemn, ridicule, or embarrass them in these situations.

- Let their children briefly know when they, their parents, have a problem (e.g. they are unwell, busy) that affects how they can respond and accounts for the way they feel.

EXAMPLES OF "I" STATEMENTS DURING GENERALIZATION

Examples of parents making positive "I" statements that may be useful for leaders to use include the following:

> Mother to child: rather than, *"I'm glad you are finally sharing"* or *"I hate it when you fight over your things with your sister,"* instead, *"It makes me proud to see you offering to let your sister use your new doll's cradle."*

> Father to child: rather than, *"I feel that if only you would listen to me, I wouldn't have to repeat things so many times,"* instead, *"I want you to listen to me. It's important to me."*

Parents, of course, do have negative feelings of their own that arise within their relationships with their children. These too may be important for parents to identify for themselves internally and to share as appropriate with their children. For example:

> Father to child: *"I'm unhappy with myself. I shouldn't have shouted at you today. I'm sorry."*

As these examples show, leaders help parents share their appropriate, positive, and, sometimes, negative feelings in daily situations. Certain parental feelings are important to convey because they are very potent relationship-building, rebuilding, and maintaining statements for parents with their children (Heard & Lake, 1997). Leaders should emphasize to parents that "I" statements should reflect these relationship aims; and should primarily be statements of positive feelings. Also, leaders should point out to parents that often highly positive feelings underlie parents' negative feelings towards their children, and that it is most productive for parents to first express their primary, positive feelings.

A relationship-building example in a difficult situation is the following:

> Mother to child: rather than, *"I am furious that you didn't call me to say you would be three hours late,"* instead, *"I am so relieved that you're here, because I was terribly worried something had happened. But I am also very disappointed that you didn't call to let me know you would be so late."*

It is important for leaders to reinforce with parents how important it is to show understanding routinely in their interactions with their children. "I" statements can be effective in the situations just illustrated, but empathy should be primary. In the last example, the mother needed to recognize and respond to her child's feelings before she stated her own feelings of worry and disappointment (e.g. *"You look upset now."*)

COMBINING "I" STATEMENTS WITH EMPATHIC RESPONDING

Leaders also want to help parents learn that "I" statements are useful when parents have the goal of influencing the outcome of a situation, especially when the parents' position is unclear or unknown to their children initially.

Example:

> Parent: *You want to keep watching TV and not take a shower tonight. You think your shower last night was enough* (empathic comments).

> Jimmy readily agrees with his parent's statement of his views!

> Parent: *I'd like to let you out of it too. But you're really dirty from playing in the garden. I don't want you to go to school that way tomorrow* ("I" statements).

> This parent may add a structuring comment, as follows, if Jimmy does not negotiate the next step for himself:

> Parent: *Take a shower now, and as soon as you are finished you can watch TV again* (structuring comment).

Developing an atmosphere of approval

In addition, leaders help parents think about how they can give positive attention more generally to their children in daily life, extending their close attention to their children's feelings and needs in play sessions to other situations at home. As well as giving positive attention, parents should be helped by leaders to introduce effective ways to give praise and reinforcement to their children in daily life. Praise and reinforcement, parents need to be told sometimes, are dependent for their effectiveness on parents developing a general attitude of approval of their children as important and loved. Leaders also need to underline for parents that praise and reinforcement are only effective when they are already paying close attention to their children's feelings and what they need, including structuring situations appropriately for them.

Alongside extending their parenting skills in showing emotional understanding and attunement to their children, parents also may need to extend their parenting skills in order to facilitate their children's practical and educational development. There are several important points, similar to the one made at the start of the program (see Chapters 4 and 5) that leaders need to make during such discussions about children's learning and competence, including the following:

- Parents have learned in their play sessions that children often are able to come up with solutions and make significant progress on their own. (Examples are helpful to use to reinforce this point.) Parents have learned during play sessions to support their children's independent learning. Examples of parents supporting children's own learning from play sessions commonly lead into some parents giving instances of their children engaging in this kind of behavior at home, and ways they have supported their children, which benefits the entire group's learning.

- Parents should not expect children to know what to do intuitively in new situations, or to carry things out immediately, once the situation is explained to them. Children need to learn steps in how to do things and may go backwards, as well as forwards, as illustrated in play sessions. Again, brief examples are useful from play sessions and then home life.

- Young children need to do things over and over again in order to establish routines for themselves, as parents have seen in their play sessions.

- Learning can be frustrating and difficult at times. Parents need to make sure they notice their children's efforts in the right direction. Parents giving positive attention to their children's learning in the right direction is more effective than pointing out and correcting mistakes for the most part.

HOW TO GIVE APPROVAL

Leaders facilitate parents in exploring how they intend to give additional approval to their children, over and above the close, positive attention they give in their home play sessions. By this point in the program, many parents are able to give ways their positive approval of their children has already increased in their daily lives. Leaders can supplement this exploration, which is most effective when led by the parents themselves, by making additional points parents may not have spontaneously thought about for themselves. In general, the discussion should include the following points, given here with illustrative examples:

- Parents should remember to give their children one-to-one attention, often without interrupting them, when their children are engaging in positive behavior.

Example. Mark and Larry are playing quietly and cooperatively with their cars. Their mother sits down and watches them play.

- Children are accustomed to using their play sessions with their parents as uninterrupted times when they can share emotionally difficult events. Many children in GFT are now able to talk about these events in daily life, especially when their parents are receptive to their emotional needs, follow their children's lead, and reflect their feelings.

Example. Frank has had a difficult day at school. His dad sits and listens to what happened, acknowledging Frank's frustration, without getting upset himself or giving advice.

- Parents need to actively show that they admire what their children do.

Example: Mary gave her sister some of her sweets. Her mother smiled at her, saying that she was happy when she saw her sharing. Her mother's praise showed Mary that her altruism was approved of by her mother.

- Children need physical affection from their parents, as well as empathic listening.

Example: Steve is working hard at his homework. His dad comes up and puts his arm around his shoulders briefly, but without distracting him from his work.

- Parents need to show respect for their children and attunement to their children's needs.

Example: Louise returns from taking her Grandma a house plant. Her mother thanks her and asks her if she would like a drink of lemonade.

- Parents need to create spaces in their lives, and the lives of their children, for having special times to be together. Parents are encouraged to start thinking together about how they may begin to do this regularly at home, anticipating that play sessions may be ending.

Example: Jason's mother said she had a walk recently with him and maybe he'd like to do that more. (Leaders can add, after eliciting parents' suggestions, that there will be more discussion soon of special times for parents who plan to end their play sessions at the end of the 20-week program.)

- Special treats and prizes are appropriate for parents to offer their children in certain situations. Parents show that they recognize and approve of their children's exceptional efforts when they give tangible rewards to their children. However, the rewards need to be suitable for "that child" in "that situation," be clearly given for specific behavior, and be made as soon as possible after the event.

Example:

> Susan, I'm so proud of you for helping me to take care of your Grandma today, and pulling up all the weeds in the garden for her. Let's go to your favorite playground to play for a while on our way home.

- Parents should examine whether they are reinforcing their children's undesirable behavior in certain situations.

Example: Marian's mother brought up her difficulties with Marian habitually putting her dirty clothes into the chest of drawers with her clean clothes:

> Up until now, I have always taken the dirty clothes away and yelled at her a lot, and grounded her. It makes me so frustrated, after I've gone to the trouble of trying to help her look nice every day. Now that we're thinking about home life, maybe I'm giving Marian attention, even though it's not very good attention, when she does this wrong, and not when she gets it right.

Some groups may need to discuss several of these points further. Commonly in our experience, some parents object to praising children for what is expected of them in the first place, and others object that they already have tried praise and rewards, but to no avail. Leaders should reflect these parents' feelings of discouragement, but also point out that the positive attention they have been giving their children in play sessions *has* been rewarding for both children and parents. Therefore, the GFT program tries to help parents use approval, acceptance, empathy, structuring, and rewards, rather than punishments in their daily parenting as much as possible. Eliciting examples of how much parents themselves like to receive praise and rewards for their own exceptional efforts are often timely during such discussions.

Negative consequences of routine punishment

Other groups may question how parenting is possible without physical punishment or other forms of punishment. Leaders may need to spend time empathizing with these parents' feelings, perhaps their feelings of confusion, lack of control, and ineffectiveness when their usual parental responses are questioned. Leaders may also wish to help parents understand that routine use of punishment can have longer term, negative consequences, even though it may result in children stopping their difficult behavior in the shorter term. Some of these negative consequences are as follows:

- This form of parenting can promote further aggression and disobedience in children.

- Relationships that are characterized by dominance and submission, with power struggles between people, often result in cycles of disobedience and punishment that are destructive and enduring.

- Children can react to serious punishment by either becoming very withdrawn or very aggressive, both inside and outside their homes.

- Children usually develop very indirect ways to get what they want, with an increase in lying and manipulation of situations and people, in order to avoid potential punishment.

Leaders also should mention to the group that there are a few cases where approval and rewarding positive behavior in children are *not* effective. In addition to the extreme behaviors leaders discussed at the beginning of the generalization training, where keeping children safe is the priority, there are a few other cases where setting limits and enforcing consequences are necessary. Leaders should remind parents that these situations will be examined last, after all the positive parenting skills, which are usually more effective, are thoroughly explored.

Generalizing the skill of structuring

Parents have experiences in play sessions with their children on which to model ways to structure events for their children in daily life. Before asking parents for examples from their play sessions (e.g. introducing home sessions to children, setting up the room at home in certain ways), leaders should remind the group that, with structuring, parents use forward thinking to plan events and circumstances in their children's lives. This planning is effective in helping children meet their parents' expectations better at the same time as having their own needs met.

Other points leaders need to include in this discussion are that planning ahead is useful for parents to do on their own, but it also can be productive to involve their children in this process, depending on the ages of their children. For example, parents may involve their 8-year-old daughter in planning out a safe route to walk to her friend's house after school on her own. Also, by giving their children information about what might happen in tricky situations, parents help their children handle these situations better.

There are numerous examples that parents frequently are able to give of new situations and how they helped their children. Perhaps they read their children books that describe the "first day at school" or ways to show their children what a dentist's office looks like, or what happens when a family moves to a new house. Or perhaps they visited a new school with their children before their first day.

Leaders also need to help parents discuss situations that occur regularly and which are more difficult. Parents and leaders can brainstorm with one another on how these situations can be structured better. For example, when a father complained that his two sons started fighting most evenings while he prepared supper, the leader suggested that the father and other parents brainstorm ways in which this situation could be improved. The father thought that his sons' underlying need was probably to be with him—and near the food when they started to get hungry. He and other parents thought together about how to structure the situation to meet the boys' need, while the father prepared supper. The father suggested he could find ways for his sons to help him prepare food; another parent suggested having them do homework or drawing at the kitchen table, while their dad made the dinner.

Leaders can use such discussions to remind parents to encourage their children to share structuring tasks whenever it is within their capacity.

In this case, the leader stated:

> *Perhaps your sons have a preference here. Maybe you could sit them down with you and decide how to set things up, giving them a couple of options to choose from, so that there is a good chance of success.*

The father then added that his sons' fighting often continued at the dinner table. Several parents suggested other structuring ideas for tackling this issue, such as seating the children apart from one another, with the father between them, while they eat. These suggestions seemed workable to this father; he offered to report back at the next meeting. The leader suggested that this type of problem was common, and asked the group for other applications of these ideas in somewhat similar situations.

Role-play is again a useful method to employ in helping parents generalize their structuring skills. For example, a leader may suggest that a parent role-play the problem raised by a parent of her 10-year-old daughter being afraid to tell her teacher that she had been ill and unable to do her homework. A role-play with the parent on how to rehearse this scenario with her daughter may be very helpful for most parents in the group.

Leaders should reinforce during these discussions on structuring that often limits are not needed as much at home when parents use structuring skills effectively. Some simple structuring techniques to review by leaders, if not raised by the parents themselves, include:

- providing alternative activities (e.g. a little sister is given some cookie dough while her big sister bakes cookies)

- adapting the home for children (e.g. putting a step near the light switch, so that a young child can turn on the light for the bathroom).

ILLUSTRATIVE EXAMPLE

The following example is an excerpt from a group discussion on generalizing the skill of structuring:

> Leader: Remember, Jackie, you said earlier that George never comes home on time. Is this still a problem, for you, or for other parents?
>
> (Several parents agree it is, including Jackie.)
>
> Leader: Let's use this problem now, when we're talking about structuring. What ideas do you have, Jackie, about how to structure things so that George is more likely to come home on time?
>
> Jackie: A watch doesn't seem to work for George. He doesn't like wearing one. I was thinking about telling him to set his cell phone alarm, so that it goes off when he needs to head for home.
>
> Leader: You've been thinking about this already. You want to have him move in the direction of taking responsibility himself.
>
> Parent 2: I tried that with Zach, but ended up telephoning his cell phone regularly because he sometimes just ignored the alarm.
>
> Leader: Remember that we talked about how difficult it can be for children to establish their own routines. You both seem to be thinking of ways to structure the situation so that your children can do this. It makes you feel impatient sometimes when they forget or ignore what they need to do, like paying attention to the alarm. It seems very important to try to persist with the method of time keeping that you think has the greatest chance of success for your child. Then it's important to show your approval when your child comes home on time, even if it doesn't always work.
>
> Jackie: I guess while George is trying out this new way of keeping track of the time with his alarm, I could phone him on his phone myself, when he doesn't show up, as long as he remembers to leave his phone on!
>
> Leader: You're realizing that there is a lot for George to remember, when he's playing with his friends, and thinking about what he's doing with them. You're doing a very good job of thinking about the situation from his point of view, and what may work for him. It certainly takes added patience on your part to help him. Has anyone else experienced something similar?
>
> Parent 3: I did with my eldest son, a few years ago, before he left home. He was constantly forgetting to tell us where he was when he was out late.
>
> Leader: You were worried about him. Do you think there was anything about what you did with your son that would be helpful to other parents?
>
> Parent 3: We never did find a good solution. It was impossible! I ended up grounding him, and then telling him off in front of his friends, but that didn't work either. It was a constant, running argument between us.

Leader: Thank you for telling us about that. You seem to be feeling regretful and still seem frustrated about that time. None of us parents get it right all the time, and what you're describing with your eldest son is a common problem. That's why we're trying to think about ways to structure the situation for George and other children now, so that we don't get into these binds that you described with your son.

This example shows one way a leader helped parents to think for themselves about structuring issues with their children, drawing on as many experiences as possible from participants in an open and accepting manner.

FOUR STRUCTURING STEPS

Leaders should review the following steps needed for successfully structuring situations with parents. The steps are as follows:

1. Decide on the exact goals (e.g. 10-year-old to do the pots and pans after dinner).

2. Anticipate what could interfere with the goal (10-year-old may not rinse the pans well).

3. Decide on ways to prevent these problems by having a positive approach (e.g. show 10-year-old how to rinse the pans).

4. Clearly say what the behavior is supposed to be, so it is clear to everyone (e.g. *"You are to wash the pans. You need to get all the food off them, rinse them, and leave them there to dry. The dishes go in the dishwasher. I will do that job while you do the pans."*)

After this review, leaders may either elicit examples in daily life from participants or, where required, use a practice example. For instance, a leader may say: *"Mary and Paul are siblings who spend most of the time in the car fighting and shouting. How can this be structured for them to ride peacefully together?"* This hypothetical example gives the group opportunities to think through the four structuring steps for themselves, and can trigger other relevant examples parents wish to address in their own lives.

Combining structuring with "I" statements

Parents may need to combine structuring statements with "I" statements some of the time. In the following example, the parent's interest in their child's views and feelings is evident. In these discussions, leaders should reinforce for parents that their attitude towards their children and positive approval of them are very important as a basis for using their structuring skills along with "I" statements. The following is an example of this:

Harry (as he rides in the car with his mother): Bobby threw something hard at me yesterday and started calling me rude names. Then I...

Parent: I want to listen to what you're telling me, but I can't do that right now. I can't listen while I am driving on this road in the snow and ice. We'll talk about it as soon as we get home.

Generalizing the skill of setting limits and consequences

After leaders are confident that parents have understood and begun to practice using all of the skills discussed earlier in daily situations, the last skill to generalize with parents is limit setting. Leaders should aim to make the following points:

- Limit setting is a skill that can be used effectively by parents when they use it judiciously and implement it within attuned and supportive relationships with their children.

- The general goal for parents is to set as few rules as possible, and use other parenting skills first.

- It is sometimes necessary for parents to use limit setting, as they have appreciated within their play sessions, because children do not automatically translate their feelings into action, and self-control develops only gradually in children.

- Parents need to keep children safe, and help children to feel safe and cared for by setting limits for them some of the time.

- Limits also are necessary for family life to run smoothly.

Leaders should review the general principles on limit setting that parents have already mastered in play sessions. They need to stress that, first of all, parents need to make certain that the expectations they have as parents are realistic ones, and within the capabilities of their children. If not, children may have to be helped regularly by parents to carry out steps in the right direction instead, rather than parents setting a rule and imposing a consequence. Parents need to be prepared to say a rule repeatedly in order to establish routines for younger children, especially for rules that have little or no meaning to them. This is because the children themselves do not have any strong motivation, other than pleasing their parents, to remember the rule. An example of a rule important to parents, but not to children, is to wash their hands before eating. (Dirt, especially invisible "dirt," does not matter to most children!)

Leaders also should ensure that parents remember that limits need to be enforced consistently, with appropriate consequences. It is useful for leaders to draw on examples from GFT play sessions of successful limit setting, with consistently delivered consequences, when generalizing limit setting, similar to the other skills. Leaders should suggest that parents share their own examples of successful limit setting in play sessions with the group.

STEPS IN RULE SETTING IN DAILY LIFE

Leaders need to give additional information to parents on steps for setting rules effectively in daily life. All of the steps leaders recommend are built on steps in limit setting carried out in play sessions, with which parents are very familiar at this point in the program. After briefly reviewing play session limit-setting steps, we suggest leaders then give the following steps on how to generalize limit-setting skills:

1. First determine whether the rule is necessary, or whether the problem can be solved another way. Limits can be avoided often by reflective listening, structuring, and engendering an atmosphere of approval, all of which parents have already learned.

2. State limits positively, clearly, and assertively. For example, instead of saying, "Don't leave your toys on the floor," a positive way of setting a rule is: "Put your toys in the box."

3. Remind children at least once or twice of the limit before imposing a consequence. The number of reminders depends on the age of the child, the importance of the limit, and the potential harm that might result if a rule is not followed.

4. Notice and approve of approximations to carrying out the rule.

5. Mention the consequence the second time (perhaps three times for young children) the rule is given but not complied with. The consequence should be directly related to the broken rule—that is, if the child will not put on boots to go out into the snow, he may not go out to play on a snowy day. Or, if the child refuses to turn off the television at the time agreed, he may not watch any more television that evening.

6. Mention the rule again, and carry out the consequence in a matter-of-fact manner.

SETTING EFFECTIVE CONSEQUENCES

Leaders need to provide parents with general ideas about consequences—what to adhere to and what to avoid—in daily life. Useful points to make are:

- A consequence should be only as severe as is necessary to enforce the limit.

- Parents should be able to carry out the consequence themselves, without undue stress on themselves.

- A consequence should follow as soon as possible after the limit is broken, in order for children to see the consequence as a direct result of their behavior.

- Rules should be stated clearly and in a respectful manner. For example, rather than name calling, such as *"You're a smelly pig, and you're having a shower,"* it is respectful and clear to say, *"You will take a shower at the end of that television program."*

- Children learn best when parents permit a natural consequence to occur. For example, a child promises to water her plant daily without help from others. She forgets for many days, and the plant dies.

- Giving a logical consequence for a broken rule is also effective and helps children learn. Logical consequences have a direct connection with the broken limit. For example, if a child does not put his mother's laptop computer back where it belongs, a logical consequence is that he loses the privilege of using the laptop for a time. Or, if a child tracks mud into the kitchen, then the child cleans it up.

- Unrelated consequences that are not connected to the rule being broken should *only* be used by parents when natural or logical consequences cannot be used or have failed. For example, *"You will not be able to watch TV after your bath because you did not come in on time."*

EXAMPLE FROM A GROUP DISCUSSION

Leader: Your son Richard is doing so well with the way you set limits in your play session now, Paul. Can you think about doing this in other parts of your life with him?

Paul: That's good to hear you say. Yes, I really want to set a limit on Richard using my tools. He just goes in when I'm not there and helps himself. Then he leaves them lying around where his little brother can get at them.

Leader: You sound frustrated, and a bit worried too, Paul. Let's think this through together; it will help everyone to hear about this. First of all, can you think of the reasons Richard has for doing this?

Paul: Well, he certainly is trying to be helpful some of the time, fixing things when I'm not there for his mom and brother. But other times he just likes to mess around with them, cutting up old bits of wood and putting screws into things.

Leader: So sometimes Richard is doing a real job, and other times he's playing.

Paul: Yeah, I guess he is playing… I never thought about it like that. I guess he is really interested in what the tools can do and enjoys learning about them. That's something we talked about together in his play sessions.

Leader: So you think both things are OK for Richard to do. It's just what he does afterwards that bothers you.

Paul: Instead of yelling at him to put the tools away and banning him from using them, I thought if I set a limit it might be better for him.

Leader: Yes, that seems reasonable to me too.

Another parent: I'm remembering how I did it with Kerry. She wanted my makeup, and would go in and get it, and drive me mad. So I bought her a makeup box and gave her some of my old makeup. She loved that. (Laughs.) I also put my good makeup well out of her way!

Leader: Yes, that's a good example of how you used structuring to change the situation for Kerry. There may be other ways to handle this for Richard too, like structuring it a bit differently.

Paul: I don't want to give him his own tools, not right now, because I am worried he will leave those around too for little Justin.

Leader: You think giving Richard his own tools and allowing him to use them in certain places might not solve the most important part of your problem, keeping Justin safe. You're thinking that a limit might be appropriate here. Let's think about how to set the limit together. A rule might be: "The tools must be put away immediately after they've been used. If they are found elsewhere, he will not be allowed to use the tools for…how long?"

Paul: I think, a week. I'll have to keep track, maybe using my calendar.

Leader: Yes, that's seems reasonable at Richard's age. I wanted to underline to everyone that Paul is on the right track. In order for parents to retain their credibility, they should keep careful track of when the time is up for consequences involving a time limit.

Another common parenting issue: telling the truth and lying

Parents often raise the issue of how to manage their children's deceitful behavior. Leaders already introduced parents to the value of approving of their children's positive behavior and avoiding punishments that give attention to bad behavior that often result in deviousness. However, children, even when given positive approval consistently, still engage in deceitful behavior occasionally. Leaders first need to acknowledge parents' positive feelings by stating that parents value honesty and want their children to be truthful. Depending on the reasons that may be presented by parents who raise this issue, leaders may wish to remind parents that it is possible that children have developed this way of behaving because of their previous experiences, and they therefore may need time to change and adapt to a new, consistent, style of parenting.

Leaders also may wish to give parents the following information. First, it is better for parents to refrain from saying that, if children tell the truth, they will not have any consequences. Sometimes children's behavior does warrant a consequence after all. Second, if parents know their children have done something wrong, it is best to say matter-of-factly that they know, rather than pretending ignorance and getting children to "confess." (If parents later find out that they made a mistake, then an apology is required.) Trapping children into admitting they have done something wrong when their parents are certain they have done so is not about truth. It commonly is a way to demonstrate parental control; parents hope that, when children get caught, they will be shamed into better behavior. In these circumstances involving shame, however, children often learn better ways of not getting caught. This often results in hostility and resentment on both sides. This in turn undermines children's confidence and self-esteem. Parents want their children to learn honesty, forgiveness, and how to repair their close relationships in positive ways; positive parental responses encourage these attitudes in children.

Prioritizing family members' needs

After covering all the parenting skills and their applications to daily life, and then addressing ways parents can combine parenting skills together, leaders need to help parents use their skills effectively when their own needs conflict with those of their children. As well as showing understanding of parents' positive feelings towards their children, and their frustrations with conflict-laden situations, leaders can normalize these dilemmas as common to family life. Practical guidelines on determining family priorities are also useful to offer to parents.

Steps for parents in determining their priorities are as follows:

1. Understand and take into account your child's viewpoint.

2. Understand and take into account your own viewpoint as a parent.

3. Think about the other issues involved in the situation, some of which may be in addition to your own or your child's viewpoints (e.g. grandparents' needs, school rules).

4. Then determine the priorities.[2]

5. The following group discussion illustrates how these steps were applied to a specific family's dilemma.

EXAMPLE

Dad: Jenny ran home from school this week and told me that she has a part in the school play. The other girl got ill, and she has the part. She was so excited! Jenny said that her teacher told her to buy a green T-shirt right away that evening and take it to school the next day... it was really upsetting for me. I was right in the middle of fixing the car, knowing I needed to get it fixed that night, so I could go to work in the morning. I'm afraid I got cross when she kept nagging me. It didn't work well at all.

Leader: It was hard on both of you. You really wanted to help her, but you had to fix the car. Let's look at how to use a lot of the skills you have developed in this situation. It might help you for the next time, if we review it now. I'm sure other parents will identify with this kind of situation themselves.

Dad: It was really clear to me afterwards that I should have just taken a minute away from fixing the car and listened to her, showing her I understood her feelings.

Leader: You were wishing that you could have done that. You are confident about reflecting her feelings now.

Parent 1: Or maybe said that you'd talk to her in a little while, if you were too worried that moment about your car. That might have given you time to think about it a bit more too, and what you wanted to do.

Father: Yes, maybe. I know what I wish I would have said.

Leader: Let's quickly pretend that I am Jenny and say it to me:

"Jenny": I got the part! I'm going to be the Green Giant! I just need a green T-shirt to take to school tomorrow.

Dad: You're so excited! I'm pleased for you too!

Leader: You're doing a good job of reflecting her feelings and giving a clear message about your feelings there. Let's look now at other feelings you had. I think a lot was going on for you.

Dad: Yes, I wanted to go get the T-shirt, but I knew I needed to fix the car. I couldn't think of how to do both of them.

---

2   Based on Guerney L. (2013).

Leader: Does anyone else have any ideas of how he might have structured the situation?

Parent 1: He might have looked at what he had at home to see if he could send anything else to school.

Parent 2: Or he might have asked someone else to go with her in their car.

Dad: I couldn't really do either of those things.

Leader: You'd already tried to think of ways to structure it differently. But you felt stuck. Did you think of bringing Jenny into it, and thinking with her about how to structure it differently?

Dad: No I didn't really see a solution. I asked her how important it was to bring in the T-shirt, and she said her teacher said it was very important.

Parent 3: Maybe it was to the teacher, but I wonder if you could have written a note to her and explained it all.

Dad: After Jenny was nagging me, and I couldn't do what she wanted and couldn't keep on fixing the car either, I just told Jenny to tell her teacher that she didn't have it. I was hoping, with the car fixed, I'd get it the next day, but Jenny was not happy at all with my promise. I had to send her to her room after a while to get some peace.

Parent 1: That happens to me too. You really wish you hadn't put in that consequence so quickly.

Dad: I can see now that if we would have talked together, and I would have shared my problem of wanting to help her, but needing to fix the car, we might have worked out a better solution together.

Leader: You have some regrets about that, but you seem to feel confident that you'd be able to manage better in the future. You really want to give Jenny what she needs as much as you can.

This example shows how supportive parents can be of one another's parenting challenges, and how important it was for the leader to allow the father and other parents to work through finding solutions themselves to the dilemma over priorities that this father raised. The leader supported the parents' exploration of alternatives, showed understanding and empathy for the father, and helped the father and group members relate their responses to the new learning about priorities that had been introduced, which is the last part of the generalization phase of the program.

When an individual family is out of sync with the group

Similar to other phases of GFT, leaders can adapt the generalization phase to individuals' needs. For example, if a family is working at a different pace from the rest of the group in their home play sessions, leaders may decide to offer those parents one or two further practice play sessions after the group ends. This family would continue to have input on generalization of skills in group meetings, but leaders would recommend that this family's generalization of skills to home life be put on hold for a while, until they appeared ready to advance. Leaders would then review parents' learning about skills generalization, and help them generalize their skills, during their extra practice sessions after the group finishes.

Or leaders may judge that a parent has not grasped the principles involved in generalizing their skills at the same pace as other group members. They may decide to hold a separate, additional, individual session for this parent before or after the group meeting, in order to help the parent keep pace with the rest of the group. However, if an additional session seems insufficient, leaders instead may recommend that the parent undertake a further parenting course that is compatible with GFT principles. In the first author's experience, when parents attend a compatible parenting course (e.g. courses using manuals such as Guerney L., 2013) after participating in GFT, their learning to use parenting skills for daily life is likely to be more successful.

Preparing the group for ending the 20-week program

Alongside helping parents generalize their skills to daily life, leaders also help parents during Meetings 17–19 to prepare for formally ending the program. The alternatives leaders and parents consider when ending GFT as a formal program are now outlined.

General considerations on ending the program

The three main options for leaders to consider are: ending the program at 20 weeks (Option 1), offering a follow-up meeting or two after the formal end at 20 weeks (Option 2), or extending the program beyond 20 weeks (Option 3), all discussed further shortly. It is important for leaders to carefully prepare parents for ending GFT, regardless of whether the program finishes at 20 weeks, or is extended beyond this. In some groups, input on ending arises spontaneously, and fits neatly into ongoing group discussions. In other groups leaders need to introduce this topic themselves, by Meeting 18 at the latest in a 20-week program, because parents need to have information beforehand on the options available for them after the formal program finishes. They need enough time to consider alternatives, to begin preparing their children for changes, and to make practical plans. During Meeting 19, leaders help each family and the group finalize the option they will choose at 20 weeks.

FACTORS INFLUENCING DECISIONS ON ENDING

Which one of the three options that is taken up is influenced by group and individual families' needs, clinical judgements by leaders, the preferences of each family, and the group's preferences. Leaders' resources and commitments after the formal end of the program, funding priorities by sponsoring organizations, and the availability of other community input also influence decision making. We recommend that leaders receive clinical supervision themselves when considering options available for families and the group as a whole. Having this outside point of reference is important when leaders weigh up their own work commitments alongside the group's and individual families' potential needs, particularly when one has to be prioritized over the other. In more complex cases, it is vital for leaders to consult their supervisor to validate their clinical judgment about termination.

EXTENDING OR ENDING CHILDREN'S SPECIAL PLAY SESSIONS

In every group, it is important for leaders to explore with parents whether their children are ready to end their special play sessions or extend them beyond the formal ending of GFT. These group discussions have several aims: first, to help parents reach an informed decision on the next step they will take with their children; second, to give all participants information on how to judge that children are ready to end; and third, how to plan and structure breaks and endings with children both in play sessions and in daily life.

Leaders already are experienced in ending CCPT with children and families; ending special play sessions has similarities to ending CCPT. However, in GFT, both individual parents and group opinions have a more essential role in making these decisions than in CCPT. Leaders need to facilitate parents' decision making by helping them and the group as a whole review the progress they and their children have made during the program.

CHILDREN CONTINUING THEIR HOME PLAY SESSIONS
FOR MAINTENANCE AND PREVENTION

The usual expectation in GFT is that home play sessions continue for parents and children after the last formal meeting for maintenance and prevention purposes. Play sessions provide families with a well-established means to maintain emotional health and prevent future difficulties. For these children and families, the play sessions conducted during the program have achieved their main therapeutic aims for the children, their parents and the family as a whole. These children and parents still find play sessions important, even though the children no longer have emotionally charged issues in their sessions.

Other indicators that children's play sessions are for maintenance and prevention are as follows:

- Children play out predominantly positive, age-appropriate themes compared with earlier sessions (see Chapter 13).

- Children's behavior and themes in sessions are reality-oriented and address current events.

- Children's family relationships and extended family relationships are largely resolved or manageable by them and their parents.

- Children's peer relationships and school issues are resolved or manageable.

- Children seem better able to manage stressful events and problematic relationships overall.

- Children show positive and sustained changes in their behavior at home and at school (adapted from Wilson & Ryan, 2005).

When play sessions come to a natural end

For some children and families, FT comes to a natural end during the last part of the program. In addition to the indicators just listed, other signs that children are ready to end special play sessions are as follows:

- Special play sessions seem less important than other activities they engage in with their parents. Some signs of this shift towards real-life activities may be children wanting to postpone their sessions or end their sessions early, while still maintaining their close relationships with their parents.

- Parents judge that their children will easily substitute another activity with their parent for home play sessions.

Most times a decision to end special play sessions after 20 weeks of GFT can be a straightforward one. As well as helping parents review the progress they and their children have made, leaders also can remind parents that, if future problems arise, they already have developed more general parenting skills. These skills may be applied to new problems in the future, and are very highly transferable. If these potential problems are minor, or if parents judge that their children may benefit from a preventative approach, parents may want to embark on a new set of home play sessions. However, leaders need to remind parents it is important that in all their fresh starts, parents line up suitable supervision and support for themselves for when this is needed.

For more serious problems, or when parents want to offer home play sessions to another child other than the children who received them during GFT (e.g. a younger sibling, a new foster or adopted child), leaders should remind parents that they will need supervision from a filial therapist, including help deciding what intervention would be best for the new child.

Substituting special times for home play sessions

Commonly, children and parents continue to look forward to their intimate time together during home play sessions, even when the sessions themselves have lost their more focused, therapeutic aims. If parents and/or children indicate that play sessions are not needed or wanted, leaders should suggest that parents substitute "special times" for home play sessions. Special times for children at the end of GFT are similar in structure to the ones offered by families with older children and teenagers, as discussed in Chapter 13. Whether children continue with home play sessions or make the switch to special times is a matter of family preference, provided that the children have finished their therapeutic work.

After leaders discuss the suitability of substituting special times for play sessions with each family considering this option, they ask parents to think about two or three activities that are both possible and sustainable at home for them and their children. Leaders and other group members may need to guide a few parents towards age-appropriate activities to offer, such as board games or football in the yard, and help them with ways they intend to involve their children in decision making on these activities. Leaders generally are able to stay in the background and merely facilitate these discussions at this point in the program; parents are usually able to support one another well and offer insightful advice. Often parents are adept at suggesting, for example, that a parent's planned special activity time sounds overly ambitious, given their experience with their own teenager's special times.

For some children who are suitable for special times, but who do not adapt to changes in routines quickly, it may be important for their parents to slot these special times into the vacated home play session time slot at the same time each week for several weeks. Other children may enjoy and benefit from a change in routine. In both cases, leaders need to review with parents the structuring messages that they intend to use with their children for this transition. Leaders may suggest concrete aids, such as a child-friendly calendar, to mark this change in household routine for school-aged children. In our experience, group members frequently make valuable contributions to one another's planning and thinking on these issues.

The day of the week and time of day for special times should be finalized during Meeting 19 for each family by leaders, as well as reviewing with them the ways special times may stretch their play session skills in certain ways. Leaders also should facilitate a discussion by participants on the importance of reflecting children's feelings about this change, rather than assuming they will have only positive feelings. It is also an opportunity for leaders to help parents generalize their discussion on ending play sessions to applications of these ideas to daily life when children end other events in their lives.

If follow-up meetings are not arranged by the group after the end of the formal program (20 weeks), leaders should have all the parents who are introducing special times with their children start them during the week before the last meeting of the program. This transition is most easily made under supervision by leaders, in case any difficulties emerge for families.

Children continuing their sessions for therapeutic reasons

For some parents and children, play sessions still have a highly therapeutic role, even at the end of the formal program. Unlike the children described earlier, these children express more difficult or unresolved play themes that do not stem primarily from recent events; their attachment and social relationships may appear problematic and stressful for them; and/or their behavior has not improved sufficiently. In these cases, leaders and parents need to decide whether these children and families need a longer time for play sessions to be effective.

Sometimes it is only one family who has much more serious problems than the rest of the group. Their difficulties may have been apparent at the outset of the program, as discussed in earlier chapters, but leaders decided to include them for other reasons. Or more serious problems may have emerged for a family during the later stages of the program. These problems may center on parent-child relationships, or they may be more intrinsic problems for the children themselves. For example, children whose previous experiences were abusive, or children with undiagnosed learning difficulties who do not experience change quickly, may need more time. Or parents themselves—for example, those with undiagnosed mental health problems, learning or attentional problems—may require more input than usual. Other times, difficult life events may have intervened to change family dynamics and the family's ability to cope with stressful life events. When children are still using their home play sessions to address deeper emotional issues, it is important that leaders encourage and facilitate their parents as much as possible to continue their home play sessions. Under these circumstances, leaders should try to schedule individually supervised FT sessions that continue after the group program finishes. Such families need closer supervision by a leader while they continue to have home play sessions, in contrast to families who opt to continue their play sessions for maintenance.

WHEN COMPROMISE ON ENDING IS REQUIRED

During any discussions on extending or ending home play sessions, leaders should emphasize that children's therapeutic needs are paramount in parents' decisions on continuing or ending sessions. In certain, more difficult, cases there may need to be compromises, with parents and/or leaders having to prioritize what is possible, rather than what is ideal in the longer run. Leaders should keep in mind that, when children still have clinical needs, and when individual FT supervision cannot be arranged, they need to move these parents too into special times with their children, rather than leaving them unsupported clinically.

In such cases, leaders need to have full discussions with parents on the advantages and disadvantages of the options available to them. Part of these discussions may be more appropriate privately, outside of group meetings, especially if leaders intend to suggest that parents attend individual therapy themselves or another form of therapy for the family. However, the group usually is aware of difficulties its members are having with home play sessions. Therefore, if leaders are respectful to parents and discuss privately with them what to say to other group members at the end of the program, issues of confidentiality need not be difficult to resolve. Sometimes in fact, the opposite issue arises and leaders need to help parents establish appropriate boundaries to personal and family issues that they share within GFT.

Children's and parents' reactions to breaks and endings

Another important group discussion topic for parents continuing their home play sessions or special times with their children is on ways to manage shorter and longer breaks. This discussion also prepares parents who are finishing their play sessions for possible reactions from their children when ending sessions and moving on to special times. As mentioned earlier in the book, ending may not be emotionally demanding for children overall because they are not ending or interrupting important adult relationships, and special times also are designed to mitigate children's negative reactions to ending, particularly when children themselves are ready to end. However, even though children's reactions are often more muted, children still can react emotionally to ending play sessions with their parents. Preparing parents for their children's—and their own—reactions to ending home play sessions is therefore an essential part of a leader's role in GFT.

Parents benefit from knowing that sometimes children can be both interesting and unpredictable when ending their play sessions. A few children may revisit earlier play themes and problem behavior before settling into accepting and adapting to ending. Other children may have mixed feelings, showing that they are glad that things are going well for them, and that they have time to do other things, yet also feeling regret, perhaps a sense of rejection, and annoyance that the times they valued are soon to be over. It is helpful for leaders also to point out that children's reactions to breaks and endings can be stronger before play sessions have fully served their therapeutic purposes, than when the sessions have run their course.

The ending phase in GFT therefore brings together and helps parents put into practice all the parenting skills that they have learned throughout the program, including their ability to generalize their skills to their daily lives. Next, the options for ending the GFT program are discussed.

Option 1: ending the program at 20 weeks

This option is chosen by groups who have resolved their children's and families' issues, or who have reached the end of their commitment to attend meetings, or who cannot attend any further meetings due to either participants' or leaders' set time limit on the length of the program. Even though the group itself ends, it is important for leaders to offer more input to individual families who continue their play sessions with their children beyond the end of the group. For the few children with clinical issues who continue home play sessions, individual, face-to-face FT supervision by a leader is essential. For children who have play sessions for maintenance and prevention, it is important that leaders offer parents indirect supervision of their additional play sessions through telephone and/or email contact. This supervision should include helping parents make the transition to special activity times when their play sessions come to a natural end.

Parents should be encouraged to contact leaders if problems arise during their extended home play sessions. Usually these contacts with leaders arise soon after the group meetings have finished, and indirect supervision is adequate to meet most parents' needs. However in rare cases—for example, when family circumstances suddenly change adversely, or important, new clinical issues outside of the scope for indirect supervision arise—leaders may need to offer face-to-face supervision to parents on an *ad hoc* basis. For children having special times with parents instead of play sessions, leaders should encourage these parents to telephone or email for troubleshooting, if significant issues or changes occur in special times after the program has ended.

Option 2: formally ending the program at 20 weeks, with follow-up meetings

Follow-up meetings seem particularly important in the first author's experience with shorter GFT programs of fewer than 20 weeks (see Chapter 16). Even with 20-week programs, it is hoped that leaders are able to offer one or two follow-up meetings to the group after the end of the formal program. In the first author's experience, follow-up meetings are usually well attended. These meetings are ideally scheduled one month apart. Leaders should explain to parents that during follow-up meetings they will review together and catch up on how special times, or further home play sessions, are going for everyone.

It is important that leaders ensure that these additional meetings are not overly structured compared with the more formal meetings during the 20-week program. Leaders want to help maintain parents' increased independence after the formal meetings end, and ensure that meetings are focused on issues *parents* raise, and on what is most useful for a particular group. In the first author's experience, in these follow-up sessions, parents typically choose to focus primarily on generalization of GFT skills for use in daily life,[3] as well as reporting on their play sessions and special times at home.

To summarize, follow-up meetings are intended to do the following:

- *Motivate parents to continue with home play sessions or special times.* When both leaders and participants have interest in the play sessions and special times conducted during the month after GFT formally finishes, many parents are more highly motivated to continue with play sessions or special times at home. Leaders can point out that this natural need to share important events with others who understand the true impact of what these events mean to the family is a very positive outcome for GFT.

- *Further solidify participants' relationships with one another.* During Meeting 20, leaders encourage members to stay in touch with one another. Follow-up meetings are another way to nurture this outcome.

- *Identify and deal with trouble spots identified by group members.* Parents may identify issues themselves—for example, that they were tired or anxious during some of the play sessions, and their children seemed to notice this. Parents may need leaders and/or other parents to make connections for them to their children's play and behavior, and then work out potential solutions together.

- *Review key skills and concepts, as needed.* Parents may already have asked leaders to review certain skills or concepts when the group agreed to attend follow-up meetings. One common skill that often needs refreshing is empathy. Parents commonly find it is more difficult to empathize with their children during daily life events than it is in play sessions. Leaders may review this skill as practiced in daily life and suggest that parents decide on a 15-minute slot during the day with their children when they can concentrate on understanding their children's viewpoint, feelings, and thoughts, even when their own opinions and feelings may differ.

- *Offer additional support with generalizing to daily life.* For a few families who have a slower pace in applying parenting skills to daily life, follow-up meetings are a way to support and bolster their progress.

Very rarely, leaders may decide to directly supervise a play session during a follow-up meeting, if another agreed time cannot be arranged or leaders did not know about a crucial issue until during the follow-up meeting itself. If, for example, a parent reports at follow-up that home play sessions have "fallen apart" after the group meetings ended, leaders may judge it timely to supervise a play session on the spot, if the child is available, in order to help the parent and child get back on track. In some cases, it will be apparent that more individual FT supervision of home play sessions is required, as discussed earlier. For less serious issues, one practice play session may suffice.

---

3   Guerney L. (2013)'s parenting skills training manual is particularly useful for leaders here.

Option 3: extending GFT beyond 20 weeks

Sometimes, despite thorough initial assessments and the skillfulness of leaders in adjusting the pace to suit the majority of the group, serious clinical issues may still be present and being actively dealt with by parents and leaders during the later meetings in a 20-week program. Leaders and the group itself know whether it is one family that is out of sync with the rest of the group, discussed earlier, or whether the majority in the group is still addressing important clinical issues in their home play sessions that require weekly input.

The number of home sessions offered during the latter part of the program and the number of follow-up meetings offered is largely a function of the severity of the problems participating families display. It also is dependent upon the motivation of the parents to continue conducting play sessions for a lengthier period of time.

In Options 1 and 2, the supervision offered by leaders to a family continues as a parallel activity to that of the group. In Option 3, leaders may decide, if logistically possible, to extend formal GFT meetings and continue to supervise home sessions in more depth for the last few meetings in the 20-week program for families, rather than beginning the generalization phase of the program. All the families in the group would then be offered two to three additional sessions on generalizing their skills to daily life afterwards, thus extending the group meetings beyond 20 weeks.

An extended example of group decision making on ending

The following example illustrates one group's discussion on ending the formal program:

> Leader 1: Let's think together about what you are planning to do when we have our last meeting of the program in a couple of weeks. Several of you already have mentioned that you'd like to have two more follow-up meetings, to keep your motivation up, and find out how other parents are doing. We hope you will want to keep on with your play sessions at home because children benefit from them so much. What are your thoughts?

> Marjorie: I've been thinking already about what to do when we finish our 20 weeks. It's quite a lot of extra work to carry on with play sessions with all three of my children, but I don't know if they're ready to end or not.

> Leader 2: You're not really sure what to do.

> Henry: You've done so much already. Maybe it would be easier for you to have special times.

> Marjorie: Special times do seem like a good idea, but I'd miss the play sessions with my children, and I think they'd miss them a lot too. Sam [her partner] does a lot of fun things with our children already, and I've really liked it that I'm doing some important playing too, not just constantly taking care of them. Plus I think all three of them are using their play sessions in their own ways, and it's very creative. Mark came home last week and was in a foul mood; he said someone pushed him around on the playground, but that he'd have been in trouble if he started fighting.

I was able to say, right then and there, that he was really frustrated. In his play session that afternoon, Mark punched the bop bag silly, then started throwing bean bags at it and asked me to join in. We ended up giggling a lot as we did it together, and it seemed to shift his mood. So even though he's 12, I think he does make really good use of this time with me.

Gemma: You must feel really useful doing the play sessions, and close to him. Tracey [her daughter] definitely is not ready to end. She is so intense when she plays with me and her dad, with all those scenes about people getting hurt. We want to help her more; she's at a different place than your children are.

Marjorie: Yes, my children's play isn't so intense, usually, even Mark's. But now that I've had a chance to think about it, I'll keep on with all the children for the next couple of months, until the summer vacation. I think I'll talk to Sam about having one-to-one time with each of them himself once a week. He might like the idea of choosing an activity with each of them.

Leader 1: You have come to a solution that works for you, Marjorie. And Gemma, we'll work something out, so that you can talk about Tracey's play sessions regularly with one of us leaders between the follow-up meetings. How about you, Henry and Lucy?

Henry: I wish I could do the same as Marjorie and Gemma, but we're coming up to a really busy time at work, when I'll have to do a lot of overtime. Lucy and I share the playtimes, but it would mean she'd have to do it all herself.

Lucy: I could do it myself, Henry, but Rob and Pat would miss their time with you a lot.

Henry: Maybe we could think about you doing the play sessions, and I could make sure I'm home for bath time and bedtime two nights a week. I think I could guarantee that. I could play with Rob in the bath first, and then have time with Pat playing in the bath, then have some time reading the boys stories before they go to sleep.

Leader 1: You both want to get it right for Rob and Pat. It's important to be realistic about what you can do, and not make plans you can't carry out, but it's also clear that you both want to make sure Rob and Pat have special times with both of you.

Stuart: I'm glad someone else feels that they can't carry on with playtimes. I just know that it will be impossible for Ruby and Jim to have more playtimes right now. We're moving soon, as some of you know…so much to do, and all our things will be packed up. I think we'll go for special times with them. I'll do something with Ruby one week and Kate will do something with Jim. Then the next week we'll swap over. If they need to start play sessions again after the move, then we'll start up again. The big question is what activities we should do together. I know it should be something that both Kate and I like to do, and something that we can keep doing every week during the move. We're a bit stuck. Any ideas for us? (Several parents then made practical and workable suggestions to Stuart and Kate, who were very responsive to their ideas.)

Leader 1: You haven't said much, Janice and Tom. How about yourselves?

Tom: We aren't as sure as everyone else what to do. Jake sometimes seems to want to stay longer for his play sessions, and other times he wants to finish early. And sometimes he just draws patterns on paper and we color them in together, or he spends a long time crashing the cars together and seems to want one of us to watch and not join in. Other times he has those stories that he wants us to play out, especially that one where he's the superhero and me or Janice are the baddy that we talked about. Jake's behavior at school is better usually, but he can get sassy with some of the teachers when he's grumpy.

Henry: I remember you talking about how important it was last week when you were the baddy, Jake was giving you some help, trying to give you a way to become a goodie, not a baddy. You and Janice are doing such a great job with Jake's play sessions, and it certainly doesn't seem easy!

Janice: Thanks, Henry. Tom and I were really hopeful after that last play session. It just seems so up and down with Jake. I guess he doesn't really seem ready to end, and I guess we just needed that encouragement you're giving us to carry on.

Leader 2: You are feeling discouraged, feeling Jake isn't as far along as you'd like him to be at this point. So hearing from Henry that you're doing a good job really is important to you both right now. (Other parents also join in with their encouragement of Jake's parents and give their views of their own children's progress.) It seems as though you see the advantage for Jake in continuing play sessions. I think I agree. He may be ready to choose to make a change to special times after a few more play sessions. However, if he should choose to continue play sessions, that would also be a good choice. It is not like going into the next grade in school, when families move on to special times. It is an option that fits the play styles of many children after some standard play sessions.

This example shows how this group of parents began deciding for themselves what was manageable for their families; it also illustrates how supportive and helpful other parents frequently are with one another in GFT.

Format for Meeting 19

The format of Meeting 19 remains the same as earlier home session meetings in having families in focus, along with a shorter discussion of all the other families' home sessions before the meeting ends. Generalization of skills also continues during this meeting, as does the topic of ending. Two additional tasks for leaders are finalizing each family's arrangements, if the group formally ends at 20 weeks, and preparing parents for the last meeting of GFT.

Finalizing each family's arrangements

Leaders finalize the group's and individual families' planned arrangements when formal meetings end. This may include thinking about how many follow-up meetings are feasible, and helping parents start special times in the week before the last meeting, if no follow-up meetings are arranged. Leaders again use the same therapeutic skills with parents on ending that they advocate parents practice with their own children. Parents' reactions, particularly in Meetings 19 and 20, may be similar to their children's—they may have mixed feelings of pride in their own and their children's progress, feelings of regret and uselessness now that their more intensive therapeutic role is ending, and anxiety along with hopefulness for the future.

It is also important for leaders to recognize that parents often have formed important relationships with one another. During group meetings, parents share common interests in a supportive and companionable way with other parents, after often beginning the program feeling isolated and demoralized. This supportive and accepting atmosphere is often difficult for parents to forego.

Preparing parents for the last meeting

With Options 1 or 2, leaders discuss with the group how they wish to mark the end of the program the following week. They guide the group towards structuring the ending of the formal GFT program, and follow parents' lead, while still maintaining their role of being a "secure base" for parents' ideas, taking into account and negotiating any potential limitations on ending plans with parents. If necessary, leaders may contribute ideas for ending themselves, such as the suggestion of a cake or an "awards" ceremony at the last meeting. In addition, leaders prepare parents for the evaluation tasks they will be asked to complete during the next meeting. Both of these topics are discussed in the next chapter.

CHAPTER 15
Ending the GFT Program
Meeting 20

Leaders usually start Meeting 20 by commenting that the contents of the GFT program are finished, as the parents know, and this last meeting is intended to celebrate their achievement. It also is a time to think about any topics that the group wishes to review. Leaders ask for suggestions from the group for topics, but also have in mind their own topics relevant for their groups. More generally, leaders aim to facilitate the group during the last meeting to have a memorable and enjoyable experience together.

Marking the ending

Some groups readily come up with suggestions during Meeting 19 on marking the ending of the program. These can range from creating certificates of achievement for leaders and other parents to sign, having an agency manager attend with agency tributes for parents, or arranging a special treat to be shared with one another. It is important that leaders facilitate the group in marking the end of GFT in a celebratory way—for example, extending the midway break and ensuring it lends itself to a shared experience, rather than being just a time for utilitarian tasks, such as making drinks.

Parent support groups and other support arrangements

Helping parents keep in touch with one another is another aim during this final meeting for leaders. They facilitate parents in discussing the valuable support they have given and received during the program from one another, and the possibilities for supporting each other after GFT ends. Experienced leaders are able to give anonymous examples from their own practice of the benefits arising from parents supporting one another after the program ends.

For example, one experienced leader mentioned to his group, explaining he was using pseudonyms, that in a follow-up meeting a mother, Harriet, described her experience of feeling very discouraged by the slow progress her daughter Penny was making in managing her bedtime routine. The mother talked to her sister about this, including her feeling that she just couldn't stand it if Penny screamed yet again for a drink before she went to sleep. Her sister simply said, *"Well your play sessions didn't work for that, then."* Harriet, feeling unsupported by her sister, then decided, even though she didn't usually take the initiative and complain to other people, to call a fellow GFT parent, Jan, who had some of these problems with her own son. When Harriet talked with Jan, she felt much better. Jan knew that she was enforcing the limits in the right way, and how hard it was to do this night after night. They even managed to laugh about how strong lunged both of their children were!

Similar experiences that leaders share with parents often illustrate effectively the potential support that can be given by fellow participants. This is because other parents often have an immediate understanding of the parent's situation because they have shared skills, shared experiences, and know one another and their children in ways that other people may not.

Sometimes more formal support arrangements are made by parents with one another spontaneously. Parents in some groups may already have exchanged contact details and arranged to meet informally without the group leaders. For other groups who are less involved or organized, leaders can encourage future contact by providing sticky labels for contact details to be written out on and exchanged with other parents during the last group meeting. Leaders may also wish to suggest an informal "buddy" system, whereby parents call or email one another periodically. A more formal buddy system is sometimes arranged, in which two or more families agree to contact one another at specified times to talk about everyday triumphs and challenges, and ways they are applying their parenting skills to daily life. For busy families, web camera, cell phone, and email contact may substitute for direct contact.

Discussing topics of interest for the group

Many groups readily suggest topics they wish to review at the last meeting, or introduce new issues that are important to discuss. Usually there is further discussion of generalizing, as parents continue to feel challenged in some situations at home with their children, and wish for additional input. Leaders should be mindful that some parents' anxiety with finishing meetings may be expressed as anxiety about their own competence, even though they felt more confident in earlier meetings. We suggest leaders again adopt the principle of helping parents to discuss their concerns and work on solutions, but also facilitate them to find positive experiences to discuss. Other parents often are able to think of positive examples for these parents to take home with them.

Supervising the transition to special times

Leaders need to supervise the progress of those families changing to special times, and discuss any issues they may raise; this benefits the entire group's learning. For example, one father found that his 8-year-old daughter, even though she had agreed to play soccer during their half hour together, was tired and bored after only ten minutes. As well as group members empathizing with his feelings of discouragement, and praising him for empathizing with her feelings despite his own feelings, the group also tackled with him the problem of how to ensure that his daughter got the most out of their time together, suggesting the options of either structuring things differently or changing the activity.

Supervising continuing home play sessions

During this meeting, leaders should allocate time to supervise the parents who continue to have home play sessions with their children, addressing not only immediate issues from their sessions, but also concerns parents may have about continuing home play sessions on their own. Many of the points made the previous week about contacting leaders if important clinical issues arise are useful to review here.

Evaluation of the program

Both informal and formal evaluations of the program are valuable for leaders to undertake with participants, including children, wherever possible.

Informal evaluation with parents during Meeting 20

Leaders should aim to provide parents with the opportunity to verbally express their views on the GFT program during the latter part of the last meeting. Leaders can introduce this topic by mentioning that it is important to have parents' honest and thoughtful feedback in order to keep things that worked the same, and to adjust the things that were not as successful. In our experience, parents often are very relaxed, forthright, and able to give their views clearly in such discussions. Leaders' openness to parents' opinions should have been evident throughout the program, but leaders may need to solicit parents' views directly on the GFT program overall. Supportive and positive comments made by parents often become treasured memories. Some of these memories may be very appropriate for leaders to share with their next group. Whether positive or not, leaders need to respond with empathy, genuineness, and non-defensiveness.

The feedback portion of the last meeting often is a way for parents to express their appreciation not just to the leaders, but more importantly to one another. If these comments do not emerge spontaneously, leaders can structure this discussion themselves with *"What is your best memory of this group?"* or ask parents to share an important memory they have with two other parents, then come back to the large group and talk about their memories in the group. Leaders' own examples of the forward movements parents have made in their responses to their children during the program also can be facilitative. For example, one leader expressed her admiration of a father who had struggled in early play sessions to reflect his son's feelings, especially during their competitive play together, and who had moved on to become adept at expressing feelings during their elaborate role-plays and their toy car chases in home play sessions.

Evaluating children's views of the GFT program

If possible, we also recommend that leaders obtain children's views of GFT with their parents' help. This can be done informally through sending out a child-friendly evaluation form through parents during Meeting 19, to be returned for Meeting 20 (e.g. *"Draw a picture of something you remember from your play sessions," "Draw a picture of your mom/dad during the first play session/last play session."*). Or parents may simply ask their children to draw or talk about the toys and play experiences in their home play sessions that have been important to them, and report these views back to the group during the latter part of Meeting 20. Alternatively, leaders may ask parents to make a short video clip of their children talking about their play sessions, if this seems clinically appropriate, to be shown during Meeting 20 to all the parents in the group. Simple questions for parents to ask their children, following Jaeger & Ryan (2007), may include:

> What did you like about playtimes? Are there things you didn't like? What didn't you like? If a friend of yours had these playtimes, what do you think they would like? Are there things they wouldn't like? If yes, what things wouldn't they like?

A more formal evaluation of children's views may also be undertaken. For example, a picture completion task for children may be designed that is similar to that of Ross & Egan (2004). And, if resources permit, leaders may decide to have a celebratory children's group separate from the parents' and leaders' group during Meeting 20. For one part of this children's group, children could be invited by the group organizer(s) to take part in a short focus group on their experiences of special playtimes. (For an example of this evaluation method, see Day, Carey, & Surgenor, 2006.)

Formal evaluation measures with parents

Formal assessment measures completed by parents at the outset commonly are administered again by leaders during the last meeting for evaluation purposes. These usually include the Parental Stress Index, the Porter Parental Acceptance Scale, and the Filial Problem List referred to in Chapter 1. Agencies and leaders also may undertake 3- or 6-month follow-up assessments, for which leaders should have prepared parents at the outset of the program. Leaders need to remind parents of any planned follow-up evaluations again during Meeting 20.

In general, when leaders are deciding on what formal measures to use for evaluation, it is important to balance the need for objective information with the need to ensure that the last meeting is an emotionally satisfying and complete one for parents. To achieve this balance, it is often more conducive to a celebratory atmosphere to ask parents to complete objective measures before the midway break, rather than towards the end of the meeting. A suggested written evaluation form for general clinical use is given in Appendix 21 for leaders' use.

Researching children's views of GFT in the UK

As part of a wider UK pilot research study (Jaeger & Ryan, in preparation), children and parents offered their own perspectives on GFT after completing a 12-week adapted program (see Chillery & Ryan adaptation in Chapter 16). Children were interviewed using a play-based evaluation technique, the "Expert Show" (Jaeger & Ryan, 2007; in preparation), in which children take the role of "experts" in the therapy they engaged in, and the interviewer adopts various children's roles, asking questions of the "expert" in a pretend TV program.

"Chris," a boy in middle childhood who had been referred to an NHS Child and Adolescent Mental Health Service (CAMHS) for conduct difficulties, gave his views on the GFT program. He was asked by a "child caller" (the interviewer) what it would be like to be watched by others (behind a one-way screen) for the first time in the playroom. He said, *"The first time you'll do it, you'll be scared. But when you get used to it, you won't be right bothered [sic]... I wouldn't worry about it."* He informed the caller that when he moved to home play sessions these were *"really good."*

When Chris was asked by another "child caller" whether he would play on his own or together with his mom or dad in play sessions, he told the caller that it was the child's choice. He expanded on this, saying: *"I like playing on my own sometimes, but **really** I like playing with my mom and dad."* In contrast to another child, who stated that both he and his mom were feeling happy in playtimes, Chris was unsure what his parents thought and felt. His response suggested a remaining level of uncertainty and insecurity in his relationships with his parents.

This interpretation was reinforced by Chris's later comments during the Expert Show interview, where children talk about their experiences directly. He spontaneously shared with his interviewer that he had stopped having home play sessions early because *"We weren't right bothered. We thought my behavior had gone up."* However, when the interviewer prompted a further response by asking how Chris felt now that home play sessions had stopped, he seemed able to clearly separate his own views from his parents:

> Chris: Well I still want to do them, but at least they've said my behavior's gone up.
>
> Interviewer: Right, so they're pleased about it.
>
> Chris: Yes, I'm pleased, but I'm not pleased.
>
> Interviewer: OK, what are you not pleased about?
>
> Chris: That we've stopped, but I am pleased that my behavior has gone up.

While shorter term GFT programs, such as the 12-week program Chris took part in, may have lasting benefits for many families, and indeed some of these benefits seem to have occurred for Chris's family, his comments serve as a poignant reminder that sometimes parents may focus on shorter term goals and over-emphasize behavioral changes in their children, rather than choosing to conduct play sessions over a longer time period to alter their parenting attitudes and relationship problems on a more fundamental level, which are two of the main aims of GFT.

Researching parents' views of GFT in the UK

In the UK pilot research, parents also were interviewed by two experienced interviewers who were filial therapists using a semi-structured interview format. Parents uniformly mentioned how important it was to be able to share their experiences of parenting with other parents. Many other aspects of the GFT experience also were noted, including changes in their own attitudes towards their children, and positive changes in their children's behavior.

Parents talked about having more understanding of their child's feelings, their increased ability to "read" their children's non-verbal communications, and their ability to communicate this to their children by the end of the 12-week program. Mary, a mother of a child with developmental delays, stated:

> I'm different now. I don't snap as quick. Sometimes it's difficult to work out what's going on for Gary, difficult to see it in his face, and he wouldn't let on. As the weeks have gone on, commenting on how he feels is good, and it's helped me understand him more, really.

Gary's father, Brian, mentioned that he'd *"never really taken much notice of his [son's] feelings"* and that his understanding had increased during GFT. He thought that his increased empathy had resulted in positive changes in his relationship with his son. He described their third home play session:

> Brian: We had a really good laugh. He had a lot of the sand in the water, and he built a bridge. I was commenting on him wanting me to fail [with bridge building].
>
> Interviewer: Would you have responded in the same way before?
>
> Brian: No we've changed that way, and [the leader] picked up on that as well, that it could be his [Gary's] way of getting rid of his inadequacies. It's different now. Before I'd be getting more frustrated with myself, and wondering why. Now I can move in there with his feelings, and I understand where he's coming from. I'm allowing it to happen.

Other parents described how they were able to generalize their parenting skills to daily life. Jane stated that she kept her son too close to her because of an accident when he was younger, which had resulted in him dying for a brief time. She believed that the group had enabled her to explore these feelings, and she began "letting go" after encouragement from other parents. She described an experience with Luke at the swimming pool:

> He absolutely loved it, and he wanted me to watch him, and he's saying, "Mum, will you watch me come down this big slide?" And I'm saying, "No, Luke, it's a bit high for you"…and I'm thinking, "I've got to let go, I've got to let go." So I'm saying, "Well, please be careful." There's no way I could have gone down that slide [with him], and he did it, and I went "You brave boy!" and it made him so happy!

All the parents interviewed reported that their children included or involved them more after the program ended. They also talked about how this involvement progressed during GFT. Becky said, *"He always included me [in his play during play sessions]. That's one thing I was shocked about."* Becky said that she felt she was closer to her son, and that he spent more time now with her; her partner, Kevin, agreed with this in his own interview. Another parent, Helen, described experiencing *"a warming sort of feeling"* directly after home play sessions with her son because:

[H]e wanted to be part of us, whereas normally he just sits on the outskirts...it was a nice warm sort of a feeling...to see that he could join in just with normal conversation, and be relaxed and be happy.

The final chapter is intended for readers who are planning to adapt the 20-session model to the requirements of the children and families they work with. It gives several adaptations of the model that adhere to the main features of GFT presented in this book, starting with the 10-week model of the first author.

CHAPTER 16

Adaptations of the 20-Week GFT Program

Various adaptations have been made to GFT to meet unique program needs. These variations demonstrate the robustness of the GFT method in helping children and families. Group program adaptations cover a wide range of populations, from programs in a number of countries worldwide, US adaptations for immigrants to the USA from Asian countries, low-income/inner-city families, racial minorities, prisoners, victims of domestic abuse, and programs aimed at children who have special needs, including those with physical and mental limitations. GFT programs also have been adapted to educational (e.g. Kinder Therapy; Child-Teacher Relationship Therapy) and residential settings, both in the USA and the UK. Readers should note that some of these programs already have been referred to in Chapter 1 in the research findings section, and in earlier chapters on the 20-week GFT program.

A few such programs, designed to meet modified time limits or other resource limitations, are included here. This chapter is not intended to be exhaustive in presenting variations of GFT. We have chosen the particular models in order to show readers the range of variations possible, and to help leaders think about adaptations that suit their populations and circumstances when delivering GFT. The programs selected here have come to our attention because they have developed to a point where GFT leaders could replicate these programs, if they work with similar populations or under similar circumstances. All of these adaptations have been used with positive results, and exist in full programmatic forms. We have provided contact information on the program designers for readers, along with brief outlines of the adaptations made in each program.

GFT criteria for adapted programs

Before innovating adaptations for themselves, readers should be aware of criteria that must be met for GFT. The variations should ensure that parents, or other significant adults in children's lives, are still the major providers of play therapy; the parents receive continued pre-instruction, feedback, and supervision from leaders; the leaders process parents' feelings throughout all meetings, along with processing those of the children; and the format does not permit a scheduled gap during the active training program (not follow-up) of more than two weeks at any point.

Shortened GFT programs

There is no question that, regardless of the number of families in a group, the 20-week model to which this book is devoted, and which the authors feel strongly is the optimal version of GFT, is the most productive and thorough version of GFT. It has been referred to as the "gold standard" of FT and should be thought of as what GFT is. The kinds of gains that can be made by parents and children in the full 20-week program yield clear qualitative differences that are not only longer lasting, but appear to permeate more into the life of the entire family.

Clinicians who wish to employ GFT should be aware that adjustments in the length of the program can be made under certain circumstances. The primary reason is a time limitation created because:

- parents cannot participate in a group that lasts the standard program length (20 weeks)

- leaders do not have 20 weeks available because of professional or personal considerations

- agency resources cannot support the full 20-week program

- insurers limit payment to approximately ten weeks

- the presenting difficulties of the child/family appear open to change in a relatively short time in a FT program (e.g. recent onset behavioral problems in school)

- the number of children and parents participating in the program is low.

Especially with shortened GFT programs, leaders need to plan very carefully to cover the basic features of the program. If, for example, a 10-week program is being considered, in our experience it is unwise to try solo leadership. The shorter time available makes it necessary for two leaders to divide the responsibilities for demos, mock and practice play sessions within the group. We start with the first author's own abbreviated 10-week program, followed by other adaptations listed in alphabetical order.

Guerney GFT 10-week program—Designer: L. Guerney

When GFT is the treatment of choice, and one or more of the earlier time-limiting conditions or circumstances are present, reducing the length of the program does not eliminate any of the essential features that make the GFT program a success.

10-week program format

For Guerney's 10-week program, it is critical that the number of participating children is kept to a maximum of six. (Resist the temptation to include seven!) The shorter program— referred to for convenience as the 10-week program—is actually somewhat variable in length, with the *average* totaling ten sessions. The reason for the variation is that the number of target children can be lower than six. The number of weeks can range from 9 to 12, in order to cover all aspects of GFT. (If time permits, a follow-up session can be included as an additional week.) A comparison of time frames for 20- and 10-week formats is given in Table 16.1.

Table 16.1 Typical distribution of sessions for 10- and 20-week formats*

Phases of the GFT program: average 10–20 weeks		
1. Introduction and training: including demos with each fully participating child and mock sessions with all parents.	2–3 weeks	5 weeks
2. Practice sessions (two per parent) and preparation for home sessions.	2–3 weeks	6 weeks
3. Home sessions.	3 weeks	4 weeks
4. Generalization (home sessions continue) and ending.	2–3 weeks	5 weeks

* Times for the first two phases for both the 10- and 20-week programs are largely a function of the number of participants. Two parents with one child each for the 10-week program require the minimum number of sessions, whereas three parents with two children each automatically take longer.

In summary, no phases of the program need to be neglected. All the goals and guidance for leaders conducting GFT remain the same. However, each phase is cut back. For example, Phases 1 and 2 are shorter because fewer children participate in demos and practice play sessions. Mock sessions are *always* included for each parent. Auxiliary siblings are provided with home sessions, and their home sessions are discussed at meetings. However, they are not included in meeting demos or practice play sessions. Leaders continue to deliver FT as a family intervention and attempt to maintain maximum contact with all family members in the face of time restrictions. If, for example, an auxiliary child develops more serious concerns, leaders may decide to include the child in practice play sessions during meetings, if time permits, or make other arrangements (e.g. individual play sessions with a leader) that would not require group time.

Evaluation of the program

While no controlled studies have been done systematically comparing Guerney's10-week programs with those that run for longer times, there is a sufficient number of studies on both the shorter and the longer programs to demonstrate that both are highly effective. Comparison of results between the 20- and 10-week formats is problematic in any case, because, when a family's problems are complex, clinicians are more likely to use the standard 20-week program. The greater time available in the 20-week program for home sessions and generalization is likely to ensure greater success.

When time is brief, clinicians often feel pressured to use behavioral approaches or use GFT and concentrate on just one child, or introduce generalization at a point earlier than what we believe is optimal. The authors feel strongly that maintaining the integrity of the original 20-week GFT program in a shortened form, as can be done in the 10-week format described here, is important. Using GFT in a proven format, whether abbreviated or the standard 20-week length, seems to serve families better than many other interventions.

Contact

Louise Guerney Ph.D., RPT-S
National Institute of Relationship Enhancement
Bethesda, Maryland, USA
(001) 301 680 8977
niremd@nire.org

Bradford UK GFT Fostering Program— Designer: P. Wilkinson

Major adaptations

The two leaders in the group are responsible for two foster families each. Children do not participate in meetings. Demos and practice play sessions are conducted with children outside of group meetings, and videos are shown in meetings of demos with each child in the program, carers' weekly practice play sessions, and weekly home play sessions. Practice play sessions and home sessions are started when individual foster carers are ready, rather than as a group. Some carers do not transfer sessions to their homes, and other carers request that a leader attends and videos their first home session in order to get established.

Target population

This program is for foster carers whose children have been referred to the UK's National Health Service (NHS) Child and Adolescent Mental Health Service (CAMHS). The local fostering service training unit also makes referrals.

Participants

There are three to four foster carers, including partners, in each group. Children in permanent and medium-term foster placements are eligible, if the outcome of their CAMHS initial assessment is for FT, along with all the other fostered and birth children in the foster families. Foster carers declaring an interest in FT also are included, if an initial assessment indicates FT, and if places are available. The foster carers volunteering themselves often offer a high level of support to foster carers who have had a child referred to CAMHS because of mental health difficulties.

Program details

After the initial CAMHS intake, a visit by a GFT leader is made to informally observe foster carers and their children playing together at home, and to introduce the idea of play sessions to children, aiming to decrease these children's hypervigilance during the home visit.

TIME FRAME

Meetings are two hours a week, for 1½ –2 school terms of 12 weeks each, along with separate, weekly, on-site play sessions for each child, until transferring to weekly home sessions. Longer term supervision of carers' and children's weekly play sessions by a leader at CAMHS premises is possible, if required by the children, instead of home sessions. "Special times" may be started afterwards. Fortnightly follow-up meetings led by leaders for foster carers who intend to continue play sessions at home after the group ends also are offered.

METHOD OF DELIVERY

One of the leaders videos demos (3–5 weeks) and practice play sessions weekly with foster carers and all the family's participating children. The leader gives carers short five-minute feedback after each play session. Videos are used for supervision and discussion during weekly meetings, along with discussions of other difficulties within placements. Generalization occurs after play session skills are internalized by carers.

Program evaluation

As an informal measure of success, most participants have opted for continuing play sessions at home after the group ends because they can attend fortnightly follow-up meetings. However, follow-up meetings are not well attended in the long term. In formal follow-up of the non-attendees, most ceased FT because they no longer were experiencing the difficulties they started with. Carers reported they had greater understanding and attachments to their children, and were able to spot in advance issues or areas that may cause their children to struggle. Some reported using FT skills more after the program ended within their daily parenting, and others have re-started play sessions when their children needed more support. The children attending the program reported that they enjoyed their play sessions and developed a positive association with CAMHS.

Other positive outcomes for CAMHS are, first, that the majority of foster children who have been through the program no longer need mental health service involvement. And second, Bradford is building up a base of therapeutically minded foster carers who use their GFT-based parenting skills with new children, as they come into placement. The program has been extended to develop a similar GFT program for families of adopted children who are referred to Bradford CAMHS.

Contact

Pam Wilkinson, Coordinator, Looked After Children's Team
Child and Adolescent Mental Health Service (CAMHS)
Bradford District Care NHS Trust
Bradford, UK
+44 (0)1274 228 300
Pam.Wilkinson@bdct.nhs.uk

Caplin & Pernet GFT 12-session program—
Designers: K. Pernet and W. Caplan

Major adaptations

The program has been shortened to 12 weeks. It can be increased for groups who require this.

Target population

This program is for low-income, inner-city families with problems such as drug abuse, split families, and hard-to-serve families with a variety of social and emotional ills, as well as for families with children in foster and adoptive placements.

Participants

Single parents and couples, also foster and adoptive parents. The age range for parents extends from some teenagers to some grandmothers across groups. There are 5–8 parents at a time in a given group.

Program details

TIME FRAME

There are 12, two-hour sessions.

METHOD OF DELIVERY

Written materials are attractive and easy reading. Parents receive a package of toys and materials for home use. The two leaders conduct demos with all the children in the program, and parents do two, ten-minute practice play sessions with each child in the family. Parents are taught four basic CCPT skills: empathy, imaginary play, limits, and structuring during Meetings 1–5, and mock play sessions with each parent include active coaching of responses by leaders. During Meetings 6–8, parents conduct ten-minute practice play sessions while the group observes, and are given feedback. Parents move play sessions home after a planning meeting, Meeting 9; practice play sessions during the remainder of the meetings may continue.

Program evaluation

Pre- and post-GFT questionnaires collected over several years indicate that parents liked the program, and reported improved relationships with their children.

Contact

1. Karen Pernet, LCSW, RPT-S, BCD
Growth Through Play Therapy
Oakland, California, USA
(001) 510 923 0520
karen@growththroughplaytherapy.com

2. Wendy A. Caplin, Ph.D. RPT-S
Growth Through Play Therapy
Philadelphia, Pennsylvania, USA
(001) 215 248 9446
wendy@growththroughplaytherapy.com
www.growththroughplaytherapy.com

Chillery & Ryan 12-week GFT program— Designers: R. Chillery and V. Ryan

Major adaptations

The program was designed for the maximum number of ten children plus auxiliaries and conducted by two experienced filial therapists. Due to the shortened time frame, groups were divided into two smaller groups for parts of several meetings during the first two phases of GFT.

Target population

In addition to clinical aims, groups also had a pilot research aim (Jaeger & Ryan, in preparation). Children who had moderate conduct and related problems at CAMHS intake clinics were assigned on the basis of geographic location (in Leeds, UK) to either Webster Stratton's Incredible Years (IY) parenting groups or to GFT groups; both were 12-week programs.

Participants

CAMHS referred families with children who had moderate to more serious conduct and related problems.

Program details

TIME FRAME

Twelve, two-hour meetings over a 13-week period. (The scheduled one-week break was to accommodate the UK half-term school holiday schedule.)

METHOD OF DELIVERY

Meetings were held in the early evening to cater for parents who worked. Couples, rather than single parents, predominated. Childcare facilities were provided at every meeting on site for all the children in participating families.

The group was divided at several points during early meetings into two subgroups, each with a leader. Meeting 1 was a large group meeting. In Meetings 2–3, parents were divided in subgroups for demos, followed by large group discussions of demos and skills training. In Meeting 4, after further skills training in the large group, parents were divided into subgroups for their mock sessions. Meetings 5–7 were devoted to practice play sessions within subgroups, then large group discussions. Meetings 8–12 on planning, home sessions, and generalization were large group meetings.

Program evaluation

Evaluation met research aims and consisted of quantitative and qualitative evaluations, including semi-structured interviews with parents post-intervention, and play-based evaluations by participating children. (See Jaeger & Ryan, in preparation. Partial interview results are given in Chapter 15.) Childcare, based on children's feedback, also was a positive experience; children's enthusiasm seemed to encourage their parents to attend weekly meetings.

Contact

Richard Chillery, General Manager, CAMHS,
Safeguarding & Healthy Child Pathway
Children and Family Services
Leeds Community Healthcare NHS Trust
Leeds, UK
+44 (0)113 305 7200
r.chillery@nhs.net

College Park GFT program—Designers: P. Higgins and S. Gold

Major adaptations

Initially, licenced therapists and interns conduct CCPT play sessions with individual children, and meet with the parents on a regular basis, until children show significant progress, and parents show readiness for FT. When learning FT, parents are permitted to observe clinicians conducting play therapy sessions with their children. Home sessions are begun on a case-by-case basis, when parents are deemed ready to conduct them. The goal is to facilitate parent-child relationships and attachments. There is less emphasis in GFT on children's problems, which have already been addressed during CCPT.

Target population

This program is for high-risk cases with many social and psychological difficulties. Many referrals come from schools and former clients, in addition to case workers.

Participants

No more than 6–8 parents, and no more than six children selected from ongoing child/family cases, are placed in a group. One or both parents from the family may attend the group. When there is a significant waiting period for the group to start, families may receive individual FT instead.

Program details

TIME FRAME

The group meets for ten weeks with one or two leaders.

METHOD OF DELIVERY

Leaders supervise parent play sessions on site with one or more children in a family through a one-way mirror. Parents are typically already aware of the value of play and how sessions are conducted when they join the group. This makes it possible for group leaders to focus more quickly on parent performance in parents' play sessions, and on generalization, than would be possible in the same short time frame for parents who had not had the same exposure.

Program evaluation

Pre- and post-GFT questionnaires indicate positive changes in child and parent behaviors. Major childhood problems, aside from relationship problems, were well controlled prior to assignment to the group. Parents give the GFT program positive ratings, and indicate that parent-child attachments are greatly strengthened.

Contact

Stacie Gold, LCSW-C, Clinical Supervisor
Youth & Family Services
College Park, Maryland, USA
(001) 240 487 3550
sgold@collegeparkmd.gov
www.collegeparkmd.gov/youth_fam_serv.htm

Landreth & Bratton 10-session GFT model: Child-Parent Relationship Therapy (CPRT)— Designers: G. Landreth and S. Bratton

Major adaptations

The CPRT 10-session model of GFT typically consists of two-hour sessions once a week, but has also been found to be effective in formats of twice a week for five weeks, every day for 10–12 days, and four weekends, to accommodate parental needs. It also can be increased, when groups require more time (Landreth & Bratton, 2006). During one intake meeting (without an FPO), a family chooses one child to participate in play sessions. If two parents participate, two children can be chosen.

No demos or practice play sessions are conducted with participating children during meetings, and no leader-parent mock sessions are conducted. Instead, demos and viewing DVD segments of the leader's play sessions, as well as role-plays with pairs of parents playing the roles of parent and child, all supervised by the leader, are vital parts of the first several training sessions before play sessions begin with children at home. All supervision is via videos of home play sessions. (Where this is not possible, parents have play sessions at the training site.) Homework assignments are given to parents throughout the program. The standard 10-week program has a scheduled follow-up meeting one month later; further meetings can turn into parent support groups run independently by participating parents. This is a one-leader model, if the leader is experienced.

Target population

Families with children showing a range of common behavioral problems and relationship issues. CPRT has been conducted and researched with a wide range of types of parent and child problems, socio-economic conditions, and ethnic groups (see Landreth & Bratton, 2006, and Chapter 1).

Participants

The number of participants recommended is a maximum of 6–8 parents, with no new group members added after the second session, and no parent able to continue with the program if more than one session is missed. (However, if an emergency situation arises, a personal training session can be arranged to cover material missed.)

Program details

TIME FRAME

Commonly ten consecutive meetings of two hours each

METHOD OF DELIVERY

Meeting 1 consists of introductions to participants, the program, and CCPT skills. Homework assignments begin here and continue throughout. A demo is conducted live with a non-participating child or via video during Meeting 2, and skills training is started.

DVD segments of leader play sessions are recommended to be shown in the first three meetings. Home sessions with the target child begin after Meeting 3. Home play sessions are supervised and discussed via video clips for families in focus during the program's meetings, and the remaining families report on their home sessions briefly. All families report on their homework assignments. Supervision, play session reports, and homework assignments continue during the last meeting, Meeting 10, and parents informally evaluate their experiences and report on any changes in their children and their relationships with them. Arrangements are made for parents who intend to continue their home play sessions.

Program evaluation

Landreth and Bratton have written both a book and a manual with session guidelines on their adaptation of GFT, CPRT (Bratton *et al.*, 2006; Landreth & Bratton, 2006). They have trained many play therapists to deliver this program. Landreth and Bratton cite numerous studies that demonstrate the effectiveness of this shortened GFT approach with diverse populations and presenting problems (see Landreth & Bratton, 2006, Ch.21, for a summary of this research), some of which have also been cited here in Chapter 1.

Contact

Sue Bratton, Ph.D., LPC, RPT-S
Center for Play Therapy, University of North Texas
Denton, Texas, USA
(001) 940 565 3864
http://cpt.unt.edu

Ortwein "Mastering the Magic of Play" program— Designer: M. Ortwein

Major adaptations

The initial training with parents is for one seven-hour day; no children are present. The program includes two, two-hour follow-up evening sessions and 4–6 supervised play sessions at the training site; 4–6 home play sessions follow, which are supervised by telephone, email, or fax.

Target population

This program is for children with a range of behavioral and emotional problems, and parent-child relationship issues. The structure is designed to accommodate working parents.

Participants

Very low-income and Child Protective Services referrals to upper-middle-class families.

Program details

TIME FRAME

16–20 hours.

METHOD OF DELIVERY

Parents are taught GFT play skills in a Saturday workshop without children present. They then have 4–6 practice play sessions at the training site individually, and 4–6 home play sessions with their children. Videos of CCPT and FT sessions are shown during training, with no live demos. Parents are taught the four main FT skills from the designer's *Mastering the Magic of Play Manual* (Ortwein, 1997). Parents are encouraged to generalize FT skills to daily life, and the program concludes with two, two-hour evening sessions for the group to help them generalize, using Louise Guerney's (2013) parenting skills course training program manual.

Program evaluation

Parent evaluations are very positive. Positive changes in children's and parents' behavior are noted from interviews with the therapist, especially for target families who had a recent divorce or remarriage.

Contact

Mary Ortwein, MS, LMFT

IDEALS of Kentucky, Institute for Development of Emotional and Life Skills

Frankfort, Kentucky, USA

(001) 502 227 0055

(001) 502 227 0055

mary@skillswork.org

www.skillswork.org

VanFleet and Sniscak GFT program for children with trauma/attachment problems— Designers: R. VanFleet and C. Sniscak*

*This program has recently been modified to the VanFleet, Sniscak and Faa-Thompson Program. Contact R. VanFleet for details.

Major adaptations

The GFT program is shortened to 18 meetings with two GFT experienced leaders, because families are often involved in multiple services. Additional educational and discussion segments are added to the program to help parents understand and respond to children's attachment- and trauma-reactive feelings and behavior. The final two meetings are held bi- or tri-weekly. Individual, family "booster" meetings and follow-up meetings are also made available.

Target population

This program is designed for foster and adoptive families whose children have more serious trauma and attachment problems. It also can be adapted for medically ill children and their families.

Participants

It is designed for 6–8 families, with up to 10–12 parents. Typically, however, groups consist of 4–7 families, including intact and single-parent families. Parents are expected to hold play sessions with most or all children in the family who are in the appropriate age range during their home play sessions.

Program details

TIME FRAME

Eighteen weeks of meetings running 2½ hours each, with a short break.

METHOD OF DELIVERY

Childcare is provided for families whose children must be present for play sessions during any given session, along with some attendance prizes consisting of toys to be used in the home FT toy kits. The group is divided at several points during meetings into two subgroups, each with an experienced leader. The didactic and discussion portions of a group are held jointly, with both leaders and all parents present. The demos and skills training portions, including two mock play sessions with each parent, and practice play sessions held during Meetings 6–12 are held in subgroups. The whole group meets to discuss the practice play sessions, watch short video clips from subgroups, and receive leaders' feedback. Each subgroup has three back-to-back, 20-minute play sessions with three different parent-child combinations. Parents have four supervised practice play sessions, or more, if needed over the course of these meetings. Final practice play sessions—and preparation for home sessions, to include all children in the family who are in the appropriate age range—take place during Meeting 13. For Meetings 14–16, families report on their home play sessions and show video clips when possible, and skills generalization begins. Meetings 17–18, held on a bi- or tri-weekly basis, continue with home session feedback and discussion, and generalization of skills, as part of a phased out ending.

Program evaluation

Pre- and post-GFT measures are collected, in addition to informal evaluation by parents during the last meeting.

Contact

Risë VanFleet, Ph.D., RPT-S
Family Enhancement and Play Therapy Center
Boiling Springs, Pennsylvania, USA

(001) 717 249 4707
rise@risevanfleet.com
www.risevanfleet.com

Walker & Wright Head Start program—
Designers: J. Walker and C. Wright

Major adaptations

This GFT program, now finished, was adapted to 12 weeks for low-income families of pre-school children with two experienced leaders. A mentor parent who attended a previous group demonstrated CCPT skills with their own child, and discussed GFT's impact. Two early meetings were devoted to making FT toys, and a follow-up meeting six months afterwards continued to help parents with their home play sessions, and generalizing their GFT skills. Videos of parent-child play sessions at the beginning and near the end of the program were made for evaluation, and also given to parents.

Target population

Head Start families and other parents from the community with children aged 3–5 living within an urban Minnesota USA county. Many parents had mental health issues and/or other cognitive and physical limitations; groups included preschoolers with special education and mental health needs, and Spanish-speaking and Hmong families. (Approximately 16 groups were run between 1998 and 2006.)

Participants

Ten very low-income families with preschool children were recruited from within the Head Start program; other families also attended from the surrounding community.

Program details

TIME FRAME

Twelve weeks, with a 6-month follow-up meeting.

METHOD OF DELIVERY

Each family who attended received transportation, dinner, and door prizes for parents' toy bags. Childcare was provided by Head Start staff. Interpreters were also provided for Hmong- and Spanish-speaking families.

Meetings 1–2 introduced participants to the program, including FT skills. In Meetings 3 and 4, toys were made with parents, to compensate for the group's lack of positive, early play experiences. Parents also were videotaped playing with their children for five minutes in parent-child dyads. Meeting 5 reviewed CCPT skills and included a demo between a mentor parent and their preschool child. Specific conversations about limit setting and where to hold play sessions at home seemed critical to ensure follow through on later home play sessions.

For Meeting 6, the group was divided into two subgroups of five parents each and a leader. Each parent practiced CCPT skills with another parent for ten minutes in both child and parent roles, while the other parents observed. Leaders actively coached the "parent" in the dyad. In the observer role, both here and in later practice play sessions, parents were assigned a specific skill to watch for and instructed to give only positive feedback to the "parent" after the ten-minute role-play. Leaders offered parents supportive and constructive feedback, when some skills needed refinement.

During Meetings 7–10, all the parents in the two subgroups conducted 15-minute practice play sessions with their children. At this time, parents also were assigned 30-minute play sessions at home with their children, which were then discussed at the beginning of each subsequent meeting. Meetings 10–11 included videotaping a five-minute play session between each parent and child using CCPT skills. Session 11 also focused on generalizing these skills to daily life and parents were assigned generalization homework for the following week.

For the last meeting, Meeting 12, parents reviewed their latest videotapes with the group and completed assessment measures; they then had a celebration dinner. Approximately six months later, the group reconvened for leaders to share outcome data and discuss parents' ability to maintain home play sessions with their children, and further generalization of skills. (These sessions were always well attended, and usually included at least 75 percent of the group.)

Program evaluation

Pre- and post-GFT outcome measures (the Parent Stress Index—Short Form and the Behavioral Assessment System for Children) were administered. They often indicated that parents continued to experience extreme stress throughout the program; however, parents also reported that they had a greater understanding of their children's behavior due to the group. (Much of their stress was reported as related to their social and economic situations.) Child behavioral issues did not significantly decrease based on these measures either. However, the attunement between parents and their children during play sessions changed. Videotaping documented changes in both parent and child behavior pre- and post-GFT. Some videos were coded and a significant positive difference was found between pre- and post-GFT tapes on the parents' ability to reflect on their children's behavior and emotional experiences. Indicatively, as seen in the videos, every parent's skills increased, and children's undesirable behaviors decreased.

Program evaluations also showed new immigrant Hmong families often dropped out of the program, and more acculturated Hmong families tended to remain. Culturally, play sessions appeared foreign in this community, and play was often seen as a luxury. Therefore, the program developed specific Hmong family parenting groups, led by a Hmong psychologist and a Hmong clinical social worker, to better meet the needs of Hmong parents.

Contact

Jason L. Walker, Ph.D., LP
Psychological Services

Children's Hospitals and Clinics of Minnesota—St. Paul
(001) 651 220 6726
Jason.Walker@childrensmn.org

Conclusion

The variations on GFT that have come to our attention and which preserve the essential features of the model have been outlined in this chapter. They will be useful to leaders, if they are unable to deliver the full 20-week program that we have set out in detail in the rest of this book, or if the families they work with seem more suitable to any of the formats given here.

On ending this book, we want to underline that the 20-week program we have presented is FT in its most complete form, a form that is very satisfying for leaders to use in helping families achieve their positive potential and hopes for their future lives together. We hope this book enables both therapists already familiar with the FT method, and those wishing to learn it, to maximize the fulfillment of therapeutic goals with GFT for all participating families.

APPENDIX 1
Recommended Resources
for Leaders

General resources

Center for Play Therapy (CPT) at the University of North Texas, *http://cpt.unt.edu.*

Family Enhancement and Play Therapy Center (FEPTC), *www.play-therapy.com.*

IDEALS of Kentucky, *www.skillswork.org.*

National Institute of Relationship Enhancement (NIRE), *www.nire.org.*

FT program resources
Video resources for Meeting 1

If a commercial video is needed, instead of a live or video demonstration with a leader, we recommend either of the following:

Filial Therapy with Eric Hatch, Ph.D. (1989). An excellent demonstration of a CCPT play session. Show the demonstration play session to parents, and *not* the FT contents. Available from the National Institute of Relationship Enhancement (NIRE), *www.NIRE/bookstore.*

Filial Play Therapy with Risë VanFleet, Ph.D. Again, show the demonstration play session to parents, and not the FT contents. Available from the American Psychological Association (APA), *www.apa.org/pubs/index.aspx.*

Resource for the generalization phase

For additional input for leaders on generalizing CCPT skills to daily life, we recommend:

Guerney, L. (2013). *Clinician's and group leader's manual for parenting: A skills training program* (5th ed.). Silver Spring, MD: IDEALS. (Available from NIRE/IDEALS, 12500 Blake Road, Silver Spring, MD 20904-2056.)

Suggested formal evaluation measures
pre- and post-GFT program

Filial Problem List (FPL) (Horner, 1974).

Measurement of Empathy in Adult-Child Interactions (MEACI) (Stover *et al.*, 1971) (primarily for researchers).

Porter Parental Acceptance Scale (PPAS) (Porter, 1954).

Parenting Stress Index (PSI) (Abidin, 1997).

Training and certification opportunities in FT

National Institute of Relationship Enhancement (NIRE).

Family Enhancement and Play Therapy Center (FEPTC).

APPENDIX 2
Setting up a New GFT Program Within an Organization[1]

The main steps towards successful organization of a new GFT program by filial therapists within an organization are set out here.

When GFT leaders are not agency staff

When GFT leaders are not regular staff members, care needs to be exercised in bringing the program into an organization that is not familiar with not only the content but also what is required of the organization to support the offering of the program. When leaders are staff members and/or the agency itself has initiated a request to have GFT programs introduced, these steps can possibly be simplified.

As in all organizing, timing is most important. The organizational steps outlined here have recommended times assigned to them, based on our experiences with larger agencies. Other settings may differ. Leaders may find that these times can be condensed somewhat after they have run the whole program a few times. The steps for organizing outlined here are designed for introducing GFT to an agency in which the leaders, unlike staff members, are not able to introduce new therapeutic programs into the agency's current services themselves.

Step 1: (approximately 4–6 months before beginning meetings)
STARTING FROM THE TOP OF THE ORGANIZATION

Leaders already need to have the director's approval for running a GFT program in their organization. This approval, depending on the organization, may already have entailed several of the steps outlined here. Once agency approval is given, the leaders then need to contact the manager(s) responsible for such programs in the organization to outline the goals, methods, and benefits of the program directly to the manager. It is important for leaders to make the case for how FT can assist the organization in its work, if this was not done earlier. For example, leaders need to underline that this program is cost effective because it can increase families' well-being as a whole, rather than simply removing a child's presenting symptoms, or just "shaping up" the most difficult "marginal" parents, thus potentially reducing re-referrals. Agencies need to understand that the therapy provided in the GFT group is likely to reduce the amount of case work needed by staff personnel more generally.

---

1   This appendix has been adapted for GFT from Guerney, L. (2013). *Clinician's and group leader's manual for parenting: A skills training program* (5th ed.). Silver Spring, MD: IDEALS, with permission from the publisher.

Leaders also need to decide with managers the best way to introduce the program to the other staff to gain their enthusiastic cooperation. In order to succeed, the program must be a unified agency or organizational effort.

REASONS FOR NOT OBSERVING GROUPS BY AGENCY STAFF

It should be made clear that staff members are welcome to contact the leaders in order to have questions answered and receive more detailed information about the program. However it also should be stressed that staff are not able to "sit in" as observers because the group has a therapeutic intent. There are issues of trust and confidentiality that may be undermined if other staff members attend some sessions. Among other things, parents may feel that they are being "checked on." Instead, leaders may wish to suggest email memos, and/or presentations with video contents to staff groups to inform them of the program in more detail. When initial intakes and assessments are conducted by professionals who will not be involved in the GFT program, more detailed information, as outlined in Appendix 3 is required. Some families have key workers or referrers assigned to them who are responsible for overall delivery of services. The key workers' or referrers' roles as "resource people" for these families, and the feedback that group leaders will provide to them, need to be clarified in more detail both with staff, including managers, and the families themselves.

Finally leaders should ensure that other staff time is approved by management (e.g. administrative support for sending out letters, making room bookings) and indicate times when this help will be needed.

Step 2: (approximately 3–4 months before starting)

STAFF COOPERATION AND INVOLVEMENT WITH THE PROGRAM

We suggest leaders offer to help the manager implement the plans that have been worked out to brief the staff. For example, a leader might write the first draft of the memo that goes to the staff, and offer to be present at the meeting in which staff members are informed of the program. These offers are not only ways of showing a spirit of cooperation: they are an opportunity for leaders to present the program in the best possible light, and an opportunity to prevent any attitudinal problems or misunderstandings that might otherwise arise. It also is a means to encourage staff members to refer families for specialist intake and assessment, and possible selection for the GFT program. However, GFT leaders should be careful to make the point that it is they who make the final decisions on group composition after the full specialist intake for GFT is complete.

Chapter 2 on intake and composition of the group addresses these issues in detail; we recommend that the chapter be read alongside this discussion. Agency initial intakes, and then specialized GFT intakes by leaders of the program, need to be conducted within a reasonable time frame for the agency involved, alongside the other tasks outlined here.

When an organization has more parents than can participate in a single group, the director and/or involved professionals, along with the GFT leaders, need to set some priorities as to whom to include in the first round of the program. Each organization, of course, will want to arrange its first group in accordance with its own priorities and situations. However, past experience in running initial GFT programs indicates that it may be wise to avoid including the most serious referral problems in the first group. This strategy is suggested in order to ease the implementation of a new program. It may be helpful to seek out group members who are reasonably adequate in their roles as parents, likely to attend sessions regularly, and whose children range between the ages of 3 and 11. This allows new group leaders an opportunity to practice delivering the program under less difficult circumstances, before conducting groups with more clinically demanding families.

CHOOSING A NAME FOR YOUR PROGRAM

Giving the program a user-friendly name may help promote interest by parents. Professionals know this program as "Filial Therapy" and "Group Filial Therapy"; these terms should be included in the description offered in the parent information leaflet. However, this labeling in our experience is overly formal for introducing the program to parents. Thinking about delivering "therapy" to their children can sometimes be unduly anxiety provoking for parents initially. For example, one GFT program was called the "Powerful Play Program" in leaflets for parents, when it was delivered by the second author and her colleague. This seemed to set a positive and less formal tone at the outset. (See Appendix 4 for an example of this leaflet.) The leaflet will need to be ready for the initial intake stage to hand out to parents.

TIME, DATE, AND LOCATION

Leaders need to determine a time that suits the leaders, participants, and the organization, taking into account all known organizational and community limitations (e.g. Wednesday night church services). Along with choosing the dates and time for the program, leaders decide on a location for their meetings.

SPACE REQUIREMENTS FOR GFT MEETINGS

Ideally the location should be a place that people associate positively with receiving help or support and which is convenient for most parents. One large room with movable chairs enables people in groups with larger numbers of participants to move out into smaller practice groups. Another smaller room, which is used for play demonstrations and parent-child play sessions, should have a video link or one-way screen. An adjoining room and/ or a kitchen for break-time refreshments is highly desirable. Children accompanying their parents to sessions also need facilities and adult supervision in a separate room. These physical arrangements are ideal. In a pinch, leaders can bring in coffee or tea to the group meeting room and breaks can be provided there, usually 30 minutes in length. Many leaders have improvised in other creative ways to allow for the necessary space needed to cover all the demands of a GFT group.

Step 3: (approximately two months before starting)

FURTHER INTAKE FOR POTENTIAL PARTICIPANTS

After an agency intake and identification of potential participants, further specialist intake of families by group leaders begins.

Step 4: (approximately one month before the first meeting)

CONFIRMATION OF A PLACE IN THE PROGRAM

Each family selected requires a confirmation letter. Again, this letter needs to be backed up with email, text/cell phone, or telephone contact. See Appendix 7 for a sample confirmation letter that leaders can use as a guide. When families have key workers or referrers assigned who are responsible for overall delivery of services (e.g. a case manager), these professionals need to be copied into the confirmation letter.

Step 5: (one week before the program starts)

FOLLOW-UP CONTACT

A phone call and email follow-up to the invitation are highly recommended. It works best in our experience if the agency or organization staff do this; leaders need to provide them with the list of names, phone numbers, and email addresses for the designated participants.

Step 6: (between the first and second weeks of the program)

NON-ATTENDANCE AT THE FIRST GFT MEETING

Sometimes parents who agreed they will attend do not come to the first meeting. Before the second meeting, leaders need to call and email these people to let them know that it is not too late to start. If a few parents have changed their minds about attending, leaders may try to find out why. At this point, leaders may add some latecomers or parents who had not been able to get into the original group, if original members make it clear that they are not continuing.

APPENDIX 3
Information for Agency Intake Professionals and Referrers who are not GFT Leaders

The following information can be adapted by GFT leaders for distribution to intake professionals and referrers who refer families onto specialist GFT intakes with filial therapists.

Introduction

The X Program *(insert the popular name of the program offered here)*, known in the therapy literature as Group Filial Therapy, is a well-integrated model of family change based on non-directive, child-centered play therapy and family therapy principles. Its basic premise is that parents or carers can be taught to have child-centered play sessions with their own children and serve as effective therapeutic agents of change for them. It is a family-based intervention—all family members are encouraged to be included, if they are willing to do so.

Is the X program an established program or a new and unproved idea?

Group Filial Therapy is very well established. There have been over 40 years of practice and research on this method, also called Filial Therapy, in the USA. There also are different ways that have been developed to carry out this approach: groups have been well researched in the USA, both shorter group models of 10–12 weeks in length and longer group models of 20-plus weeks in length. The other way in which families are helped is in individual Filial Therapy. For these programs, a 10–20-week training and supervised practice period is the usual length of time for moderate clinical problems. Filial Therapy is increasingly practiced worldwide.

Filial Therapy has improved parent-child relationships when there have been a wide range of difficulties reported by parents and teachers, or when there have been family problems. For example, children with attentional difficulties and behavior problems, children who have had traumatic experiences, and children who have had depression and other anxieties have been helped by Filial Therapy. Also, children and parents who have had difficulties in their relationships due to a variety of causes (e.g. late adoption after maltreatment by birth parents; divorce and separation) have been helped.

Who is included in the X program?

Children and parents who… *(insert the program's inclusion criteria here)*. All children between the ages of 3 and 11 are eligible and their parents or carers. Because Group Filial Therapy is a family-based program, later in the program parents are helped to spend special playtime or activity time with their younger (under 3 years) and older (over 11 years) children. Parents are encouraged to begin conducting special playtimes with all of their children ranging in age from 3 to 11, and not just the child referred. If both parents in a two-parent family are unable to participate, parents unable to actively take part are encouraged to come along for the training and introductory meetings in order to be able to give active support to the parent who is participating and carrying out the program.

How long is the program?

The set program is 20 weeks long *(insert dates of program meetings here, including any breaks)*. Parents need to be motivated and committed to attending each week, and bring their children along for practice play sessions during some of the meetings. If the group decides they wish to continue further, there is the option of… *(insert any planned additional meetings here, if already known)*.

Where and when will the program be held?

The meetings will be on *(insert day of week)* for 2.5 hours from *(insert time)* at *(insert venue)*.

What happens during the X program?

This program is well structured to ensure that families are helped as a dynamic unit. It trains parents to deliver special playtimes to their children. The program assumes that children communicate their emotions most effectively and earliest through their play, and that play is both empowering and enjoyable for children and their parents. The X program teaches parents the basic skills of child-centered play therapy, a well-recognized approach, and helps them to conduct these play sessions under supervision and then independently under indirect supervision at home. It does not train parents to become therapists! Parents conduct play sessions only with their own children.

The entire group learns together to conduct special play sessions, concentrating on four skill areas. Group leaders demonstrate these play skills with each child in the program; they hold group discussions and parents have practice opportunities. When the initial training has been completed, parents have practice play sessions with their own children, supervised by the group leaders and observed by the rest of the group. After parents' play skills are established, they transfer play sessions to their own homes. During later group meetings, parents receive more help in consolidating their skills, and in understanding the underlying meaning of their children's play and their own reactions. The final phase of the program helps parents transfer their child-centered skills to their daily lives.

Please note that this training is a skills-based approach; it is a step-by-step process; parents are helped to practice special play skills under supervision *before* they transfer these skills to their homes and daily lives.

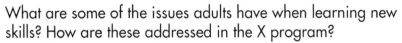

What are some of the issues adults have when learning new skills? How are these addressed in the X program?

The anxieties adults feel in new situations usually disappear quickly when they realize that the approach used by the program leaders is very supportive. Leaders assume that adults learn best when their strengths are pointed out, and the skills they already have are built on. Group leaders employ ways to learn for adults that are enjoyable, and emphasize ways group members can support and encourage one another. The group leaders appreciate that parents are the main people who are important to their children, and who should have the greatest understanding of them already. The leaders want to help parents find the best ways of helping their children, and they take a collaborative approach with them.

How will participants be selected for the program?

When intake professionals or referrers decide Filial Therapy is an option for a family, they give the family general information on the program, set out in the leaflet given to parents (see Appendix 4). If parents express an interest in considering the X Program, a referral is then made to the filial therapists conducting the program to arrange further intake appointments with the family. Filial therapists will contact the family to explain the next steps in the intake process further. Intake professionals explain to families that the filial therapist will contact the family to arrange a time that the family comes in again to play together; then the adults talk with the therapist about what occurred and the X Program.

General Leaflet on the X Program for Interested Parents

Is the ·················· Program right for you and your child?

Do you have a child or children between the ages of 3 and 11 years old?

Do you find yourself arguing and shouting at your child more often than you would like to?

Do you feel you have lost touch with what your child thinks and feels?

Do you sometimes feel that your child is the one in charge, rather than the other way round?

Would you be willing to learn to improve your parenting and relationship with your child?

PARENTING CAN BE CHALLENGING!

WE ALL KNOW THAT

WE ALSO KNOW THAT...

YOU ARE THE MOST IMPORTANT PERSON IN YOUR CHILD'S LIFE

We want to help...

(Insert name of organization)

Tel. ··························

POWERFUL PLAY

Information for parents of children under 12 years of age

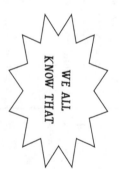

The .... Program is for parents and their children

Its aim is to help parents learn proven skills for communicating with and disciplining their children by means of special (healing) play methods that parents learn and later apply at home.

Play is "pleasant to swallow" and rewarding for both parents and children. Play is a very good way to develop more positive and closer relationships between parents and children.

It is a family program: all the children in your family between the ages of 3 and 11 years old can take part. And if your children have two significant parent figures in their lives, both are urged to come along and participate.

WHAT IS THE .... PROGRAM?

The .... Program (also called Filial Therapy) is a week group program (with .... additional, optional weeks afterwards). It helps parents learn some of the same skills Play Therapists use to help children who have problems. The group leaders in the .... Program can help parents be as effective professionals in helping their own children.

You and your children will be given direct help in group meetings before you take these skills home with you.

These are some of the skills you will be learning:

• Limiting setting.
• How to get your children to listen to you.
• How to listen to your children.
• How to be more in charge and in control as a parent.

By the end of the .... week program, you will see a real difference in:

• Your relationship with your children.
• Your children's behavior.
• Your confidence and competence in your parenting skills.

When is the program held?
(Insert day of week, time of day and length of program.)
Childcare is available on site for all the children of families who attend (or give other childcare arrangements)

Where are the meetings held?
(Insert information here.)

What is the group like?
You will meet with other parents to learn new skills to become more effective parents. First the leaders help you practice skills together. Then they supervise parents having special play times with their children. Afterwards parents will be able to apply them at home.

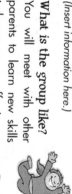

Who are the group leaders?
(Insert names of leaders.) They are qualified Play Therapists who specialize in Filial Therapy. They plan to make these group meetings as relaxed and enjoyable as possible for everyone.

How do I register?
You will be invited to participate by the Assessment Team at your local .... Service.

APPENDIX 5
Letter Arranging the GFT Assessment Phase for Interested Families

(Insert letterhead of agency)

(Insert date) ....

Dear *(insert names of parents)* ....

Thank you for your expressed interest in the X Program. You have already been given the general leaflet on the program, and we discussed in our telephone call recently what the next appointments are for. I am writing to confirm the two appointments with me to decide on the program's suitability for your family: *(Insert dates, times, and venue for meetings here.)*

Since it is important for all family members to attend this first meeting, we have set it up so that it is possible for everyone to attend together. It also would be useful for you to bring along a supportive adult to mind your children during the second half of the appointment. There will be 20–30 minutes at the beginning of this appointment when I watch your family play or do an activity together. For the second part of this time, I meet with you parents separately, so that we can talk together about what happened.

The second appointment is all about the X Program, and is only for the parents to attend. You will receive further information on the program, or have another option for services proposed to you, as well as having all your questions arising from these meetings addressed.

We realize that you will want to tell your children what the first meeting they attend is about. We suggest that you give children who are old enough to understand the following brief explanation:

> *Our family wants to get along better together and we are going to see (name of place or organization) for some help. (Name of leader) wants to watch how our family does some playing together. All you need to do is play almost any way you want with the toys in the room. You do not need to perform in any way. Just have fun. Whatever we all do will be fine with them.*

Parents may also add, for children who need further explanation:

> *Nobody else will be with us, but (name of leader) will be able to watch through an observation window (if available, or on a video) all the things we've been doing. (Name of leader) would like to see how we do things together as a family. They would like us to enjoy our time together. Then we parents will talk it over with (name of leader) and decide in a little while what comes next. You will be waiting for us for a short time with .... (caretaker) while we talk.*

Thank you again for your interest in the X Program. Please confirm your attendance with our administrator *(insert name and contact details)*. And please call, or email me personally, if you have any questions about these next two meetings.

Sincerely,

.... (filial therapist's name and contact details)

APPENDIX 6
Family Play Observation Hypotheses Suggestions for Leaders

Below are suggestions for leaders in organizing their hypotheses during FPOs. The first areas to consider are from a family therapy perspective and the second areas are from a child therapy perspective.

Family therapy perspective

- Parenting styles and the strength of the parenting alliance.

- Family structure and unresolved family dynamics issues.

- Attachment styles within family dyads (Stollack, Barley, & Kalogiros, 2000).

Additional family play dynamics

Attuned play: Are participants joining together for the same intent? Are the affective states similar? Are physical rhythms the same and participants in close physical proximity?

Expressive momentum: Does the play activity become more elaborate and include new ideas and creative movement over time? Is this expressive momentum shared? Is it enjoyed, and is it flexible?

Flow/break: How, by whom, and when is the momentum broken? Is one participant changing the rules, emotional states, etc. quickly?

Form and energy balance: Can boundaries and focus be established? How can rules, planning, redirecting, and verbalizing help this or hinder this?

Play metaphors and imagery: What verbal or play images are repeated in the play? Which ones suggest strong emotional themes? Are these expressed together by family members or in isolated play? Are these themes actively addressed or resolved?

Parent-child roles: Are parents primarily facilitators and children players (the usual roles)? Do parents follow their children's leads? When parents introduce contents, can they return easily to a supportive role (Harvey, 2000)?

Kinds of interactions between each child and each parent (attuned or misattuned).

Interactions between target child and siblings: (separately for each pair, if more than one sibling is present).

Level of interaction among all participants. Note degree of interaction among all family members present, any absence of relating among subsets, and if certain types of interactions tend to prevail until a parent or another child enters in.

Locus of control in the family; locus of control among the children in sibling groups.

Methods used by parents to control their children (Rye & Jaeger, 2007; Guerney L., undated handout). Smith's (2000) 9-point scale categories, used for structured observations of parent-child dyads, also may be of general interest to leaders, but see our cautions against using checklists during FPOs.

Parent's affect: from "no affect" to "free range of affect and pleasure in play."

Parent's intrusiveness: from "continually structured" to "non-directive."

Parent's praise: from "no praise, negative comments" to "good amount for effort and completion of tasks."

Parent attention: from "ignored child" to "attended to positives and ignored negatives."

Parent's developmental sensitivity: from "almost all interactions over- and/or under-estimated child's development" to "high sensitivity to developmental level."

Parent's responsiveness to child's interactions: from "parent did not respond or engage child" to "parent highly responsive."

Parent-child involvement: from "no interaction to high level of verbal and non-verbal interaction."

Child's social responsiveness: from "completely withdrawn from toys and parent" to "child friendly, social and inviting."

Child's attention to activities: from "activity for <1 minute" to "sustained interest in most activities."

Child's activity level: from "overly active" to "no excessive movements."

Child's aggressiveness: from "argumentative, destructive, aggressive frequently" to "never aggressive, etc."

Child's responsiveness to parent's interaction: from "no response to parental attempts" to "responded almost all the time."

Child's responsiveness to questions: from "did not respond to parent's questions" to "responded to all questions."

Child therapy perspective

The following areas may be relevant to consider during FPOs for referred children and their siblings:

- Attachment style.

- Emotional and social development.

- Cognitive and language development.

- Play development.

- Physical development.

- Verbal and non-verbal affective expressions of the child.

- Neurological or unusual signs (speech difficulties, attentional problems, etc.) (Rye & Jaeger, 2007).

APPENDIX 7
Sample Confirmation
Letter to Parents

(Insert letterhead of agency)

(Insert date) ....

Dear *(insert names of parents)* ....

At our last meeting, we agreed you will attend the X Program. We are looking forward very much to having you in the program. We are now confirming this in writing. As you know, the first meeting will be held *(insert date, time, and venue details here)*. It is important that you attend this meeting. You will meet the other parents, along with the other leader, and we will begin the program contents.

If you cannot attend the first session for some reason, it is important to let us know right away. We will try to work out ways to accommodate you and the group in your absence for this meeting, and to catch you up to attend the second meeting. *(If there is an incentive prize, or attendance certificate, mention that here.)*

Please contact us as soon as you become aware of a problem. *(Contact details for both leaders to be inserted here.)*

Sincerely,

....

GFT leaders

APPENDIX 8
Creating an Informal Group Atmosphere at the Outset[1]

1. Generally, circular or horseshoe seating arrangements work out well because they "include" everyone more or less equally. However, as time goes on, leaders may find that a different arrangement works better for some groups.

2. Use members' first names from the beginning, and encourage parents to call you by your first name. This is particularly important if there is someone in the group of high social status (e.g. doctor, lawyer, county commissioner). Establishing a first-name basis with everyone creates an equalizing effect that encourages the shy to participate and allows higher social status people to feel comfortable, even when they make mistakes.

3. While leaders want participants to view the GFT program as an educational approach, and to appreciate the advantages of being taught skills for improving communications with their children, they do not want to make the experience seem too much like "school." Leaders promote this unnecessary association if they distribute too much written material during the first meeting. Suggestions are given in Chapter 5 on the handouts needed by parents and their placement during the first meeting.

4. Jargon-free language and a vocabulary suitable for all group members should be used in order to make the contents as user-friendly as possible.

5. Have the coffee/tea/juice ready, so people can get some immediately, if they wish.

6. Remember to inform participants about venue rules and layout (e.g. toilets, fire, smoking). If smoking is permitted, describe where parents may go to smoke at break time.

7. During this first meeting, leaders may want to circulate a list for volunteers to sign up to supplying snacks for the coffee break held midway through each meeting. Leaders need to supplying a simple snack for the first meeting themselves.

---

1   Excerpted from Guerney, L. (2013). *Clinician's and group leader's manual for parenting: A skills training program.* (5th ed.). Silver Spring, MD: IDEALS, with permission from the publisher.

APPENDIX 9
Sample GFT Videotaping Consent Form

I have parental responsibility for:

(Insert name[s]) ....
....

I understand that the professionals viewing the tapes agree to keep the information confidential.

I understand that the tapes and this form will be kept by the group facilitators in a locked file when not in use.

YES/NO *(circle one)* I agree to the videotaping of my play with my child for intake purposes at *(insert the venue)*.

Section 1: Videoing for clinical supervision

I agree that the following can be videotaped and used for the facilitators' clinical supervision:

YES/NO *(circle one)* Demonstrations of play skills with my child/children by the group facilitators *(insert names of leaders)* at *(insert the venue)*.

YES/NO *(circle one)* My practice play sessions at *(insert the venue)* during the X Program meetings.

YES/NO *(circle one)* My sessions at home, where video equipment is available.

Section 2: Videoing for training and teaching purposes

I agree that the following can be used by the facilitators for teaching and training purposes with professionals:

YES/NO *(circle one)* Demonstrations of play skills with my child/children by the group facilitators *(insert names of leaders)* at *(insert the venue)*.

YES/NO *(circle one)* My practice play sessions at *(insert the venue)* with my child/children during the X Program meetings.

YES/NO *(circle one)* My sessions at home, where video equipment is available.

Signed..Date ....

APPENDIX 10
Participating Children's Leaflet

Children's booklet

Hi, our names are
(*insert names of leaders and their photos*).

You came with your family to play and met one of us.

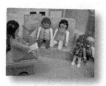 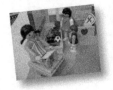

Then one of us watched your family play.

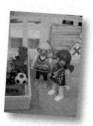

Your parents are coming more times to see us, with other parents, so that everyone in your family learns to have more good times together. The parents are all learning to do special play times with their children.

You will come more times too. The first time you come will be to play with one of us for a short time. All the parents will watch us play, and then talk about what it was like. You can do most things while we play. No one will tell you what you have to play.

You will come more times after your parents learn more about special play times. They will have short play times with you, while we watch and learn more. Later on, your play times will be longer with your parents.

If you have brothers and sisters, they may have special play times too, all by themselves, just like yours will be.

?

You might have questions about what will happen. Your mom or dad can talk to you about it all. If they don't know the answers, they can ask us next time.

APPENDIX 11
Overview of Filial Therapy

The aims of Filial Therapy

Filial Therapy has been shown to be an effective program for numerous reasons. It is beneficial for children in many ways, including helping them to develop a better understanding of their own and others' feelings, and learning to express their needs and feelings more appropriately. Usually children's presenting problems decrease because in special playtimes they can work through difficult experiences and conflicts they have had with others, and find ways to work things out for themselves. This increases their self-confidence and they also learn to trust their parents more.

The program benefits parents as well because they understand their children's feelings, motives, and development better, learn firsthand the importance of child-centered play, and expand the ways they communicate with their children and promote their trust. Parents learn effective ways to enhance their authority with their children too. All of these things lead to less frustration in parents and more competent parenting.

Families as a whole benefit also; the program tries to involve all family members. It has been shown to improve ways families communicate and cope with difficult events, as well as helping them find more enjoyable ways of being together.

The sequence for Filial Therapy

- Initial evaluation of the children and family.

- Discussion of the rationale, content, and process of Filial Therapy.

- Demonstrations of child-centered play sessions with children while parents observe and then discuss.

- Skills training and "mock" sessions.

- Practice play sessions, followed by feedback from leaders and discussion.

- Home-based sessions and discussion (practice play sessions may continue during meetings).

- Generalization of Filial Therapy principles to daily life.

- Evaluation of the program and ending.

Important principles for conducting GFT play sessions by parents

- Parents develop warmer relationships with their children.

- Parents accept their children exactly as they are.

- Parents establish a feeling of permissiveness in their play sessions, so that children feel free to express their feelings completely.

- Parents are alert to recognizing the feelings their children are expressing, and reflect those feelings back to them in such a manner that the children understand their behavior better.

- Parents maintain a deep respect for their children's ability to solve their own problems, if they are given the chance to do this. Children are the ones to make choices and change themselves.

- Parents follow their children's lead and do not direct their children's actions or conversation.

- Children set the pace of the play sessions. Sometimes change is a gradual process for children that is respected by their parents.

- Parents set minimal rules in play sessions; these are the ones to help their children feel safe and accepted. The way parents set rules promotes their children's ability to develop self-control.[1]

Home play sessions

After training and practice during meetings, parents conduct their weekly play sessions independently at home, with additional supervision and extra practice from filial therapists during meetings when they are needed.

Selecting toys for home sessions

Filial therapists help parents select specific toys and materials that are needed for their home play sessions. Toys for special play sessions are intended to help children express their feelings and they lend themselves to interactive and imaginative play.

---

1   Modified from Axline, V. (1947) *Play therapy: The inner dynamics of childhood.* Boston, MA: Houghton Mifflin.

APPENDIX 12
Handout for Parents on the Structure of the GFT Program

MEETING 1 Introductions to the program and one another. Summary of GFT's aims and objectives. Brief demo (live or video) of CCPT with a non-participating child. Overview of basic child-centered play skills.
MEETINGS 2–5 Demo of a play session with each participating child by leaders. Discussion of the skills used and feedback from parents. Skills training with parents. "Mock session" training.
MEETINGS 6–10 Practice play sessions by parents with each of their participating children. Feedback by the group leaders and discussion. Additional skills training.
MEETINGS 11–12 Planning for home play sessions. Processing of each parent's first home session.
MEETINGS 13–15 Practice play sessions by parents, either weekly or occasionally. In-depth supervision of selected families' home play sessions. Group reports of home play sessions. Discussion of play themes.
MEETINGS 16–19 Practice play sessions by parents, weekly or occasionally. In-depth supervision of selected families' home play sessions. Group reports of home play sessions, including play themes. Generalization of skills to daily life.
MEETING 20 Ending and evaluation of the program by participants.
OPTIONAL FOLLOW UP MEETING(S) Discussion of issues for parents who continue home play sessions/special times.

APPENDIX 13
Leaders' Agendas for Each Meeting of the 20-Week Program

Meeting 1: Introduction to the program
Aims for Meeting 1

- Begin to develop group support.

- Help parents effectively manage their anxieties over both their group membership and their skills as parents.

- Introduce Filial Therapy skills on a general level.

- Prepare parents for the whole of the program.

- Prepare parents for the next meeting.

Pre-meeting tasks for leaders

1. Final checks on venue, break arrangements, and participants' list.

2. Room and equipment ready for video recording group meetings.

3. Demo (optional) arranged; room and equipment ready for conducting a live session with a child outside the group, or for playing a DVD.

4. Parents' manual and handout on preparing children for the GFT program copied and ready for distribution near the end of the meeting.

5. Copies of program structure, along with dates for meetings, ready for distribution near the end of the meeting.

Agenda for leaders during Meeting 1

1. Leaders introduce themselves and briefly address confidentiality and recording issues.

2. Introduction of group members to each other, including what parents' personal goals are.

3. Brief overview of GFT's effectiveness, program goals, and contents, and parents' role in program, along with rationale for play sessions and how the method will relate to the desired goals of the parents.

4. Introduction of rationale for demos with each child in the program and logistics for observing and discussing demos.

5. Leader shows a video or conducts a demo for parents live.

6. Leaders conduct discussion with parents about what they observed when watching the session.

7. Coffee break.

8. Handout "Introduction to the four basic CCPT skills" introduced to parents and each skill discussed; brief introduction to toys and materials used.

9. Preparing parents for next meeting's agenda, including demos with their own children; skills learning.

10. Parents preparing their children for the program; handout on this topic distributed.

11. Working out a demo schedule.

12. Distributing the Parents' Training Manual, to be read by next week and brought along each week.

13. Leaders give handout on the program structure and meeting dates, then end the meeting positively.

NB: If there are any pre-GFT measures to be filled out, these may be finished at the end of the group, while demos are finalized, or given to parents to take home and return.

Post-meeting tasks

1. Debrief with co-leader.

2. Receive supervision.

3. Decide on how demos and post-demo discussions will be divided between two leaders during next several meetings, and how teaching components will be divided.

Meeting 2: Beginning demos and skills learning
Aims for Meeting 2

• Continue to develop positive group support.

• Show parents during demos the skills they are being taught for their own play sessions.

• Help parents begin to view their children in more objective terms during demos.

• Motivate parents to continue to participate in the program and begin thinking about the main CCPT skills in action.

• Foster parents' interest in conducting play sessions.

Pre-meeting tasks for leaders

1. Administrator to remind parents whose children are participating in demos, and remind all parents of next meeting's time and date.

2. Room and equipment for live demos, observation by parents, and recording of demos set up.

3. Finalize childcare arrangements for children coming in for demos.

4. Make extra Parent's Training Manuals available for each meeting.

Agenda for leaders during Meeting 2

1. Leader conducts demos with children in program, and other leader gives brief *sotto voce* comments to parents observing.

2. Discussion of parents' reactions to their children in the demos.

3. Coffee break.

4. Discussion of leaders' CCPT skills shown in demos, and answering of parents' questions regarding skills shown.

5. If fortuitous moments arise early, begin formal teaching of skills of structuring or empathic responding.

6. Briefly preparing parents for next meeting's demos and skills training, including reminding parents of the children scheduled for future demos.

7. Ending the meeting.

Post-meeting tasks

1. Debrief with co-leader, including reviewing order of demos, shared teaching plans, and success of childcare arrangements.

2. Receive supervision, as needed.

Meeting 3: Continuing demos and skills learning
Aims for Meeting 3

- Maintain group support and cohesion.

- Continue to show parents during demos the skills they are being taught for their play sessions.

- Continue to help parents to view their children in more objective terms during demos.

- Motivate parents to continue to participate in the program.

- Begin training parents in "showing understanding" skills.

- Foster parents' interest in conducting play sessions.

Pre-meeting tasks for leaders

1. Remind parents whose children are participating in next week's demos.

2. Leaders to prepare packets of toys and play scenario cards for "showing understanding" skills practice.

3. Leaders to collect their own small toys to use during skills training, preparing toy packets and scenarios on cards for pairs to use for all the skills training in the next two meetings.

Agenda for leaders during Meeting 3

1. Leader conducts demos with children in program, and other leader gives brief *sotto voce* comments.

2. Discussion of parents' reactions to their children in the demos.

3. Coffee break.

4. Discussion of leaders' CCPT skills shown in demos, and answering of parents' questions regarding skills shown.

5. Beginning of formal teaching on skill of empathic responding: large group exercise, and first role-play exercise.

6. Discussion of the role-play exercise.

7. Briefly preparing parents for next meeting's demos and skills training, including reminding parents of children participating in demos.

8. Ending the meeting.

Post-meeting tasks

1. Debrief with co-leader, including demos, success of shared teaching arrangements, and parents' reactions to early skills training.

2. Receive supervision, as needed.

Meeting 4: The final demos and more skills learning
Aims for Meeting 4

- Maintain group support and cohesion.

- Show parents during the final demos the skills they are being taught for special play sessions.

- Continue to help parents to view their children in more objective terms during demos.

- Motivate parents to continue to participate in the program.

- Train parents in following children's lead, structuring, and limit-setting skills.

- Foster parents' interest in conducting play sessions.

- Prepare parents for next meeting's mock sessions.

Pre-meeting tasks for leaders

1. Administrator to remind parents whose children are participating in demos.

2. Leaders have packets of toys and play scenario cards on remainder of skills available during meeting for skills practice.

Agenda for leaders during Meeting 4

1. Leader conducts demos with children in program, and other leader gives brief *sotto voce* comments.

2. Discussion of parents' reactions to their children in the demos.

3. Coffee break.

4. Briefer discussion of leaders' CCPT skills shown in demos and answering of parents' questions regarding skills shown.

5. Formal teaching on skill of following children's lead: leaders' input, illustrative examples, and leaders' role-play of this skill.

6. Parents' role-play in pairs of following children's lead.

7. Group discussion of role-play.

8. Formal teaching on skill of structuring: leaders' input and modeling, followed by practice by parents.

9. Teaching steps of limit setting.

10. Parents verbally rehearse limit setting.

11. Leaders help parents think of limits for their play sessions.

12. Leaders role-play limit setting, followed by parents' role-playing this skill.

13. Discussion of the role-play exercise.

14. Brief preparation of parents for next meeting's mock sessions.

15. Ending the meeting.

Post-meeting tasks

1. Debrief with co-leader, including demos, success of skills training, and parents' reactions to skills training.

2. Debrief with co-leader on preparation of parents for mock sessions.

3. Receive supervision, as needed.

Meeting 5: Mock sessions and preparation for first practice play sessions

Aims for Meeting 5

- Strengthen group support and cohesion.

- Help any parents with performance anxieties.

- Motivate parents to feel successful at skills learning.

- Train parents to put all the skills they are learning into practice.

- Foster parents' interest in conducting play sessions.

- Prepare parents for next meeting's first practice play sessions.

Pre-meeting tasks for leaders

1. Leaders decide on which skills to practice with individual parents during mock role-plays.

2. Leaders decide on what type of "child" to play out and scenarios.

3. Leaders decide on how mock session role-plays are divided up between them.

4. Leaders decide on general schedule of families for group's first practice play sessions, which begin the following week.

Agenda for leaders during Meeting 5

1. Introduction of parents to mock sessions practice.

2. Leaders take turns conducting mock play sessions with every parent in the group.

3. Coffee break, including informal debriefing by parents with one another.

4. General group discussion of mock session practice, including parents' ideas on what they want more practice on.

5. Leaders give more detailed feedback to each parent, following GFT guidelines on feedback for mock and practice play sessions.

6. Additional skills training for the group, as required.

7. Preparation of parents for next meeting's first practice play sessions, including finalizing the selection of the first families, and working out a schedule for the following few weeks.

8. Providing additional training and rehearsal to families scheduled for next meeting's play sessions, as required.

9. Helping parents prepare their children for practice play sessions.

10. Ending the meeting.

Post-meeting tasks

1. Debrief with co-leader, including success of mock sessions and any needs for additional skills training.

2. Debrief with co-leader on preparation of parents for first practice play sessions.

3. Receive supervision, as needed.

Meeting 6: Beginning practice play sessions
Aims for Meeting 6

- Strengthen group support and cohesion.

- Help any parents with performance anxieties.

- Developing parents' basic level of skills proficiency during practice play sessions.

- Increase the group's skills competencies.

- Prepare parents who are conducting next meeting's first practice play sessions.

Pre-meeting tasks for leaders

1. Decide on how supervision of individual parents will be divided between two leaders during the next several meetings.

2. Discuss further skills training that may be needed.

Agenda for leaders during Meeting 6

1. Selected parents conduct practice play sessions with their children in the program; a leader gives brief *sotto voce* comments to observing parents.

2. Coffee break and informal debriefing of first sessions by parents with one another.

3. Supervision of each parent's first play session by a leader in front of the group.

4. Processing other parents' reactions to observing first play sessions.

5. Further skills training.

6. Preparing parents who are starting their first practice play sessions the following week.

Post-meeting tasks

1. Co-leaders decide on which skills parents need further practice in.

2. Debrief with co-leader on group's reactions to sessions observed.

3. Debrief with co-leader on progress and supervision of the parents who had their first practice sessions.

4. Receive supervision, as needed.

Meeting 7: Continuing first practice play sessions
Aims for Meeting 7

- Strengthen group support and cohesion.

- Help any parents with performance anxieties.

- Increase the group's skills competencies.

- Prepare parents who are conducting next meeting's first practice sessions.

Pre-meeting tasks for leaders

1. Decide on how supervision of individual parents will be divided between two leaders during the next several meetings, if not yet agreed.

2. Discuss further skills training that may be needed.

Agenda for leaders during Meeting 7

1. Selected parents conduct practice play sessions with their children in the program; a leader gives brief *sotto voce* comments to observing parents.

2. Coffee break and informal debriefing of first sessions by parents with one another.

3. Feedback on each parent's first play session by a leader in front of the group.

4. Processing other parents' reactions to observing first play sessions.

5. Further skills training.

6. Prepare parents who are starting their first practice sessions the following week.

Post-meeting tasks

1. Debrief with co-leader on further skills training offered, and group's reactions to sessions observed.

2. Debrief with co-leader on progress and supervision of the parents who had their first practice sessions.

3. Receive supervision, as needed.

Meeting 8: Starting second practice play sessions
Aims for Meeting 8

- Strengthen group support.

- Help parents reflect on their children's play during their sessions.

- Develop parents' basic level of skills proficiency during play sessions further.

- Increase the group's skills competencies.

- Keep the group together overall on skills attainment.

- Motivate parents to conduct home play sessions.

- Prepare parents who are conducting next meeting's practice sessions, when required.

Pre-meeting tasks for leaders

1. Review first and second practice play session schedule for the group to ensure all parents are moving on to their second ones.

2. Review any training needs of individuals and the group as a whole.

3. Copies needed of toys and materials handout for parents.

Agenda for leaders during Meeting 8

1. Selected parents conduct practice play sessions with their children in the program; a leader gives brief *sotto voce* comments to observing parents.

2. Coffee break and informal debriefing of sessions by parents with one another.

3. Feedback on each parent's second play session by a leader in front of the group. (NB: This may include finishing supervising one or two parents' first practice play sessions.)

4. Discussion of other parents' reactions to observing these play sessions.

5. Brief discussion of parents' reflections on the meaning of children's play in sessions.

6. Further skills training, as required.

7. Preliminary discussion of toys and materials for home play sessions and video recording of home sessions; handout given to parents.

8. Prepare parents who are having practice play sessions the following week, as required.

Post-meeting tasks

1. Debrief with co-leader on further skills training offered, and group's reactions to sessions observed.

2. Debrief with co-leader on progress and supervision of the parents who had their practice sessions.

3. Receive supervision, as needed.

Meeting 9: Continuing second practice play sessions
Aims for Meeting 9

- Maintain group support and foster more independence.

- Help parents reflect on their children's play during their sessions.

- Develop parents' basic level of skills proficiency during play sessions further.

- Increase the group's skills competencies.

- Keep the group together overall on skills attainment.

- Motivate parents to conduct home play sessions.

- Prepare parents who are conducting next meeting's practice sessions, when required.

Pre-meeting tasks for leaders

Co-leaders review further skills training needed by individuals and the group.

Agenda for leaders during Meeting 9

1. Selected parents conduct practice play sessions with their children in the program; a leader gives brief *sotto voce* comments to observing parents.

2. Coffee break and informal debriefing of sessions by parents with one another.

3. Feedback on each parent's second play session by a leader in front of the group.

4. Discussion of other parents' reactions to observing these play sessions.

5. Further skills training, as required.

6. Brief discussion of parents' reflections on the meaning of children's play in sessions.

7. Prepare parents who are conducting practice sessions the following week, as required.

Post-meeting tasks

1. Debrief with co-leader on further skills training offered and group's reactions to sessions observed, including their understanding of children's play.

2. Debrief with co-leader on progress and supervision of the parents who had their practice sessions.

3. Receive supervision on parents' readiness to start home sessions and any other group issues, especially in complex cases.

Meeting 10: Finishing second practice play sessions
Aims for Meeting 10

- Maintain group support and foster more independence.

- Finish second practice play sessions.

- Help parents reflect on their children's play during their sessions.

- Develop parents' basic level of skills proficiency during play sessions further.

- Keep the group together overall on skills attainment.

- Motivate parents to conduct home play sessions.

- Continue to prepare parents for home sessions, returning to the discussion of toys and materials.

- Prepare parents for the next meeting's different agenda.

Pre-meeting tasks for leaders

1. Leaders discuss further skills training that may be needed by individual parents and the group.

2. Leaders check their schedule to ensure that all parents are now finishing their second practice play sessions, or other provisions have been made.

Agenda for leaders during Meeting 10

1. Selected parents conduct practice play sessions with their children in the program; a leader gives brief *sotto voce* comments to observing parents.

2. Coffee break and informal debriefing of sessions by parents with one another.

3. Feedback on each parent's second play session by a leader in front of the group.

4. Discussion of other parents' reactions to observing these play sessions.

5. Brief discussion of parents' reflections on the meaning of children's play in sessions.

6. Further skills training, as required.

7. Further discussion of toys and materials for home play sessions and video recording of home sessions.

8. Prepare parents for next meeting on preparing fully for home play sessions.

Post-meeting tasks

1. Debrief with co-leader on further skills training offered, group's reactions to sessions observed, group's progress on skills attainment, and readiness for home sessions.

2. Debrief with co-leader on progress and supervision of the parents who had their practice sessions.

3. Plan catch-up sessions for parents, when required.

4. Receive supervision, as needed.

Meeting 11: Transition to home sessions
Aims for Meeting 11

- Increase the group's skills competencies.

- Motivate parents to conduct home play sessions.

- Maintain group support.

- Prepare parents psychologically for home play sessions.

- Prepare parents for practical home sessions issues.

- When home session videos will be used, verify compatibility of parents' video equipment with meeting equipment.

Pre-meeting tasks for leaders

1. Discuss the readiness of each parent for home sessions.

2. Copies needed of handout, "Home play session notes."

Agenda for leaders during Meeting 11

1. Consolidation of skills; psychological and practical preparations for home sessions.

2. Preparation of parents for next meeting's supervision of home sessions, including video recordings, when chosen, and write-ups of home sessions. Final check for compatibility of parents' home video equipment with meetings equipment.

3. Rehearse with parents any challenging issues anticipated in their home play sessions.

4. Review each family's practical arrangements for their home sessions.

Post-meeting tasks

1. Discuss possible first home session issues for families.

2. Plan catch-up sessions for parents, when required.

3. Receive supervision, as needed.

Meeting 12: First home sessions
Aims for Meeting 12

- Help parents begin to conduct home play sessions effectively.

- Motivate parents to continue their home play sessions, troubleshooting any problems that have arisen.

- Maintain group support and cohesion.

- Consolidate skills development.

- Prepare parents for the next meetings.

Pre-meeting tasks for leaders

1. Ensure parents' video recordings are compatible with electronic equipment at meeting, when video used.

2. Decide on each leader's responsibility for video equipment or verbal feedback with each parent.

3. Work out a possible flexible schedule for supervision (live or video) of families in focus from Meeting 13 onwards.

Agenda for leaders during Meeting 12

1. Begin to supervise each parent's first home session from their written reports and videos, and troubleshooting any issues arising.

2. Coffee break, with leaders reviewing their possible families in focus schedule for subsequent meetings in light of parents' experiences.

3. Supervision of remaining parents' first home session from their written reports and videos, troubleshooting any issues arising.

4. Selection of families in focus for next meeting's detailed supervision of their home sessions, and live sessions during meetings (where video not used).

5. Working out a flexible timetable for families in focus for the next few meetings.

6. Rehearsal for any parents who will conduct their first home sessions during the following week, when required.

7. Preparation of parents for next meeting's and subsequent meetings' agendas.

8. Verifying compatibility of video equipment with that at meeting for any remaining parents.

Post-meeting tasks

1. Debrief with co-leader on progress and reactions of parents to first home sessions.

2. Iron out any scheduling issues for home session and live supervisions during subsequent meetings.

3. Plan catch-up sessions for parents, when required.

4. Receive supervision, as needed.

Meeting 13: Early home sessions
Aims for Meeting 13

- Help parents continue to conduct home sessions effectively.

- Motivate parents to continue their home play sessions, troubleshooting any problems arising.

- Maintain group support and cohesion.

- Consolidate skills development.

- Review parents' reports of home sessions.

Pre-meeting tasks for leaders

1. Decide each leader's responsibility for video or verbal feedback with each parent.

2. Revise flexible schedule for supervision of families in focus, either video or live supervision, as required.

Agenda for leaders during Meeting 13

1. In-depth supervision of home sessions of families in focus, including their written reports and videos, with detailed feedback after each video. When no video is used, live supervised sessions during the meeting and detailed feedback after all the live sessions finish.

2. Coffee break.

3. Supervision of remaining home sessions of families, including their written reports and videos.

4. Addressing of skills issues arising from live or home sessions.

5. Developing more skills competence in parents.

6. Supervision of remaining parents' home play sessions.

7. Preparation of families in focus for next meeting's detailed supervision of their home sessions, and live sessions during meetings (when video not used).

8. Continue to work out a timetable for families in focus for subsequent meetings.

9. Rehearsal of any parents who will conduct their first home sessions during the following week, as needed.

10. Brief preparation of parents for next meeting.

Post-meeting tasks

1. Debrief with co-leader on progress and reactions of parents to home sessions.

2. Iron out any scheduling issues for home session and live supervision during subsequent meetings.

3. Plan catch-up sessions for parents, when required.

4. Receive supervision, as needed.

Meeting 14: Early home sessions
Aims for Meeting 14

- Help parents continue to conduct home sessions effectively.

- Motivate parents to continue their home play sessions.

- Maintain group support and cohesion.

- Consolidate skills development.

- Prepare parents of toddlers and teens who are ready for short play sessions/special times.

Pre-meeting tasks for leaders

1. Ensure parents' video recordings are compatible with electronic equipment at meeting, when video used.

2. Designate the leader responsible for video or verbal feedback with each parent.

Agenda for leaders during Meeting 14

1. In-depth supervision of home sessions of families in focus, including their written reports and videos, with detailed feedback after each video. When no video is used, live supervised sessions during the meeting and detailed feedback after all the live sessions finish.

2. Coffee break.

3. Supervision of remaining home sessions of families, including their written reports and videos.

4. Addressing skills issues arising from live or home sessions.

5. Developing more skills competence in parents.

6. Preparing parents for short home play sessions/special times with toddlers and teens.

7. Supervision of remaining parents' home play sessions.

8. Preparation of families in focus for next meeting's detailed supervision of their home sessions or live sessions during meetings (when video not used).

9. Brief preparation of parents for next meeting.

Post-meeting tasks

1. Debrief with co-leader on progress and reactions of parents to home sessions.

2. Iron out any scheduling issues for home session and live supervision during subsequent meetings.

3. Plan catch-up sessions for parents, when required.

4. Receive supervision, as needed.

Meeting 15: Continuing home sessions
Aims for Meeting 15

- Help parents continue to conduct home sessions effectively.

- Motivate parents to continue their home play sessions.

- Maintain group support and cohesion.

- Continue more advanced skills development.

- Begin to focus on play themes in more depth.

Pre-meeting tasks for leaders

1. Discuss the group's level of skills attainment and intended focus on play themes.

2. Decide each leader's responsibility for video or verbal feedback with each parent.

Agenda for leaders during Meeting 15

1. In-depth supervision of home sessions of families in focus, including their written reports and videos, with detailed feedback after each video. When no video is used, live supervised sessions during the meeting and detailed feedback after all the live sessions finish, including supervision of their home sessions.

2. Begin to use play themes to parents in feedback and discussion for in-depth understanding of their children's play.

3. Coffee break.

4. Address skills issues arising from live or home sessions and developing more advanced skills competence in parents.

5. Supervision of remaining parents' home play sessions, including supervision of parents who offered short home play sessions/special times with toddlers and teens.

6. Preparation of families in focus for next meeting's detailed supervision of their home sessions, and live sessions during meetings (when video not used).

7. Brief preparation of parents for next meeting.

Post-meeting tasks

1. Debrief with co-leader on progress and reactions of parents to home sessions and to play themes.

2. Iron out any scheduling issues for home session and live supervision during subsequent meetings.

3. Receive supervision, as needed.

Meeting 16: Later home sessions
Aims for Meeting 16

- Help parents continue to conduct home sessions effectively.

- Motivate parents to continue their home play sessions.

- Maintain group support and cohesion.

- Continue more advanced skills development.

- Continue to focus on play themes.

- Introduction of generalization of skills to daily life.

Pre-meeting tasks for leaders

1. Discuss the group's level of skills attainment, understanding of, and applications of play themes.

2. Discuss group's readiness for generalizing their skills to daily life.

3. Decide on each leader's responsibility for video or verbal feedback with each parent.

Agenda for leaders during Meeting 16

1. In-depth supervision of home sessions of families in focus, including their written reports and videos, with detailed feedback after each video. When no video is used, live supervised sessions during the meeting and detailed feedback after all the live sessions finish, including supervision of their home sessions.

2. Continue to use play themes with parents in feedback and discussion for in-depth understanding of their children's play.

3. Coffee break.

4. Address skills issues arising from live or home sessions and developing more advanced skills competence in parents.

5. Introduction of generalizing skills to daily life: empathy and "I" statements in daily life, as relevant to group; developing an atmosphere of approval, and structuring.

6. Supervision of remaining parents' home play sessions, including supervision of parents who offered short home play sessions/special times with toddlers and teens.

7. Preparation of families of focus for next meeting's detailed supervision of their home sessions, and live sessions during meetings (when video not used).

8. Brief preparation of parents for next meeting.

Post-meeting tasks

1. Debrief with co-leader on progress and reactions of parents to home sessions, play themes and introduction to generalization.

2. Iron out any scheduling issues for home session and live supervision during subsequent meetings.

3. Receive supervision, as needed.

Meeting 17: Later home sessions
Aims for Meeting 17

- Help parents continue to conduct home sessions effectively.

- Motivate parents to continue their home play sessions.

- Maintain group support and cohesion.

- Continue more advanced skills development and focus on play themes.

- Continue generalization of skills to daily life.

- Begin preparation of parents for ending the 20-week program.

Pre-meeting tasks for leaders

1. Discuss the group's level of skills attainment, understanding of and applications of play themes, and generalizing their skills to daily life.

2. Discuss options available for ending from funders', leaders', and parents' viewpoints.

3. Decide on each leader's responsibility for video or verbal feedback with each parent.

Agenda for leaders during Meeting 17

1. In-depth supervision of home sessions for families in focus, including their written reports and videos, with detailed feedback after each video. When no video is used, live supervised sessions during the meeting and detailed feedback after all the live sessions finish, including supervision of their home sessions.

2. Continue to use play themes with parents in feedback and discussion for in-depth understanding of their children's play.

3. Coffee break.

4. Address skills issues arising from live or home sessions; develop more advanced skills competence in parents, when required

5. Continue generalization of skills to daily life: review empathy, "I" statements, developing an atmosphere of approval, structuring, introduction of limit setting and consequences, and prioritizing family members' needs as appropriate for the group.

6. Supervision of remaining parents' home play sessions.

7. Preparation of families in focus for next meeting's detailed supervision of their home sessions, and live sessions during meetings (when video not used).

8. Brief preparation of parents for next meeting and for ending the 20-week program.

Post-meeting tasks

1. Debrief with co-leader on progress and reactions of parents to home sessions, play themes, and generalization.

2. Iron out any scheduling issues for home session and live supervision during subsequent meetings.

3. Review parents' preferences for post-group meeting sessions.

4. Receive supervision, as needed.

Meeting 18: Later home sessions
Aims for Meeting 18

- Help parents continue to conduct home sessions effectively.

- Motivate parents to continue their home play sessions.

- Maintain group support and cohesion.

- Continue more advanced skills development, focus on play themes, and generalization of skills to daily life.

- Continue preparation of parents for ending the 20-week program.

Pre-meeting tasks for leaders

Decide on each leader's responsibility for video or verbal feedback with each parent.

Discuss any outstanding issues regarding home play sessions, generalization, and ending the program.

Agenda for leaders during Meeting 18

1. In-depth supervision of home sessions of families in focus, including their written reports and videos. When no video is used, continue with live sessions and supervision of home sessions.

2. Continue to use play themes with parents in feedback and discussion for in-depth understanding of their children's play.

3. Coffee break.

4. Address skills issues arising from live or home sessions, with the goal of developing more skills competence in parents.

5. Continue generalization of skills to daily life: review empathy, "I" statements, developing an atmosphere of approval, structuring, limit setting and consequences, and prioritizing family members' needs as appropriate for the group.

6. Supervision of remaining parents' home play sessions.

7. Preparation of families of focus for next meeting's detailed supervision of their home sessions, and live sessions during meetings (when video not used).

8. Brief preparation of parents for next meeting and for ending the 20-week program.

Post-meeting tasks

1. Debrief with co-leader on progress and reactions of parents to home sessions, play themes, and generalization.

2. Iron out any scheduling issues for home session and live supervision during the next meeting.

3. Review ending options discussed.

4. Receive supervision, as needed.

Meeting 19: Later home sessions
Aims for Meeting 19

- Help parents continue to conduct home sessions effectively.

- Motivate parents to continue their home play sessions.

- Maintain group support and cohesion.

- Continue more advanced skills development, focus on play themes, and generalization of skills to daily life.

- Continue preparation of parents for ending the 20-week program.

Pre-meeting tasks for leaders

1. Decide on each leader's responsibility for video or verbal feedback with each parent.

2. Discuss any outstanding issues regarding home play sessions, generalization and ending the program.

Agenda for leaders during Meeting 19

1. In-depth supervision of home sessions of families in focus, including their written reports and videos, with detailed feedback after each video. When no video is used, live supervised sessions during the meeting and detailed feedback after all the live sessions finish, including supervision of their home sessions.

2. Continue to use play themes with parents in feedback and discussions for in-depth understanding of their children's play.

3. Coffee break.

4. Address skills issues arising from live or home sessions.

5. Continue generalization of skills to daily life: review empathy, "I" statements, developing an atmosphere of approval, structuring, limit setting and consequences, and prioritizing family members' needs as appropriate for the group.

6. Supervision of remaining parents' home play sessions.

7. Finalizing each family's arrangements for special activities/continued home play sessions after the program formally ends.

8. Preparation of parents for last meeting's agenda in the 20-week program.

Post-meeting tasks

1. Debrief with co-leader on progress and reactions of parents to home sessions, play themes, and generalization.

2. Review the ending options discussed with each family.

3. Receive supervision, as needed.

Meeting 20: Ending the program
Aims for Meeting 20

- Help parents continue to conduct home sessions effectively.

- Motivate parents to continue their home play sessions and/or special times.

- Maintain group support and cohesion.

- Mark the ending of the 20-week program with parents.

- Help parents evaluate the GFT program.

Pre-meeting tasks for leaders

1. Discuss any outstanding issues regarding home play sessions, generalization, and ending the program.

2. Prepare formal evaluation tools for distribution.

3. Prepare practical arrangements to mark the ending, if leaders have this task.

Agenda for leaders during Meeting 20

1. General comments from leaders on the ending of the program.

2. Facilitate support and contact arrangements post-program.

3. Facilitate discussion of issues arising for the group on ending.

4. Supervision of families who introduced special activity times during the last week.

5. Supervision of families continuing to have home play sessions during the last week.

6. Evaluation of the program: any formal evaluations to be completed here.

7. Extended coffee break.

8. Evaluation of the program: informal evaluation.

9. Future contact arrangements reviewed and goodbyes facilitated.

Post-meeting tasks

1. Debrief with co-leader on group progress and ending meeting.

2. Evaluate the 20-week program informally with one another and with supervisor.

3. Congratulate one another on completing the program together!

APPENDIX 14
Information for Parents on Preparing their Children for the X Program[1]

The week before demonstration play sessions start with your children, we suggest that you go through the children's leaflet with them. This introduces us leaders and the program. This extra handout is for children who want more information.

What do I tell my children if they ask more about the demonstrations the leaders will be doing with them?

We suggest the following:

> The leaders for our meetings are [first name] and [first name]. Here are their photos. One of the leaders will be taking you to a room with toys in it so that all the parents at the meeting can see how special playtimes are done. Children can do most things they want in there. And each child will have a turn all by themselves. We will be behind the mirror in the next room watching the leader play with you. We'll all be quiet so that we can hear and watch what's happening.

If there is a camera in the room, then we suggest saying the following:

> There will be a camera in the room with you, so that we can film and then watch what happened later with the leaders.

Add the following sentence, if required:

> The camera is there because it helps parents to learn more, before they start to do special playtimes with their own children.

What do we tell our children if they ask more about practice play sessions we will be doing ourselves?

It is useful to introduce the idea that parents will do the same things as the leader does during the demonstration session, and that this will be after parents have had more meetings and all the children have had a demonstration playtime with a leader. Therefore, we suggest that parents refer to the next step in the program very briefly, in a matter-of-fact way:

> When all the children have had a special playtime with a leader, then parents will start to do their own playtimes with their children. It will work the same way. The leaders and the other parents will watch from behind the mirror (and the camera

---

1   To be handed out during the first meeting, along with the children's booklet.

will be there). The leaders and parents will talk about these special playtimes afterwards. Once everyone learns how to do these playtimes, then we will be doing them at home [as well as at the meetings, where this option is chosen].

What if my child doesn't listen to any of this information?

Children may have a variety of reasons for not listening to everything parents want to say about the special playtimes. Sometimes it is simply too much information to take in at one time. If that is the reason, and it is especially so for younger children or children with attentional or cognitive difficulties, then we suggest parents break it down into smaller bits of information, and repeat the information when it's needed. If children fail to absorb this information because they are anxious about what it may lead to for them, or for other reasons, then ideally parents would find the right moments to share very small pieces of information at times their children can absorb it.

Any further tips?

This program teaches parents to help their children understand and plan for new situations. Too much information shared at the outset may not be useful for children. You will be able to judge as parents who know your own children well whether to give them information when each new phase of the program unfolds, or whether your children want to know the overall plan well ahead of time. You will be able to discuss this with your group leaders and other group members as you take part in the program.

It is important for parents to emphasize that it is the leader first of all and then the parents who are being watched and learning new ways of being with their children. This is because some children who have low self-esteem, who are very shy, or who believe others think they are exceptionally bad children, may become very anxious about adults watching them. These children sometimes may either be very reluctant to take part in these play sessions or may become very inhibited as they try to be on their very best behavior.

For the above reasons and for other reasons, we urge parents not to coach their children on how parents wish they would behave during play sessions with leaders and themselves. The more spontaneous children are during play sessions, the more leaders are able to offer helpful suggestions to parents on how to handle situations and children's reactions. In fact, these things may be the very reasons parents decided to attend this program! We are sure parents will be very interested to see what their children will do during these playtimes, even though parents sometimes are a little bit nervous about what they might see. Leaders are sure this program is going to help families get along better together. We leaders are eager to share this interesting and effective program with all of you and everyone in your families!

APPENDIX 15
Parents' Training Manual
for Play Sessions

This manual serves as a guide and is useful to you for learning and for home play sessions. However it is not a stand-alone guide. We will provide ample opportunities during our meetings for everyone to raise questions and discuss all of the points in this manual.

Why play sessions?

Play sessions are recommended for children 3–11 years old who have problems with their own feelings and/or difficulty in relationships with others. Children often misperceive parents' intentions and feel unhappy, insecure, or mistreated for very little apparent reason. Children may not be aware of their own needs and feelings, and thus parents cannot always help their children in their usual ways. Communication between parents and children about their deeper needs is, therefore, insufficient or incomplete.

One purpose of play sessions is to create a situation in which your children may become aware of feelings that they have not allowed themselves to recognize. In the presence of their parents, your children have an opportunity to communicate their feelings through play. It is essential that, as parents, you accept your children's feelings during special play sessions. This helps your children come to a better understanding of how to cope with their feelings, as they experience, or re-experience, difficulties during their play sessions.

Another purpose of play sessions is to build your children's feelings of trust and confidence in you as parents. If you respond to your children in the manner prescribed for play sessions, it increases their trust that they can communicate with you more fully and honestly about their experiences and feelings. This should eventually lead to more moderate and mature ways of expression, and less use of extreme and immature forms of emotional expression. Children will have less fear that, by being open with you, they will lose your respect or your affection.

A third purpose is to build your children's confidence in themselves. Just as we expect you will eventually feel that your children trust you more, your children also should experience your sense of trust in them. One goal is for children to feel more secure in making their own decisions, when that is appropriate. Often children need to learn to be less fearful of making mistakes. It is important for them to learn that they have choices, and are themselves responsible for much of what befalls them. This is very important for any children who have a problem to overcome. This means being free to make choices (including making mistakes) and experiencing the consequences, good or bad. By allowing your children freedom of choice in their play sessions, and by allowing them to experience the consequences of free choice, you build their sense of confidence. You also build their confidence by giving them your complete and exclusive attention in play sessions. This leads to your children seeing themselves as more worthwhile and likeable people, which are key ingredients, not only to self-confidence, but also good adjustment.

What parents do in play sessions

You will be learning to have one-to-one play sessions with each of your children in the program. The skills you will be learning are discussed next.

1. Follow children's lead

The role of parents in a play session is to establish an atmosphere of free play and acceptance of their children. This means that you have to take a very unusual attitude towards your child—very different from the way you usually relate to other people, especially children. You set the stage by limiting the duration of the play session, and establishing a few basic rules. But what children do with the toys, and what they say in the session are strictly up to them (some parents may want to set one or two personal limits, to be discussed later in the program). Children may use the toys to explore feelings they have not been able to express adequately before, or to convey things they often communicated in less appropriate ways.

Children who have more extreme behavior may want to use the time to be aggressive, or they may want to sit and stare at the wall—unwilling to involve themselves at all—or they may wish to leave after a few moments. However, most children are very eager to participate and spend time with their parents one to one.

Parents need an open mind and willingness to follow their children's lead. Therefore, it is important that parents avoid the following in order not to influence their children's play and responses:

- Criticism.

- Questions, leads, or invitations.

- Suggestions, advice, or persuasion.

- Interruptions or interference.

- Information giving—unless directly requested by your child.

- Teaching, preaching, or moralizing.

- Initiating an activity.

- Praise, approval, encouragement, or reassurance.

You will notice that several of these responses would be positive in real life with your children, but in play sessions they can influence their behavior, sometimes because children want to gain adult approval. In short, it is important for you to establish a setting in which your child, and your child alone, sets the agenda.

2. Parents set the stage

Children are helped by parents to know what play sessions are about and how long they last. Parents learn the following introductory and departing messages:

INTRODUCTORY MESSAGE

> *[Name of child], this is a very special room [time, place, depending on the space you are using]. You can do ALMOST anything you want.* If you cannot do something, I will tell you.*

* This statement may include the optional statement: "You may say anything you want in here." Personal limits will be discussed further during meetings on limit setting. A few additional personal limits requested by parents can be negotiated.

DEPARTING MESSAGE

Give two time warnings as the session ends. One time warning is given five minutes before the end of the playtime, and the last warning is given one minute before the end. For example: *"Johnny, we have (five, then one) minute(s) more to play today."* At the end of the playtime, firmly, but pleasantly, say: *"Our time is up for today. It's time to leave now."*

WHEN CHILDREN RESIST ENDING

If children are reluctant to leave the room, parents reflect their feelings and restate that the session is ending. You will be learning how to do this, using your body and voice to stress your message and conviction, and reflecting your child's feelings, before attempting to enforce leaving. You will learn to:

- Stand straight up from your position at your child's level.

- Place your hand on your child's shoulder and guide them in the direction of the door.

- Go directly to the door and open it.

- Change the tone of your voice from acceptance to a firm and clear intention.

3. Children receive parents' full attention

Equally important, you must be fully involved with your child, giving full attention to everything your child says, does, and feels. You will be attentive to your child's mood, and note very carefully all the feelings your child is willing to reveal. This gives children the go-ahead to begin to uncover more of their deeper feelings. If you are asked to participate in an activity, you should engage fully. But attention should be focused primarily on how your child wants you to participate, following your child's direction, and showing you understand your child's feelings. Your child's play in the session need not be conventional. For example, a child may like to cheat at cards or make new rules. In these circumstances, you should reflect only your child's strong need to win, or your child's desire to have things go their way, or the means your child uses to have things go their way. These feelings are reflected in an uncritical, warm, and supporting tone. In the training you do, you will learn how to reflect feelings and show understanding in your play sessions.

4. Parents focus on children's feelings and actions

You can best demonstrate to your children that you accept and understand their feelings by reflecting their expressed feelings and actions. This takes the form of noting aloud what your child seems to be feeling: for example, *"You're disappointed it didn't hit the target." "That makes you mad." "You're very upset when I don't answer your questions right away." "It feels good when it goes together the way you want it to."*

Your child's actions are also accepted by your manner and verbal comments: for example, *"You're really beating him up." "You're going to kick him around." "You're sitting on my lap." "You're aiming very slowly, so it will be sure to hit."*

These are all appropriate comments by parents in their play sessions. Complete silence on the one hand, or merely sociable conversation on the other, are discouraged. Children may fear disapproval when their parents are very silent, so it is important to comment, letting them know that your attitude is continuously accepting. With regard to social conversation, it leads most children to feel that they should answer questions, or talk about what their parents want to talk about, rather than take the initiative themselves.

More important than any technique, however, is the spirit under which this time with your children is undertaken. It is important that you try not to be mechanical, stilted, or artificial. You can avoid this best by bending all your efforts towards trying to put yourself in your children's place, and understanding the world as they see it, not as you see it, and not as you wish them to see it. You try to understand your children's feelings through what they are doing and saying. Also, you leave your own worries or reactions out of it as much as you can. Sometimes, it will be difficult. But you simply try to understand what your children are trying to express, and communicate to them that you understand—that you know what they are feeling, and that it's all right with you.

You may find that some of the things your child does are distasteful or worrisome. You need not permit such behavior during any other time outside of the play session. However, it is essential to be very giving and accepting of any and all behavior in the play session (except the limits mentioned later). Children quickly pick up the idea that what goes in the play session may or may not be allowed out of the play session. Outside the session in your daily life, you can continue to be very firm about prohibiting some of the activities that are permitted in the session. Tell your children in daily life that such things are not allowed; they are only allowed in the play session (e.g. use of bad words, berating their parent).

5. Limits on children's behavior

There are a few restrictions on your child's activity in the play session; our term for these is "limits." A limit is a rule for children's behavior. Children need help from parents to be clear about boundaries to their behavior. They then feel safe, and are able to explore their environment and try out more mature behavior. In play sessions, rules or limits are clearly stated at the time of the first infraction. Rules are never given before an infraction. The consequence is imposed after children choose to break the limit again. Children learn that what happens to them is a direct consequence of their behavior. They can begin to take responsibility for their actions when parents learn to use limits and consequences in playtimes.

Some guidelines to consider before making a limit are:

- Is this limit necessary for the safety of my child?

- Is this limit necessary for the safety of others?

- Is this limit necessary for the protection of valuable property?

- Is this limit enforceable?

REASONS FOR SETTING AS FEW LIMITS AS POSSIBLE IN PLAY SESSIONS

Children cannot be expected to remember a great number of rules. If few boundaries are set, children know what these are; they can then explore the situation, and can lead the way within these boundaries.

Since consistency is vital—you want to be viewed as a person who does what they say—the fewer the limits imposed, the more likely it is that you will enforce the limits every time they are broken.

SPECIFIC LIMITS

Determine if a limit is necessary. Usual limits for play sessions are for child and parent safety, with children not being allowed to hit, kick, hurt, or endanger themselves or their parents in any way, safety and protection of property (e.g. nothing should be thrown at the mirrors, camera, windows, or other spots to be protected both during meetings and at home), and one or two personal limits needed by parents also may be negotiated. In addition, except under unusual circumstances, children do not leave the room during play sessions, except for one trip to the bathroom and one drink for the child.

COMMUNICATING AND ENFORCING LIMITS

You will learn that it is vital, whenever it is not an emergency, to empathize with your child's desire to break a limit, and then follow the steps now outlined.

Step 1. Stating the limit: Phrase the limit in a forceful but pleasant tone. Change your voice from an accepting tone to one of authority. Be brief and clear.

In the following order: catch your child's attention, reflect their desire to do the prohibited action, and state the limit. NB: no reason is provided initially. For example:

> *Johnny, you want to shoot the darts at the mirror. Remember, I told you if there was something you couldn't do, I would tell you? One of the things you may not do is shoot the darts at the mirror.*

If children persist in asking why, reflect their wish to know why, and then reflect their annoyance or confusion about the rule. For example:

> *You don't see why we have this rule." "You don't like it." (Or) "You don't like it, if you don't know why.*

Occasionally, there is a child who simply cannot let go of the "why" question without an answer. In such an instance, provide a simple reason—for example, *"Clay leaves marks."* And be prepared to move onto additional challenges from an occasional child who says, *"You can get those marks off."* In this instance, do not provide more reasons "from your side." Instead, address the underlying feeling. For example, *"You don't think that it's a good reason."* Rarely does a child continue beyond this point, when feelings are followed and acknowledged acceptingly.

Step 2. Warning: If your children break a limit you have just set (i.e. it is the second time this occurs in a session), remind them of the rule and state what will happen if the limit is broken again. A warning is given so that your children know beforehand what will happen if the limit is broken, and then can decide whether to risk the consequence. For example:

> *Johnny, you want to do that again. Remember I told you that you couldn't shoot the darts at the mirror? If you shoot the dart at the mirror again today, we will have to end the playtime today.*

Step 3. Enforcement of the consequence: If your children break the rule again, after the consequence has been given, restate the rule and follow through with the consequence you warned your children about. Use a firm but pleasant tone. Perhaps stand up immediately or guide your children to the door to help them clearly recognize your insistence on leaving now because of the broken limit. For example:

> *Johnny, you still want to shoot the darts. Remember I told you if you shot the mirror again, you would have to leave the playroom for today? Since you shot the mirror, we have to leave right now, for today. We will play again next time.*

When rules are set and enforced this way, children begin to learn that they are responsible for what happens when they make a choice to break a limit—after having been warned previously and knowing what the result will be. For each subsequent session, when a rule has already been set in a previous play session, parents start at the warning step, and omit Step 1. They progress to Step 3, enforcement of the consequence, only if the rule is broken again. The only exceptions to this are:

- If your child is very young or learning impaired, the rule itself (Step 1) should be restated, if a week or more has gone by since stating it first. Follow the next two steps, if your child breaks the rule again in the same session.

- For children of any age, the rule is restated if it is broken after a long period (a month or more) has passed since the original rule was given.

Setting up play sessions at home

Once your initial training and practice is complete, and both you and your leaders feel confident about transferring play sessions with your children to your home, leaders help every parent finalize play session arrangements that maximize their success. You and your leaders will discuss the following together:

1. *Setting aside a time* (approximately one half hour every week) for a home play session with your child. Hopefully, this will be at a time and place where you are completely isolated from the rest of the family, and can guarantee no interruptions. Your uninterrupted attention and your reliability in making sure the sessions happen weekly are some of the most important conditions for fruitful play sessions. If a change is absolutely necessary, it should be discussed in advance with your child, and an alternative arrangement offered. Once you begin play sessions, you should consider your availability to your child as a form of contract that you cannot break.

2. *Selecting a room for play* where there will be least concern if things get spoiled or broken. Water may be spilled, play dough smeared, or toys dropped and broken. Least preferred is your child's own playroom, where other toys might be distracting.

3. *The choice of toys* is important to the success of the play session. Primarily, the toys should be inexpensive and unbreakable, and lend themselves to expressive, interactive, and imaginative play. The toys are especially selected in order to help your child release feelings, such as nurturance and aggression, and to re-enact feelings in relation to family members, other children, etc. in a safe and accepted place. Other toys may be added depending on your child's preferences. For older children (9+), other items (e.g. interactive games for older children) probably would be needed. These toys are reserved for use by your child only in play sessions with a parent. Your child may not take or use the toys out of the session (drawings or paintings are an exception). A list of toys to collect that are suitable for home play sessions will be distributed prior to starting home play sessions.

4. *What to tell your children.* It is not necessary to go into a long explanation with your children about their home play sessions. You may simply say you want to spend more time with each of them. Older children may insist on further details. In this case, place the emphasis on your wanting to spend time alone with your children in a special play setting. Not that you want to help them, but that you want to be together, have fun, and improve your relationship. There is usually very little difficulty in getting your children to participate.

Children's reactions to home play sessions can be a very rewarding experience for both parents and their children. Some children move quickly in a direction opposite to the way they have been behaving earlier; some at first behave like themselves, but in an exaggerated or more forceful manner. Some children become very aggressive, some very quiet, some may revert to very baby-like behavior, some like to order the parent around—taking complete control of the situation. Other children are unable to express their feelings in the beginning. Some, at first, act as though they have only negative feelings. Others may want the parent to make decisions, and they may do things just to please their parents to make sure they continue to have parents spend this time alone with them.

You try to reflect any of these feelings your children express in play sessions as they occur, rather than giving explanations or making the choices for your children. You should learn a great deal about how your children feel at times towards their families and themselves. You probably will also learn more about your own feelings towards your children. Home play sessions, along with group meetings, will enable you to move towards more positive relationships in your family life, and, once home play sessions are well under way, leaders will help you apply these and other parenting skills to your daily lives more fully.

Revised from Guerney, L., Stover, L. & Guerney, B. *Training manual for play sessions.* (Unpublished document.) Pennsylvania State University, PA. Reprinted in C. E. Schaefer (Ed.). (2002). *The therapeutic use of child's play: Basic readings (2nd ed.)* (pp. 216–227). New York, NY: Jason Aronson.

APPENDIX 16
Form for Leaders' Direct Supervision Notes of Practice Sessions

This form is suggested for leaders' use during ongoing note taking and feedback for live or videoed play sessions that are supervised in detail during meetings.

Order of activities	Positive feedback	Suggested improvements
Two to three word description with order of events and child's responses.	What worked and when for parents—give brief examples to illustrate; note when to give feedback on skills (first or last?).	Where skills lacking or misapplied—select the most relevant.

APPENDIX 17
Suggested Materials
List for Home Sessions

Family-related materials

Doll family (mother, father, brother, sister, baby, and any other relevant dolls).

Family of cloth puppets.

Dollhouse or house box and doll furniture.

Baby doll and doll's equipment (optional; e.g. small doll's blanket).

Real baby bottle.

Cups and saucers, toy pan, pretend food.

Soft, cuddly animal (e.g. teddy bear).

Dress-up materials

Dress-up clothes (hats, pieces of fabric, purse, comb, doctor's bag, rings, etc.).

Gun with "bullets" to shoot (e.g. bullets made of non-harmful materials).

Two pretend cell phones.

Pretend money.

Flexible rubber knife.

Small toys

Small plastic cars, trucks, rescue vehicles to push around.

Plastic soldiers, knights, dinosaurs.

A small amount of Lego® or a similar construction toy, blocks.

Interactive games

Deck of cards.

Ring toss.

Other materials

Inflated plastic bop bag (preferably 4ft high) or a pillow with hand-drawn face.

Non-hardening modeling material, rolling pin, shapes, and cookie tray.

Crayons, paints or paint sticks, drawing paper.

Pan or plastic bowl for water and cup, pitcher, scoop for water play.

Small tray with sand and small figures.

Mat for messy play.

Video camera and other equipment for home recordings.

APPENDIX 18
Form for Parents' Written Recording of Home Sessions

Home play session notes

Name of parent ....

Name of child..

Date of session .... Time ....

Session .... Duration of session ....

The main activities during this play session were: *(please give the activities in order)*

....

....

....

....

....

The parts of the play session that went well for me were:

....

....

....

....

....

The parts of the play session that were challenging/harder for me were:

....

....

....

....

....

The main issues in my child's play were *(for later home play sessions)*:

....

....

....

....

The main feelings my child expressed were:

....

....

....

....

My main feelings about the play session were:

....

....

....

....

Issues from this play session I want to discuss during the next meeting are:

....

....

....

....

APPENDIX 19
Leaders' Checklist for Home Play Session Arrangements

Name of family ....

Composition of family ....

Names of parent(s) planning to deliver home play sessions and/or special activities

....

....

Names of children starting play sessions ....

Names of teens and tots for later play sessions or special activity times with parent(s)

....

....

Play material (circle as appropriate):

                        Complete   Not complete

Comments

....

....

....

Storage of FT materials at home:

Comments

....

....

....

Home space used and position of video camera (when used):

Comments

....

....

....

Time of day and day of week:

Comments

....
....
....

Childcare arrangements:

Comments

....
....
....

Type of recording (circle as appropriate):

                Video and written   Written only

Type of video

....

Comments

....
....
....

APPENDIX 20
Parents' Report Form
on "Special Times"

Home "special times" notes

Name of parent ....

Name and age of child ....

What date and time of day did this special activity take place?

....

How long did this interaction last? ....

Where did it take place? ....

What activity did you share? What took place in the session?

....

....

....

....

....

Make note of verbal exchanges. Were there any things said by your child that you think should be noted? If possible, quote some of your verbal responses. What play session skills were you able to use (e.g. empathy)?

....

....

....

....

....

How positive was the overall experience for you and your child? Please explain why.

....

....

....

....

What, if any, difficulties did you encounter?

....

....

....

....

How did this interaction compare to other day-to-day interactions with your child?

....

....

....

....

APPENDIX 21
A Suggested Evaluation Form for Ending the GFT Program

Parents' comments on the filial training program

Name (optional) ....

Date ....

Instructions: Part A

Please complete the sentences with a brief comment. Answer only what is appropriate.

1. I think this program helped me to:

    ....

    ....

2. I think the activities used by the group leaders were:

    ....

    ....

3. It would have been better if the leaders had:

    ....

    ....

4. I would like to have had more:

    ....

    ....

5. The part of the program I liked the best was:

    ....

    ....

6. The main thing I would change in the program is:

    ....

    ....

7. Since taking part in this program my relationship with my child has:

....

....

8. The training materials used were:

....

....

9. The thing I liked best about the leader was:

....

....

Instructions: Part B—Personal preference section

Each statement has three alternatives. Mark each alternative for each statement with a number 1, 2, or 3. Use number 1 for the alternative you feel is best. Use number 2 for the alternative that is moderately good. Use number 3 for the alternative you like the least:

EXAMPLE:

The time of the day that is best for me to attend classes is:

☐ morning

☐ afternoon

☐ evening

Additional comments:*

....

....

....

*If you think none of the alternatives are appropriate or if you want to suggest alternatives that are more appropriate, please write such information in the "Additional comments" space below each item.

10. The most useful method used by the leader was:

☐ group discussion

☐ lecture

☐ videos

Additional comments:

....

....

....

11. I feel the leaders were:
    ☐ very understanding and accepting
    ☐ somewhat understanding and accepting
    ☐ not understanding and accepting

Additional comments:

....
....
....

12. The thing I learned the most from the program was:
    ☐ to communicate better with my children
    ☐ to be more aware of the special problems of my children
    ☐ to understand child development better

Additional comments:

....
....
....

13. The play sessions I did at home were:
    ☐ easy to do
    ☐ a little hard
    ☐ much too hard

Additional comments:

....
....
....

14. Doing the play sessions at home:
    ☐ improved the quality of my play sessions
    ☐ helped me in using the skills at home
    ☐ didn't make any difference

Additional comments:

....
....
....

15. The leaders really seemed to know what they were talking about:
     ☐ most of the time
     ☐ some of the time
     ☐ hardly ever

Additional comments:

....
....
....

16. I felt comfortable in my group:
     ☐ from the beginning
     ☐ after a few sessions
     ☐ never

Additional comments:

....
....
....

17. My child really got a lot out of the play sessions:
     ☐ all of the time
     ☐ some of the time
     ☐ rarely

Additional comments:

....
....
....

18. Please make any other comments below:

....
....
....
....
....
....
....
....

References

Abidin, R. R. (1997). Parenting Stress Index: A measure of the parent-child system. In C. P. Zalaquett & R. J. Wood (Eds), *Evaluating stress: A book of resources* (viii, pp. 277–291). Lanham, MD: Scarecrow Education.

Ackerman, N. W. (1966). *Treating the troubled family.* New York, NY: Basic Books.

Andronico, M. P., Fidler, J., Guerney, B. G., & Guerney, L. F. (1967). The combination of didactic and dynamic elements in Filial Therapy. *International Journal of Group Psychotherapy, 17*, 10–17.

Axline, V. (1947). *Play therapy: The inner dynamics of childhood.* Boston, MA: Houghton Mifflin.

Baruch, D. W. (1949). *New ways in discipline.* New York, NY: McGraw Hill.

Baumrind, D. (1971). Current patterns of parental authority. *Developmental Psychology Monograph, 2,* 1–103.

Baumrind D., & Black, A. (1967). Socialization practices associated with dimensions on competence in pre-school boys and girls. *Child Development, 38,* 291–328.

Beck, A. T. & Emery, G. (1985). *Anxiety disorders and phobias: A cognitive perspective.* New York, NY: Basic Books.

Bifulco, A. (2003) *Lifespan Attachment Style Interview (ASI).* London, UK: Royal Holloway, University of London.

Bratton, S. (1998). Training parents to facilitate their children's adjustment to divorce using the filial/family play therapy approach. In C. E. Schaefer & J. M. Briesmeister (Eds), *Handbook of parent training: Parents as co-therapists for children's behavior problems* (2nd ed.) (pp. 549–572). New York, NY: Wiley.

Bratton, S., & Landreth, G. (1995). Filial therapy with single parents: Effects on parental acceptance, empathy, and stress. *International Journal of Play Therapy, 4,* 61–80.

Bratton S., Landreth, G., Kellam T., & Blackard, S. (2006). *Child parent relationship therapy (CPRT) treatment manual.* New York, NY: Routledge.

Bratton, S., Ray, D., & Motif, K. (1998). Filial/family play therapy: An intervention for custodial grandparents and their grandchildren. *Educational Gerontology, 24,* 391–406.

Bratton S., Ray, D., Rhine, T., & Jones, L. (2005). The efficacy of play therapy with children: A meta-analytic review of the outcome research. *Professional Psychology: Research and Practice, 36,* 375–390.

Carkhuff, R. R. (1969). *Helping and human relations. A primer for lay and professional helpers. Volume II: Practice and research.* New York, NY: Holt, Rinehart & Winston.

Ceballos, P. (2008). School-based child parent relationship therapy (CPRT) with low income first generation immigrant Hispanic parents: Effects on child behavior and parent-child relationship stress. *Dissertation Abstracts International, 69*(8-A), 3042.

Celaya, E. (2002). *A preventative program: Filial therapy for teen mothers in foster care. Dissertation Abstracts International, 63*(01-B), 564.

Chau, I., & Landreth, G. (1997). Filial therapy with Chinese parents: Effects on parental empathic interactions, parental acceptance of child and parental stress. *International Journal of Play Therapy, 6,* 75–92.

Clark, K. (1996). The effect of Filial Therapy on child conduct behavior problems and the quality of the parent-child relationship. *Dissertation Abstracts International, 57,* 2868.

Cochran, N. H., Nordling, W. J., & Cochran, J. L. (2010). *A practical guide to developing therapeutic relationships with children.* Chichester, UK: Wiley.

Coopersmith, S. (1967). *The antecedents of self-esteem.* San Franciso, CA: Freeman.

Costas M., & Landreth G. (1999). Filial therapy with non-offending parents of children who have been sexually abused. *International Journal of Play Therapy, 8*(1), 43–66.

Day, C., Carey, M., & Surgenor, T., (2006). Children's key concerns: piloting a qualitative approach to understanding their experience of mental health care. *Clinical Child Psychology and Psychiatry, 11*(1), 139–155.

Dorfman, E. (1976). Play therapy. In C. Rogers (Ed.), *Client centered therapy* (pp. 235–278). London, UK: Constable.

Drewes, A. and Mullen, J. A. (Eds). (2008). *Supervision can be playful.* Lanham, MD: Jason Aronson.

Eardley, D. (1978). An initial investigation of a didactic version of Filial Therapy dealing with self-concept increase and problematic behavior decrease. (Unpublished doctoral dissertation.) Pennsylvania State University, PA.

Erikson, E. (1977) *Childhood and Society.* London, UK: Triad/Granada.

Eyburg, S., & Pincus, D. (1999). *Eyburg Child Behavior Inventory and Sutter-Eyburg Student Behavior Inventory—Revised.* Odessa, FL: Psychological Assessment Resources.

Fuchs, N. R. (1957). Play therapy at home. *Merrill-Palmer Quarterly, 3,* 89–95.

Gil, E. (1991). *The healing power of play: Working with abused children.* New York, NY: Guilford Press.

Ginsberg, B. (1989). Training parents as therapeutic agents with foster/adoptive children using the filial approach. In C. E. Schaefer & J. M. Briesmeister (Eds), *Handbook of parent training: Parents as co-therapists for children's behavior problems* (2nd ed.) (pp. 442–478). New York, NY: Wiley.

Glazer-Waldman, H., Zimmerman, J., Landreth, G., & Norton, D. (1992). Filial therapy: An intervention for parents of children with chronic illness. *International Journal of Play Therapy, 1,* 31–42.

Glover, G. & Landreth, G. (2000). Filial therapy with Native Americans on the Flathead reservation. *International Journal of Play Therapy 9*(2) 57–80.

Gordon, T. (1970). *Parent effectiveness training.* New York, NY: Peter Wyden.

Grskovic, J., & Goetze, H. (2008). Short-term Filial Therapy with German mothers: Findings from a controlled study. *International Journal of Play Therapy, 17,* 39–51.

Guerney, B. G. (1964). Filial therapy: description and rationale. *Journal of Consulting Psychology, 28*(4), 303–310.

Guerney. B. G., & Flumen, A. B. (1970). Teachers as psychotherapeutic agents for withdrawn children. *Journal of School Psychology, 8*(2), 107–113 (NIMH Report 1826401).

Guerney, B. G., & Stover, L. (1971). Filial therapy: Final report on NIMH grant 1826401. (Available from NIRE/IDEALS, 12500 Blake Road, Silver Spring, MD 20904–2056.)

Guerney, B. G., Stover, L., & DeMeritt, S. (1968). A measurement of empathy for parent-child interaction. *Journal of Genetic Psychology, 112,* 49–55.

Guerney, L. F. (1975). Brief follow-up study on Filial Therapy. Paper presented at the April meeting of the Eastern Psychological Associates, New York. Silver Spring: IDEALS. (Available from NIRE/IDEALS 12500 Blake Road, Silver Spring, MD 20904–2056.)

Guerney, L. F. (2000). Taking Filial Therapy into the 21st century. *International Journal of Play Therapy,* *9*(2), 1–17.

Guerney, L. F. (2003). Filial play therapy. In C.E. Schaefer (Ed), *Foundations of play therapy* (pp. 99-142). Hoboken, NJ: John Wiley and Sons.

Guerney, L. F. (2013). *Clinician's and group leader's manual for parenting: A skills training program* (5th ed.). Silver Spring, MD: IDEALS. (Available from NIRE/IDEALS, 12500 Blake Road, Silver Spring, MD 20904–2056.)

Guerney, L. F. and Guerney, B. G. (1987). Integrating child and family therapy. *Psychotherapy, 24*(35), 609–614.

Guerney, L. F. & Guerney, B. G. (1989) Child relationship enhancement: Family therapy and parent education. Special issue: *Person-centered approaches with families. Person-Centered Review,* 4, 344–357.

Guerney L. F., & Guerney, B. G. (1994) Child relationship enhancement family therapy and parent education. In C. Schaefer & L. Carey (Eds), *Family play therapy* (pp. 127–138). Northvale, NJ: Jason Aronson.

Guerney, L. F., Stover, L. & Guerney, B. G. Training manual for play sessions. (Unpublished document.) Pennsylvania State University, PA. Reprinted in C. E. Schaefer (Ed.). (2002). *The therapeutic use of child's play: Basic readings (2nd ed.)* (pp. 216–227). New York, NY: Jason Aronson.

Harris, Z. & Landreth G. (1997). Filial therapy with incarcerated mothers: A five week model. *International Journal of Play Therapy, 5*(2), 59–79.

Harvey, S. (2000). Dynamic play approaches in the observation of family relationships. In K. Gitlin-Weiner, A. Sandgrund & C. E. Schaefer (Eds.), *Play diagnosis and assessment* (2nd ed.) (pp. 457–573). Chichester, UK: Wiley.

Heard, D. & Lake, B. (1997) *The challenge of attachment for caregiving.* London, UK: Routledge.

Hobbs, N. (1962). Sources of gain in psychotherapy. *American Psychologist, 17,* 741–747.

Hobbs, N. (1963). Strategies for the development of clinical psychology. *American Psychology Association, Division of Clinical Psychology Newsletter, 16*(2), 3–5.

Horner, P. (1974). Dimensions of child behavior as described by parents: A monotonicity analysis. (Unpublished master's thesis). Pennsylvania State University. PA.

Jang, M. (2000). Effectiveness of Filial Therapy for Korean parents. *International Journal of Play Therapy, 9*(2), 39–56.

Jaeger, J. & Ryan, V. (2007) Evaluating clinical practice: Using play-based techniques to elicit children's views. *Clinical Child Psychology and Psychiatry, 12*(3), 437–450.

Jaeger, J. & Ryan, V. (2011) Integrating attachment theory and non-directive play therapy to treat children with more serious attachment problems. In A. Drewes, S. Bratton & C. E. Schaefer (Eds), *Integrative play therapy* (pp. 265–296). Hoboken, NJ: John Wiley and Sons.

Jaeger, J. & Ryan, V. (in preparation) Parents and children's views of Group Filial Therapy: A pilot study.

Joseph, J. (1979). *Joseph pre-school and primary self-concept screening instructional manual.* Chicago, IL: Stoelting.

Johnson, M. T. (2006). Filial therapy with Asian American families. Paper presented at the Association for Play Therapy International Conference, October. Toronto, Canada.

Kale, A. L., & Landreth G., (1999). Filial therapy with children experiencing learning difficulties. *International Journal of Play Therapy, 8,* 35–56.

Kidron, M. and Landreth, G. (2010). Intensive child parent relationship therapy with Israeli parents in Israel. *International Journal of Play Therapy, 19*(2), 64–78.

Kot, S. (1995). Intensive play therapy with child witnesses of domestic violence. (Unpublished doctoral dissertation.) University of North Texas, TX.

Kraft, A. (1973). *Are you listening to your child? How to bridge the communication gap through creative play sessions.* New York, NY: Walker.

Landesberg, S. & Snyder, W. (1946). Nondirective play therapy. *Journal of Clinical Psychology, 2,* 203–213.

Landreth, G. (2012). *Play therapy: The art of the relationship* (3rd ed.). New York, NY: Routledge.

Landreth, G. & Bratton, S. (2006). *Child parent relationship therapy (CPRT): A 10 session Filial Therapy model.* New York, NY: Routledge.

Landreth, G. & Lobaugh, A. (1998). Filial therapy with incarcerated fathers: Effects on parental acceptance of child and parental stress and child adjustment. *Journal of Counseling and Development, 76,* 157–165.

Lazarus, A. A. (1971). *Behavior therapy and beyond.* New York, NY: McGraw Hill.

Leventhal, T., & Stollack, G. (1965). *Problem list.* Eatontown, NJ: Children's Psychiatric Center.

Levine, E. (1977). Training elderly volunteers in skills to improve the emotional adjustment of children in a daycare center. (Unpublished doctoral dissertation.) Pennsylvania State University, PA: 7803393.

Moore, R. (1964). *DesMoines child guidance center maladjustment index: Parent rating scale.* DesMoines, IA: Child Guidance Center.

Morrison Bennett, M. O. & Bratton, S. (2011) The effects of child teacher relationship training on the children of focus: A pilot study. *International Journal of Play Therapy, 20*(4), 193–207.

Moustakas, C. E. (1951). Situational play therapy with normal children. *Journal of Consulting Psychology, 15,* 225–230.

Ortwein, M. C. (1997). *Mastering the magic of play: Training manual for parents in Filial Therapy.* Silver Spring, MD: IDEALS. (Available from NIRE/IDEALS, 12500 Blake Road, Silver Spring, MD 20904–2056.)

O'Sullivan, L. & Ryan, V. (2009). Therapeutic limits from an attachment perspective. *Clinical Child Psychology and Psychiatry, 14*(2), 215–235.

Oxman, L. (1971). The effects of Filial Therapy: A controlled study. *Dissertation Abstracts International, 32*(B1), 1.

Parpal, M., & Maccoby, E. E. (1985). Maternal responsiveness and subsequent child compliance. *Child Development, 56,* 1326–1334.

Porter, B. M. (1954). Measurement of parental acceptance of children. *Journal of Home Economics, 46,* 176–182.

Rogers, C. R. (1951). *Client-centered therapy.* Boston, MA: Houghton Mifflin.

Ross, N., & Egan, B. (2004). "What do I have to come here for; I'm not mad?" Children's perceptions of a child guidance clinic. *Clinical Child Psychology and Psychiatry, 9*(1), 107–115.

Ryan, V. (2004). Adapting non-directive play therapy interventions for children with attachment disorders. *Clinical Child Psychology and Psychiatry, 9*(1), 75–87.

Ryan, V. (2007a). Non-directive play therapy with abused children and adolescents. In K. Wilson & A. James (Eds), *The child protection handbook* (3rd ed.) (pp. 414–432). London, UK: Bailliere Tindall.

Ryan, V. (2007b). Filial therapy: Helping children and new carers to form secure attachment relationships. *British Journal of Social Work, 37,* 643–657.

Ryan, V. (2009). Play therapy: psycho-social approaches to trauma and emotional problems in young children. In K. Stagnitti & R. Cooper (Eds), *Play as therapy: Assessment and therapeutic interventions* (pp. 187–204). London, UK: Jessica Kingsley.

Ryan, V. & Bratton, S. (2008). Child-centered/non-directive play therapy for very young children. In S. Kelly-Zion, C. E Schaefer, J. McCormick, & A. Ohnogi (Eds), *Play therapy for very young children* (pp. 25–66). Lanham, MD: Rowman and Littlefield.

Ryan, V. & Courtney, A. (2009). Therapists' use of congruence in child-centered/non-directive play therapy and Filial Therapy. *International Journal of Play Therapy, 18*(2), 114–128.

Ryan, V. & Edge, A. (2012). The role of play themes in non-directive play therapy. *Clinical Child Psychology and Psychiatry, 17*(3), 354–369.

Ryan, V. & Needham, C. (2001). Non-directive play therapy with children experiencing psychic trauma. *Clinical Child Psychology and Psychiatry, 6*(3), 437–453.

Ryan, V. and Wilson, K. (1995).Non-directive play therapy as a means of recreating optimal infant socialisation patterns. *Early Development and Parenting, 4*, 29–38.

Ryan, V. & Wilson, K. (2000/1996). *Case studies in non-directive play therapy*. London, UK: Jessica Kingsley.

Ryan, V. & Wilson, K. (2005). Using non-directive play therapy with emotionally troubled adolescents. In C. E. Schaefer & L. Gallo-Lopez (Eds), *Adolescent play therapy* (pp. 96–120). New York, NY: Jason Aronson.

Rye, N. & Jaeger, J. (2007). Filial therapy: Assessing families for Filial Therapy. *British Journal of Play Therapy, 3*, 32–37.

Schore, A. N. (2000). Attachment and the regulation of the right brain. *Attachment and Human Development, 2*, 23–47.

Sensue, M. (1981). Filial therapy follow-up study: Effects on parental acceptance and child development. *Dissertation Abstracts International, 42*(1), 0148B.

Sheely-Moore, A. & Bratton, S. (2010). A strengths-based parenting intervention. *Professional Schools Counseling, 13*(3), 175–183.

Smith, D. T. (2000) Parent-child interaction play assessment. In K. Gitlin-Weiner, A. Sandgrund & C. E. Schaefer (Eds), *Play diagnosis and assessment* (2nd ed.) (pp. 340-370). Chichester, UK: Wiley.

Solomon, M., Pistrang, N., & Barker, C. (2001). The benefits of mutual support groups for parents of children with disabilities. *American Journal of Community Psychology 29*(1), 113–32.

Stagnitti, K. (1998). *Learn to play: A practical program to develop a child's imaginative play skills*. Victoria, Aus.: Coordinations Publications.

Stollack, G. E. (1968). The experimental effects of training undergraduates as play therapists. *Psychotherapy, Theory, Research and Practice, 5*, 77–80.

Stollack, G. E., Barley, A., & Kalogiros, J. D. (2000). Assessment of the child and family in play contexts. In K. Gitlin-Weiner, A. Sandgrund & C. E. Schaefer (Eds), *Play diagnosis and assessment* (2nd ed.) (pp. 474–513). Chichester, UK: Wiley.

Stover, L., & Guerney, B. G. (1967). The efficacy of training procedures for mothers in Filial Therapy. *Psychotherapy: Theory, Research and Practice 4*(3), 110–115.

Stover. L., Guerney, B. G., & O'Connell, M. (1971). Measurements of acceptance, allowing self-direction, involvement, and empathy in adult-child interaction. *Journal of Psychology, 77*, 261–269.

Sywulak, A. E. (1979). The effect of Filial Therapy on parental acceptance and child adjustment. *Dissertation Abstracts International, 38*(12), 6180B.

Tew, K. L., Landreth, G., Joiner, K. D., & Solt, M. D. (2002). Filial therapy with chronically ill children. *International Journal of Play Therapy 11*(1), 79–100.

Tyndall-Lind, A. (1999). A comparative analysis of intensive individual play therapy and intensive sibling group play therapy with child witnesses of domestic violence. *Dissertation Abstracts International, 60*(5-A), 1465.

VanFleet, R. (1992). Using Filial Therapy to strengthen families with chronically ill children. In L. VandeCreek, S. Knapp, & T. Jackson (Eds), *Innovations in clinical practice: A source book*, (Vol. 11, pp. 87–970). Sarasota, FL: Professional Resource Exchange,.

VanFleet, R. (2013). *Filial therapy: Strengthening parent-child relationships through play* (3rd ed.). Sarasota, FL: Professional Resource Press.

VanFleet, R., Ryan S., & Smith, S. (2005). Filial therapy: A critical review. In L. Reddy, T. Files Hall & C. E. Schaefer (Eds), *Empirically-based play interventions for children* (pp. 241–264). Washington DC: American Psychological Association Press.

VanFleet, R., Sywulak, A. E. & Sniscak, C. C. (2010) *Child-centered play therapy*. New York, NY: Guilford Press.

Walker, K. F. (2008). Filial therapy with parents court-referred for child maltreatment. *Dissertation Abstracts International, 68*(8A), 3300.

Wall, L. (1979). Parents as play therapists: A comparison of three interventions into children's play. *Dissertation Abstracts International, 39(11),* 5597.

Wenar, C. & Kerig, P. (2006). *Developmental psychopathology: From infancy through adolescence* (5th ed.). London, UK: McGraw Hill.

Wilson, K., & Ryan, V. (2005). *Play therapy: A non-directive approach for children and adolescents* (2nd ed.). London, UK: Elsevier Science.

Wolpe, J. (1969). *The practice of behavior therapy.* New York, NY: Pergamon Press.

Yuen, T., Landreth, G., & Baggerly, J. (2002). Filial therapy with immigrant Chinese families. *International Journal of Play Therapy, 1,* 63–90.

Subject Index

Author Index